# Literary Medicine: Brain Disease and Doctors in Novels, Theater, and Film

# Frontiers of Neurology and Neuroscience

## Vol. 31

Series Editor

J. Bogousslavsky Montreux

# Literary Medicine: Brain Disease and Doctors in Novels, Theater, and Film

Volume Editors

J. Bogousslavsky Montreux
S. Dieguez Fribourg

49 figures, 9 in color, and 8 tables, 2013

KARGER Basel · Freiburg · Paris · London · New York · New Delhi · Bangkok · Beijing · Tokyo · Kuala Lumpur · Singapore · Sydney

**Frontiers of Neurology and Neuroscience**
Vols. 1-18 were published as Monographs in Clinical Neuroscience

**Julien Bogousslavsky, MD**
Center for Brain and Nervous System Diseases
GSMN Neurocenter, Clinique Valmont
CH–1823 Glion/Montreux (Switzerland)

**Sebastian Dieguez, MD**
Laboratory for Cognitive and Neurological Sciences
Neurology Unit
Department of Medicine
CH–1700 Fribourg (Switzerland)

Library of Congress Cataloging-in-Publication Data

Literary medicine : brain disease and doctors in novels, theater, and film / volume editors, J. Bogousslavsky, S. Dieguez.
p. ; cm. -- (Frontiers of neurology and neuroscience, ISSN 1660-4431 ; v. 31)
Brain disease and doctors in novels, theater, and film
Includes bibliographical references and index.
ISBN 978-3-318-02271-1 (alk. paper) -- ISBN 978-3-318-02272-8 (e-ISBN)
I. Bogousslavsky, Julien. II. Dieguez, S. (Sebastian) III. Title: Brain disease and doctors in novels, theater, and film. IV. Series: Frontiers of neurology and neuroscience ; v. 31. 1660-4431
[DNLM: 1. Brain Diseases. 2. Medicine in Literature. 3. Physicians. W1 MO568C v.31 2013 / WZ 330]
R836.A1
612.8'22--dc23

2013003768

Bibliographic Indices. This publication is listed in bibliographic services, including Current Contents® and Index Medicus.

Disclaimer. The statements, opinions and data contained in this publication are solely those of the individual authors and contributors and not of the publisher and the editor(s). The appearance of advertisements in the book is not a warranty, endorsement, or approval of the products or services advertised or of their effectiveness, quality or safety. The publisher and the editor(s) disclaim responsibility for any injury to persons or property resulting from any ideas, methods, instructions or products referred to in the content or advertisements.

Drug Dosage. The authors and the publisher have exerted every effort to ensure that drug selection and dosage set forth in this text are in accord with current recommendations and practice at the time of publication. However, in view of ongoing research, changes in government regulations, and the constant flow of information relating to drug therapy and drug reactions, the reader is urged to check the package insert for each drug for any change in indications and dosage and for added warnings and precautions. This is particularly important when the recommended agent is a new and/or infrequently employed drug.


www.karger.com
Printed in Switzerland on acid-free and non-aging paper (ISO 9706) by Reinhardt Druck, Basel
ISSN 1660–4431
e-ISSN 1662–2804
ISBN 978–3–318–02271–1
e-ISBN 978–3–318–02272–8

# Contents

# Preface

For most people, including neurologists and psychiatrists, the first contacts with brain disease and its consequences take place in reading novels or watching movies. Another initiation may also be through personal experience with a family member afflicted by a specific disorder, but a more scholarly experience is usually delayed until the academic years for future physicians and health professionals. Classical and modern literature is indeed full of patients with interesting neurological, cognitive, or psychiatric diseases, oftentimes including detailed and accurate descriptions, suggesting that the authors were inspired by observations made on real individuals.

In many cases, these literary portrayals of diseases even predate their formal identification by medical science. For instance, one of the best and most vivid reports of acute progressing stroke was written by Marcel Proust in *In Search of Lost Time* about the fatal disease of the narrator's grandmother. Proust was the son of a famous physician and had heard the daily reporting of medical cases during the family meals from a very young age. Alexandre Dumas probably provided the first precise description of a locked-in syndrome in the case of Mr. Noirtier in *The Count of Monte Cristo*, and William Shakespeare's plays are a source of a surprising number of various neurological and psychiatric cases. In *Louis Lambert*, Honoré de Balzac may have written the first accurate report of schizophrenia, several decades before Kraepelin and Bleuler provided the first modern descriptions of the condition.

In previous books devoted to neurological diseases in famous artists, writers, and musicians [1–3], we mentioned fascinating self-reports by famous novelists, such as Charles-Ferdinand Ramuz's own account of his stroke in his diary, or the first known report of a transient ischemic attack by Stendhal in his correspondence to Fiore. However, fictional literature is much richer and encompasses nearly all kind of disorders affecting the nervous system, with certain favorites, such as memory loss and behavioral syndromes. There are even unique observations, which cannot be found in scientific and clinical literature, because of the lack of appropriate studies. A striking example is the extraordinary description of the instable psychological condition immediately preceding the acute entrance into chronic psychosis, reported in André Breton's novel *Nadja* and in the correspondence of Léona Delcourt, i.e. Nadja herself.

Not only does literature offer a creative and humane look at disorders of the brain and mind, but just as authors have been inspired by medicine and real disorders, clinicians also have much to gain from literary depictions of the disorders they encounter in their daily practice. While the present coverage of literary medicine obviously is partial, it provides an amazing and fascinating look at conditions, patients, and doctors, in a way which is both reminiscence and novelty.

*Julien Bogousslavsky*, Montreux
*Sebastian Dieguez*, Fribourg

## References


1 Bogousslavsky J, Boller F (eds): Neurological Disorders in Famous Artists. Front Neurol Neurosci. Basel, Karger, 2005, vol 19.

2 Bogousslavsky J, Hennerici MG (eds): Neurological Disorders in Famous Artists – Part 2. Front Neurol Neurosci. Basel, Karger, 2007, vol 22.

3 Bogousslavsky J, Hennerici MG, Bäzner H, Bassetti C (eds): Neurological Disorders in Famous Artists – Part 3. Front Neurol Neurosci. Basel, Karger, 2010, vol 27.

Bogousslavsky J, Dieguez S (eds): Literary Medicine: Brain Disease and Doctors in Novels, Theater, and Film.
Front Neurol Neurosci. Basel, Karger, 2013, vol 31, pp 1–9 (DOI: 10.1159/000343238)

# Madness in Blaise Cendrars' Novels: Moravagine and Company

Laurent Tatu[a,b] · Julien Bogousslavsky[c]

Departments of [a]Neuromuscular Diseases and [b]Anatomy, CHU Jean-Minjoz, University of Franche-Comté, Besançon, France; [c]Center for Brain and Nervous System Diseases, GSMN Neurocenter, Clinique Valmont, Glion/Montreux, Switzerland

**Abstract**

The literary work of Blaise Cendrars (1887–1961), né Frédéric Sauser, one of the major French-speaking authors of the 20th century, is imbued with references to neuropsychiatry. This theme is a constant presence in his writing as a result of his involvement of the First World War and his personal experiences, which were punctuated with neurologic and psychiatric events. Cendrars' own particular ideas on the genesis of mental disorders went against the more traditional views on psychiatry. He remained skeptical about hysteria and did not subscribe to psychoanalysis. His ideas were enriched by his experience with the war-related neuropsychiatric problems developed by soldiers. He thus proposed the notion of 'pathological fear' surrounding these disorders. There are a number of characters suffering from 'borderline' mental disorders in Cendrars' work, including two shocking, mad murderers, Moravagine and Fébronio. The character Moravagine, a neurology patient suffering from a brain tumor, enabled Cendrars to delve into the grey areas that can exist between neurologic and psychiatric diseases. Fébronio, a real psychotic, enabled Cendrars to explore ethnopsychiatry.



Blaise Cendrars (1887–1961), né Frédéric Sauser, was one of the great French-speaking authors of the 20th century (fig. 1). Cendrars was born in La Chaux-de-Fonds in Switzerland. He acquired French nationality in 1916 following his voluntary enlistment in the French Foreign Legion during the First World War.

His work is full of references to neuropsychiatry. This theme is a constant presence in his writing owing to his involvement in the Great War. It results in part from his personal experiences, which were punctuated by neurologic and psychiatric events.

Cendrars' neurologic journey was marked by phantom limb syndrome following the amputation of his right forearm after a war injury, and by two strokes, which deprived him of the use of his limbs and then his speech at the end of this life [1].

His personal psychiatric experience really began after the death of his mother. Then aged 20, he entered a period of considerable psychiatric difficulty, which may

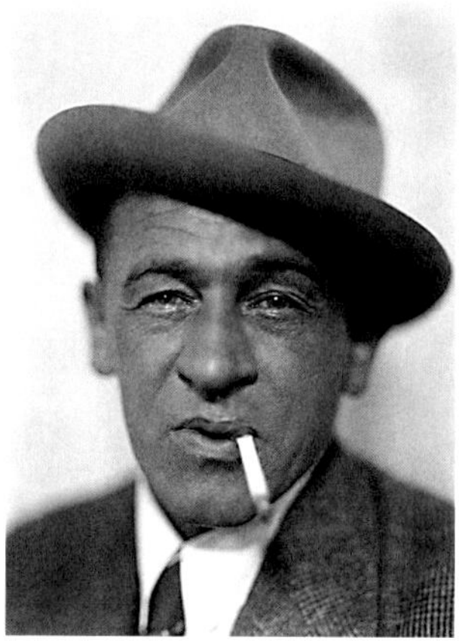

**Fig. 1.** Blaise Cendrars at the time of publication of *Moravagine*. ©Martinie/Roger Viollet. Reprinted with kind permission.

have resulted in him being hospitalized [2]. His failing psychological state is evident in his correspondence [3]:

> I have finally dared to understand all the emptiness in my current life. . . I am forced to recognize all the pointlessness, the absurdity of my life. . . there are days when I feel at the peak of my life. . . from the top of my sunny peak, I throw myself into the abyss of the night! So I do not know what stops me and prevents me from pulling the trigger I have clenched between my teeth!

A few months later, Cendrars began studying medicine in order to gain a better understanding of psychiatry and nervous disorders. He enrolled at the Faculty of Medicine in Bern for the summer semester of 1908 and chose a placement at La Waldau psychiatric clinic. The experience was cut short as Cendrars was disappointed by the teaching and ideas on disease put forward by the psychiatrists [4]. 'Psychiatric deception' was certainly not his only reason for abandoning his medical studies, as he states: 'It's really funny being a medical student. It could last a lifetime, as you never stop learning, studying the mystery that is man. But then there's the faculty, exams. . . I've had enough!' [5].

## Madness according to Cendrars

Cendrars' first contact with mental illness shaped his singular ideas on psychiatry, which are expressed in the very first pages of *Moravagine*. He believed that mental illness was not necessarily caused by a pathological state, but that it could be part of the normal variations in an individual's state of health:

> Before investigating and examining the mechanism of the morbid causes, they [the authors] consider the 'disease in itself', condemn it as an abnormal, harmful state and indicate first and

foremost the thousand and one ways to fight it, disrupt it, suppress it, by defining health as a 'normal', absolute, fixed state... [Diseases] are a transient, intermediate, future state of health. They are perhaps health itself [6].

This perception of mental health was partly inspired by the ideas of Ricciotto Canudo (1879–1923) expressed in *Les libérés, mémoire d'un aliéniste,* published in 1911. Canudo, who dedicated a copy of his work to Cendrars, wrote in 1918: 'My experience leads me more and more to not always considering madness as an illness or as an ill state – but sometimes as a profuse state of health' [7].

Therefore, for Cendrars, the boundary between madness and reason was indistinct and changeable. Many of the characters in his work are unpredictable, disturbed individuals who would nowadays be characterized as 'borderline'. He also believed that normal subjects could experience hallucinatory or delirious phenomena. In *Moravagine*, the psychiatrist Raymond-la-Science is a victim of this type of phenomenon during his train journey to Twer station [8].

In opposition to more traditional psychiatric concepts, Cendrars displayed his unique views in the very first drafts of the *Moravagine* manuscript in 1917: 'issue a terrible indictment against the psychiatrists and experimentally determine their psychology' [9]. He nevertheless entered into the psychiatric debates at the beginning of the 20th century with his ideas on hysteria and rejection of psychoanalysis:

Hysteria, the Great Hysteria, was then in fashion in medical circles. After the preliminary work by the schools of Montpellier and La Salpêtrière who, in a manner of speaking, had only gone so far as determining, situating the object of their study, several foreign men of science, particularly the Austrian, Freud, had taken up the problem, had gone into it more amply, more profoundly, had lifted it, extracted it from its purely experimental and clinical domain to make of it a kind of pataphysics of social, religious and artistic pathology, in which it was not so much a question of coming to know the climacteric of this or that obsession born spontaneously in the farthest regions of consciousness and determining the simultaneity of the 'auto-vibrism' of sensations observed in the subject, but rather of creating, or forging an entire system of sentimental (supposedly rational) symbolism of acquired or innate slips of the subconscious, a kind of key to dreams for use by psychiatrists, as codified by Freud in his works on psychoanalysis... [10].

Cendrars exposed his nonallegiance to psychoanalysis on several occasions:

If psychoanalysis had interested me, I could have written a great paper or a brochure to popularize this theory in France. But I didn't believe in it. Upon my return from Germany, where I was able to observe its devastating effects first hand amongst intellectuals in Vienna and Munich... I said just enough to Guillaume Apollinaire to provide him with the material for a long section in his column, La Vie Anecdotique, for the Mercure de France. Until proof of the contrary, I believe I can affirm that it's in this column that the term 'psychoanalysis' was printed for the first time in France, at least in the non-medical press (winter 1911–12) [11].

These ideas about mental disorders led Cendrars to adopt a negative attitude towards the issue of their treatment:

They (the alienists) use blackmail, trickery, sequestration and commit terrible extortions. They impose ether, opium, cocaine, by restrictions and by doses. Everything is based on a scale established according to irrevocable statistics. When you combine showers, poisons, you can anticipate nervous prostration and exaltation of sensitivity [12].

## War Neuroses and 'Pathological Fear'

The First World War brought Cendrars, who volunteered to serve in the French Foreign Legion, into contact with other types of psychic dysfunction. The conflict indeed caused nervous disorders with no visible injuries, called 'war psychoneuroses'. They appeared in the form of mental disturbances and previously unseen neurological signs such as camptocormia. These soldiers were quite quickly considered to be potential malingerers who were seeking to escape their duty of defending the homeland. Whether or not the war was responsible for the onset of these disorders remained a matter of debate for a long time [13].

The influence of the war, its violence and horrors, on the mental state of the soldiers left no doubt in Cendrars' mind: '. . . in less than three months, the first horrors of the war had already marked a number of adolescents with a stigma worse than any gaping wound or scar, and I had seen more than one face among our young comrades close like a mask on an intolerable, painful secret' [14]. Cendrars, who was personally affected by the moral repercussions of the war, showed lenience towards the soldiers presenting inappropriate behavior: 'I do not condemn them. As, ultimately, what made me myself go out alone on patrol? The taste for risk? Bravado? The desire to get myself killed? No, quite simply the blues. I was just as broken and profoundly unwell as they were' [15].

For Cendrars, the ultimate violence of the Great War, which had never before reached this scale, produced quite wise patients. The bloodthirsty madmen in his works are not products of the war. He reports several examples of depressed, confused, or amnesic soldiers like Souriceau: 'He was a poor madman who had lost his regiment to the war, who had lost reason to the war, who had lost everything, he was a madman, a poor madman' [16]. The old dispute over masculine hysteria re-emerged in a military form. Cendrars approached the issue with the example of the soldier Lang: 'He was a lousy soldier. When the blues got hold of him, he was more annoying than a woman at that time of the month. He'd get a migraine, would brood, was frankly unbearable and had acute neurasthenia. Another hysteric. God, these big strapping fellows are such cowards' [17].

According to Cendrars, fear, a drug that could incite action, was the key factor encompassing all these nervous disorders and explained their onset. He thus incorporated the theories of the neuropsychiatrist Paul Voivenel (1880–1975), who, with his concept of 'pathological fear' was the true precursor of the understanding of war psychoneuroses and posttraumatic stress syndrome. Voivenel differentiated between soldiers who became ill from their abnormal fear and cowards who refused to fight [18]. In line with this idea, Cendrars developed the example of the soldier Faval: 'The fear of dying. I've never seen anyone as scared as Faval' [19]. Fear causes Faval to take desperate action in an attempt to escape the front. Together with another soldier called Tarasa, he thinks up a strategy to be evacuated owing to a false injury. Despite the risk of ending up in front of the war council and a firing squad, they decide to injure each other with their guns. Faval shoots Tarasa first, but once injured, Tarasa does not have the strength to shoot his comrade in return. Tarasa dies in hospital from an infected wound and the corporal Cendrars protects Faval from prosecution: 'He shot because he was afraid. He was afraid of dying. A soldier who has never been afraid on the front is not a man. I don't like military judges who send a man to Biribi due to a weakness. A soldier has the right to be afraid. That's why I hushed up this ridiculous business' [20].

Cendrars did not have the same lenience for soldiers who used firearms to injure themselves out of pure deception in order to escape the war, i.e. those who exhibited a 'coward's fear' rather than 'pathological fear'. After the armistice, he met Uri, an old soldier from his squadron who had only stayed on the battlefield for a few days:

> Were you injured or are you a deserter? – I was discharged, he replied. Look! And Uri showed me his right hand, which was missing three fingers. He laughed cynically. – I'm not stupid, he said. – Bastard, I said, you blew up your hand! – So? he said. – You are a right scoundrel, I said. That was the first time I met a guy from the squadron with whom I didn't want to go for a drink [21].

War psychoneuroses led to an excess of treatments like electric psychotherapy, renamed 'torpillage' in its military version, which sometimes involved torture [22]. Those in favor of experimental and aggressive treatments for war neuroses justified their use by the contagious nature of the disorders presented by soldiers considered as malingerers. Cendrars confirmed the contagious nature of the disorders that sometimes led to desertion: 'It was a curious epidemic, of a mental nature, like what should occur on a raft of shipwrecked people when, one after another, the survivors let themselves slip into the water much more out of desperate vanity than because they are exhausted by the deprivations and suffering they have endured' [23]. However, he ruled out any notion of malingering in these soldiers, the most seriously affected of whom ended up in centers for intractable psychoneuroses:

> The madmen institutionalized there are definitely not malingerers, nor sufferers of fatigue, or neurasthenia: they have all earned their insanity stripes in the different military neurology centers where they stayed, were observed, underwent lengthy interrogation and were selected and sorted by numerous expert committees [24].

## The Mad Murderers: Neurology and Ethnopsychiatry

In the work of Cendrars, the two most detailed cases of mad murderers are those of Moravagine and Fébronio. Moravagine kills and mutilates young girls. Declared insane, he is locked up in the Waldensee asylum, a fictional transcription of La

Waldau asylum in Bern. He escapes with the complicity of his psychiatrist to embark on escapades around the world punctuated by serial murders. An aviator during the Great War, Moravagine ends his life in 1917 in a military neurology center while writing an account of his travels on the planet Mars.

A number of psychiatric patients were proposed as models for Moravagine's character. Adolf Wölfli (1864–1930), a schizophrenic and rapist of young girls and a prominent figure in 'Art Brut' institutionalized in La Waldau, was one of them, as was Joseph Fessler, a delinquent with whom Cendrars exchanged correspondence [25]. The Swiss writer, Jacques Chessex (1934–2009), even proposed Favez, the heroic mental patient in his novel *Le vampire de Ropraz*, as a literary model for Moravagine by imagining a fictional encounter between Favez and Cendrars [26].

This multiplicity of possible psychiatric models must not overshadow the fact that Cendrars presents Moravagine as a neurology patient suffering from a tumor of the third cerebral ventricle. He thus tackles, in his own way, the somewhat hazy separation between psychiatry and neurology, between mental disorders and organic nervous system lesions.

The long explanation of Moravagine's clinical observation and the results of his autopsy in the novel are a faithful reproduction of an article published in the journal *La presse médicale* on July 23, 1917 under the title: 'Infundibular syndrome in a case of tumor of the third ventricle' [27]. The authors of the article, Henri Claude (1869–1945) and Jean Lhermitte (1877–1959), were reputable neurologists who were recruited to work in a military neurology center. Cendrars reproduced this article, replacing the biographical data of the soldier under observation with those of Moravagine. He also changed the name of the neurology center, which became Centre 101 bis. Finally, he replaced the name of Mademoiselle Loyez, collaborator of Henri Claude, with that of Germain Soyez, the nurse who cared for Moravagine (fig. 2).

The search for neurological models for Moravagine's character was more difficult and less dramatic. However, it should be noted that in *J'ai saigné*, Cendrars reports his encounter with a patient suffering from right-sided hemiplegia and aphasia following trepanning during his stay at the Châlons-sur-Marne military hospital in October 1915. Cendrars was involved in speech rehabilitation and recounts his long recovery when he was recovering from the amputation of his right forearm.

Another example of a mentally ill murderer is the Brazilian Fébronio. With this character, there was no question of a brain tumor. Fébronio, a real person whose murders made a big impact in Brazil in the 1920s, is presented by Cendrars as a purely psychiatric case. The final text published by Cendrars is based on four articles published in *Paris-Soir* in May and June 1938 under the title 'Les pénitenciers des noirs'. Cendrars reports a conversation with Fébronio in his prison, but it is more likely that he worked from press extracts and documents rather than actually meeting him [28].

Fébronio attacked young men, whereby he raped, killed, mutilated, and tattooed them with cabalistic signs in a ritualistic manner. He was arrested in 1927 in Rio de Janeiro, and quickly revealed himself to be a serious psychotic convinced that he was

**LE SYNDROME INFUNDIBULAIRE**

**DANS UN CAS DE TUMEUR DU TROISIÈME VENTRICULE**

**Par MM. Henri CLAUDE et J. LHERMITTE**

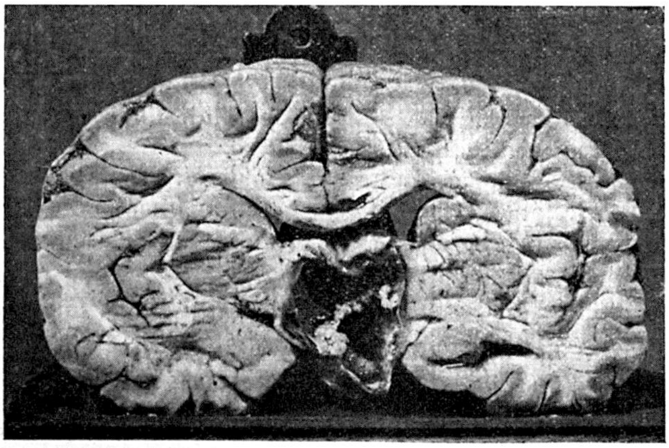

Fig. 2. — **Cerveau,** coupe transversale montrant la dilatation du 3[e] ventricule et la tumeur kystique remplissant le ventricule et notamment la région infundibulaire.

**Fig. 2.** Blaise Cendrars adapted Moravagine's autopsy report [27].

the prophet of a new religion. He said he was obeying visions and voices falling from the skies. He recorded his delusions in a book that remained hidden for a long time (fig. 3).

There is a plethora of similarities between Moravagine, the product of Cendrars' creative mind, and Fébronio, a real person: mental illness, serial killings, memoires, Brazil, etc. The two characters are also presented as incurable. Moravagine relapses by killing a young girl within minutes of escaping the asylum. Cendrars also claims to have spoken to Fébronio: ' *"Say, if you were released today, would you start again?"* – *"I would start again!"*' he replied with a smile of morose delectation' [29]. Moravagine, a fictional character, who was the burdensome double of Cendrars for many years, thus found his own double in Fébronio, a real person.

Cendrars' use of the case of Fébronio is a clear example of ethnopsychiatry. His crimes were the result of his uprooting and his forced acceptance of the mentality of whites and the inhibition of his instincts:

> The criminality of colored, not to say primitive, folk who are in daily contact or grappling with modern civilization and who have more or less, willingly or by force, undergone, adopted, imitated, learned, feigned, and often to the point of inhibition of their instincts and their most natural reflexes, the mentality and the prejudices of their masters and of their white superiors, has always greatly interested me as I consider it as a short circuit, a backlash [30].

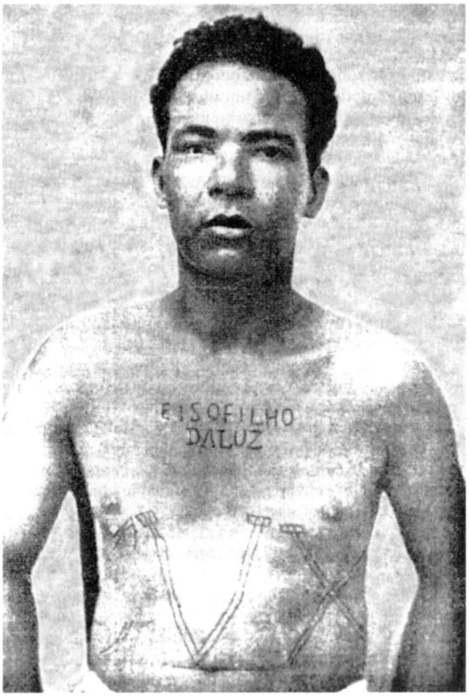

**Fig. 3.** Fébronio in 1927 (origin unknown).

For Cendrars, Blacks who became Christians did not forget their deep roots, and the explosion of their mystic ancestral terror could result in the most hateful of crimes:

> In my eyes, Fébronio is the distant descendent of a great African shaman and, like all the Blacks of Brazil who can no longer drink from the fountains of African mysticism and are lost children, of mixed-race despite his deep coloration, that is to say a negro-Christian bastard whose intelligence and spirituality exhaust and sink to the other side of the pantheistic tradition and the animist religion of his race [31].

La folie est le propre de l'Homme
(Madness is the human condition)
*Blaise Cendrars* [32]


## Acknowledgements

We would like to give particular thanks to Miriam Cendrars for her invaluable help and for providing information on her father's medical history; Marie-Thérèse Lathion, curator of the Blaise Cendrars collection at the Swiss National Library (Bern) for her time and availability, and Christine Le Quellec Cottier, director of the *Centre d'études Blaise Cendrars (CEBC)* at the Swiss National Library (Bern) for her helpful advice.

## References


1 Tatu L: The missing hands of Blaise Cendrars; in Bogousslavsky J, Hennerici MG, Bäzner H, Bassetti C (eds): Neurological Disorders in Famous Artists – Part 3. Front Neurol Neurosci. Basel, Karger, 2010, vol 27, pp 143–159.

2 Hugues R: Sauser avant Cendrars. Revue Neuchateloise, No 89, 1979.

3 Lettre à Agnès et Georges Sauser. 12 avril 1909. Inédits secrets 1969 page 37–38.

4 Miriam Cendrars: La vie, le verbe, l'écriture. Paris, Denoël, 2006, pp 148–157.

5 Blaise Cendrars: Premier entretien avec Michel Manoll. Tout autour d'aujourd'hui – œuvres complètes tome 15. Paris, Denoël, 2006, pp 7–8.

6 Blaise Cendrars: Moravagine. Tout autour d'aujourd'hui – œuvres complètes tome 7. Paris, Denoël, 2003, p 13.

7 Ricciotto Canudo: Les libérés, mémoire d'un aliéniste. Paris, Fasquelle, 1911.

8 Blaise Cendrars: Moravagine. Tout autour d'aujourd'hui – œuvres complètes tome 7. Paris, Denoël, 2003, pp 102–113.

9 Fonds Blaise Cendrars des archives littéraires suisses (Berne). Dossier Moravagine O 67.

10 Blaise Cendrars: Moravagine. Tout autour d'aujourd'hui – œuvres complètes tome 7. Paris, Denoël, 2003, p 12.

11 Blaise Cendrars: L'homme foudroyé. Tout autour d'aujourd'hui – œuvres complètes tome 5. Paris, Denoël, 2002, p 353.

12 Blaise Cendrars: Moravagine. Tout autour d'aujourd'hui – œuvres complètes tome 7. Paris, Denoël, 2003, p 15.

13 Tatu L, Bogousslavsky J: La folie au front. La grande bataille des névroses de guerre (1914–1918). Paris, Éditions Imago, 2012.

14 Blaise Cendrars: L'homme foudroyé. Tout autour d'aujourd'hui – œuvres complètes tome 5. Paris, Denoël, 2002, p 22.

15 Blaise Cendrars: L'homme foudroyé. Tout autour d'aujourd'hui – œuvres complètes tome 5. Paris, Denoël, 2002, p 22.

16 Blaise Cendrars: Moravagine. Tout autour d'aujourd'hui – œuvres complètes tome 7. Paris, Denoël, 2003, p 201.

17 Blaise Cendrars: La Main coupée. Tout autour d'aujourd'hui tome 6. Paris, Éditions Denoël, 2002, p 21.

18 Paul Voivenel: Sur la peur morbide acquise. Annales Médico-Psychologiques 1918;9:283–308.

19 Blaise Cendrars: L'homme foudroyé. Tout autour d'aujourd'hui – œuvres complètes tome 5. Paris, Denoël, 2002, pp 29–31.

20 Blaise Cendrars: L'homme foudroyé. Tout autour d'aujourd'hui – œuvres complètes tome 5. Paris, Denoël, 2002, p 27.

21 Blaise Cendrars: La Main coupée. Tout autour d'aujourd'hui tome 6. Paris, Éditions Denoël, 2002, pp 275–276.

22 Tatu L, Bogousslavsky J, Moulin T, Chopard JL: The 'torpillage' neurologists of World War I: electric therapy to send hysterics back to the front. Neurology 2010;75:279–283.

23 Blaise Cendrars: L'homme foudroyé. Tout autour d'aujourd'hui – œuvres complètes tome 5. Paris, Denoël, 2002, p 20.

24 Blaise Cendrars: Moravagine. Tout autour d'aujourd'hui – œuvres complètes tome 7. Paris, Denoël, 2003, p 202.

25 Christine Le Quellec Cottier: Devenir Cendrars. Paris, Éditions Champion, 2004, pp 239–241.

26 Jacques Chessex: Le vampire de Ropraz. Paris, Grasset, 2007, pp 107–110.

27 Henri Claude, Jean Lhermitte: Le syndrome infundibulaire dans un cas de tumeur du troisième ventricule. Presse Médicale 1917;23 juillet:54–62.

28 Judith Traschel: Sous le signe de Fébronio. Continent Cendrars 1991–1992;N°6-7:54–62.

29 Blaise Cendrars: Premier entretien avec Michel Manoll. Tout autour d'aujourd'hui – œuvres complètes tome 15. Paris, Denoël, 2006, p 13.

30 Blaise Cendrars: Fébronio. Tout autour d'aujourd'hui – œuvres complètes tome 8. Paris, Denoël, 2003, p 236.

31 Blaise Cendrars: Fébronio. Tout autour d'aujourd'hui – œuvres complètes tome 8. Paris, Denoël, 2003, p 242.

32 Blaise Cendrars: Bourlinguer. Tout autour d'aujourd'hui – œuvres complètes tome 9. Paris, Denoël, 2003, p 200.



Professor Laurent Tatu
Department of Neuromuscular Diseases
CHU Jean-Minjoz, Boulevard Fleming
FR–25030 Besançon Cedex (France)
E-Mail laurent.tatu@univ-fcomte.fr

Bogousslavsky J, Dieguez S (eds): Literary Medicine: Brain Disease and Doctors in Novels, Theater, and Film.
Front Neurol Neurosci. Basel, Karger, 2013, vol 31, pp 10–34 (DOI: 10.1159/000345527)

# Balzac's *Louis Lambert*: Schizophrenia before Kraepelin and Bleuler

Sebastian Dieguez

Laboratory for Cognitive and Neurological Sciences, Département de Médecine, Hôpital de Fribourg, Université de Fribourg, Fribourg, Switzerland

**Abstract**

Honoré de Balzac (1799–1850) is well known for his penetrating observations and descriptions of the burgeoning social life and emerging modernity of 19th century France. This chapter focuses on the novel *Louis Lambert*, first published in 1832. It is argued that its main character provides the first complete and convincing description of schizophrenia – 69 years before Kraepelin fully developed the concept of *dementia praecox* and 76 years before Bleuler coined the word 'schizophrenia'. We consider the history of the concept of schizophrenia and the intriguing possibility that it is a recent disease. Indeed, if schizophrenia had always existed, it would seem odd that Balzac's novel should be the very first convincing and complete literary account of the disease. This claim is examined by a thorough description of Louis Lambert's symptoms as they appear in the text, and compared to other claims of priority (namely, Shakespeare's *King Lear* and Gogol's *Diary of a Madman*). The chapter also provides some background on Balzac's relationship with mysticism, mental illness, and the world of psychiatry. We conclude with remarks regarding influences of *Louis Lambert*, the case for the priority of the novel as the princeps case of schizophrenia, and its relevance to the recency hypothesis of schizophrenia.



The French writer Honoré de Balzac (1799–1850) is well known for his extraordinary gifts of observation and description. Among his many talents and interests, he devoted a fair share of his monumental œuvre *La comédie humaine* (The Human Comedy) – a lifetime project encompassing close to 100 interlinked novels – to medical, philosophical, and psychological issues. Because of the author's prominence in 19th century intellectual circles, these particular writings are of great interest to historians of neurology and psychiatry. Scholars have often been struck by the accuracy and precision of his descriptions of doctors and patients, and could also gather in his works a great deal of information about the social representations of illness and medicine of his time [1, this vol., pp. 225–235].

There is, however, one specific character that became especially noteworthy to psychiatrists, and indeed to Balzac himself: Louis Lambert (fig. 1). First introduced in *Notice biographique sur Louis Lambert* (1832), later reworked as *Histoire intellectuelle de Louis Lambert* (1833), and then simply *Louis Lambert*, this character, although a minor one in the overall structure of *La comédie humaine*, has raised a considerable number of medical interpretations [1–7]. Despite its rather short appearance in Balzac's career, *Louis Lambert* served him by embodying his deepest beliefs about the nature of the human mind and the structure of reality, his fascination with – and fear of – insanity, his conception of the notion of genius, and furthermore is the only novel written in the first-person. Balzac was clearly aware that *Louis Lambert* stood apart from his other works. It reads almost like a medical case report, offering perspectives from the patient himself and from external observers, and was also conceived as a personal statement of the author against those who thought he was crazy. Moreover, Balzac had intellectual ambitions extending far beyond being acclaimed as a great writer. For him, *Louis Lambert* could serve to 'someday guide science into new directions', and the novel was explicitly directed at a medical and scientific readership.

Quite apart from its spiritual and mystical theories (see below), the story was indeed praised for its prescient, penetrating, and convincing description of the symptoms of schizophrenia, decades before the disease was formally recognized, described, and documented by psychiatrists. The portrayal is so strikingly reminiscent of real-life clinical cases that many have assumed Balzac must have known such an individual. This might well be the case, but no Louis Lambert persona or analogue could demonstrably be traced in Balzac's biography. Rather, Lambert might be a composite of Balzac himself, persons he had actually met, case descriptions he had read in the medical literature, anecdotes told to him by doctors and friends, an embodiment of ideas he'd gathered from mystically inclined writers such as Swedenborg, or perhaps simply a result of Balzac's prophetic gifts and fine knowledge of the human mind. Be that as it may, it remains that as early as 1832 Balzac described the signs of early and late psychosis so meticulously in *Louis Lambert* that the psychiatrists Devic and Morin [4] wrote in 1927 that they were 'all in there'.

Before we proceed to describe Lambert's psychiatric history, we need to consider the history of the concept of schizophrenia itself. A very general overview will serve to put Louis Lambert's biography into medical perspective, and raise the intriguing (and unsolved) question of whether schizophrenia existed prior to the 19th century. The last sections will provide an outline of Balzac's relationship with mysticism, mental illness, and the world of psychiatry, as well as some final remarks highlighting the ambiguity regarding influences for *Louis Lambert*, marshaling the case for the priority of the work as the princeps case of schizophrenia, and speculating on its relevance to the recency hypothesis of the condition.

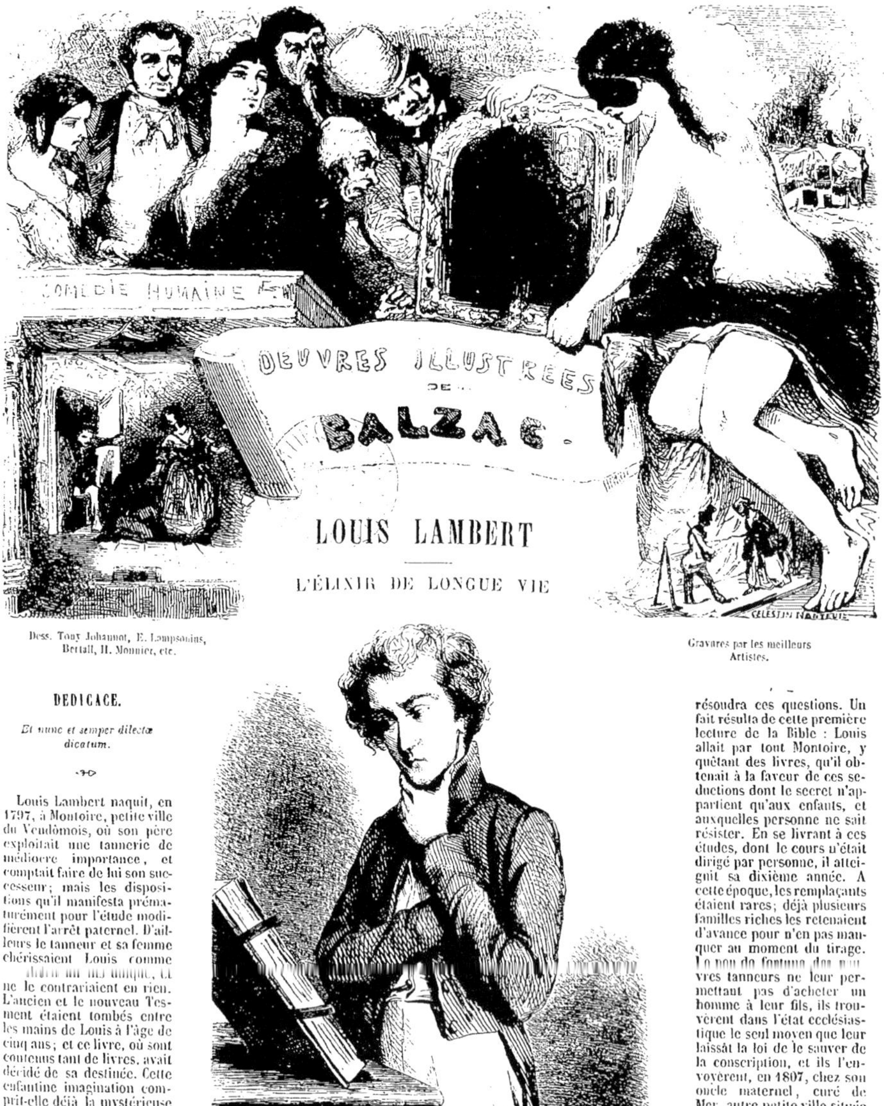


LOUIS LAMBERT

L'ÉLIXIR DE LONGUE VIE

Dess. Tony Johannot, E. Lampsonius, Bertall, H. Monnier, etc.

Gravures par les meilleurs Artistes.

DEDICACE.

*Et nunc et semper dilectæ dicatum.*

Louis Lambert naquit, en 1797, à Montoire, petite ville du Vendômois, où son père exploitait une tannerie de médiocre importance, et comptait faire de lui son successeur; mais les dispositions qu'il manifesta prématurément pour l'étude modifièrent l'arrêt paternel. D'ailleurs le tanneur et sa femme chérissaient Louis comme [illegible] et ne le contrariaient en rien. L'ancien et le nouveau Tesment étaient tombés entre les mains de Louis à l'âge de cinq ans; et ce livre, où sont contenus tant de livres, avait décidé de sa destinée. Cette enfantine imagination comprit-elle déjà la mystérieuse profondeur des Écritures? pouvait-elle déjà suivre l'esprit saint dans son vol à travers les mondes? s'éprit-elle seulement des romanesques attraits qui abondent en ces poëmes tout orientaux? ou, dans sa première innocence, cette âme sympathisa-t-elle avec le sublime religieux que des mains divines ont épanché dans ce livre? Pour quelques lecteurs, notre récit

Un grand penchant l'entraînait vers les ouvrages mystiques. — PAGE 2.

résoudra ces questions. Un fait résulta de cette première lecture de la Bible : Louis allait par tout Montoire, y quêtant des livres, qu'il obtenait à la faveur de ces séductions dont le secret n'appartient qu'aux enfants, et auxquelles personne ne sait résister. En se livrant à ces études, dont le cours n'était dirigé par personne, il atteignit sa dixième année. A cette époque, les remplaçants étaient rares; déjà plusieurs familles riches les retenaient d'avance pour n'en pas manquer au moment du tirage. [illegible] vres tanneurs ne leur permettant pas d'acheter un homme à leur fils, ils trouvèrent dans l'état ecclésiastique le seul moyen que leur laissât la loi de le sauver de la conscription, et ils l'envoyèrent, en 1807, chez son oncle maternel, curé de Mer, autre petite ville située sur la Loire, près de Blois. Ce parti satisfaisait tout à la fois la passion de Louis pour la science et le désir qu'avaient ses parents de ne point l'exposer aux hasards de la guerre. Ses goûts studieux et sa précoce intelligence donnaient d'ailleurs l'espoir de lui voir faire une grande fortune dans l'Église. Après être resté pendant environ trois ans chez

85 Paris. - Imprim. de Schneider, rue d'Erfurth, 1.

1

**Fig. 1.** Frontispiece of *Louis Lambert*. The text reads: 'A strong bias drew his mind into mystical studies' [51].

## Schizophrenia through the Ages

*Schizophrenia: The Early Years*

As is well known, the word 'schizophrenia' was first introduced by the Swiss psychiatrist Eugen Bleuler in a 1908 article [8] and then in his 1911 book *Dementia Praecox or the Group of Schizophrenias*. The term served as an improvement on the earlier notion of 'dementia praecox', a term introduced in 1860 by French alienist Bénédict Augustin Morel in his *Traité des maladies mentales* to refer to cases of young patients whose condition seemed to mimic the impairments usually seen in senile dementia, namely emotional disorders, lack of will and energy, and progressive dissolution of the personality. Emil Kraepelin later used the concept more comprehensively; by 1899, in the sixth edition of his *Textbook of Psychiatry*, he presented dementia praecox as a general heading encompassing cases of hebephrenia and catatonia (both concepts introduced by Karl Ludwig Kahlbaum in the 1860s), as well as paranoid dementia (first described by Charles Lasègue in 1852 as 'delusion of persecution'), as he thought all three conditions were really manifestations of the same underlying illness. To this, he added a number of symptoms: flattened or inappropriate emotional responses, stereotyped behavior, catatonic postures, disorders of attention, hallucinations, delusional beliefs, and an irreversible deterioration of intellectual functions [9, 10].

Although rather successful, the concept was criticized for its overinclusiveness and superficiality. Bleuler was informed by Freudian psychoanalysis and saw the value of investigating the very thought processes of such patients. He also pointed out that the term dementia praecox was misleading, as on the one hand it implied the notion of a progressive and irreversible deterioration, and on the other hand it unnecessarily restricted its application to the young. His conception was far ranging in phenomenological details; the core of schizophrenia, he thought, was 'the dislocation of varied psychic functions', namely a dissociation between cognition, memory, emotions, perceptions, and identity.[1] This led to the identification of the main problem of schizophrenic patients as being an impairment in the capacity for 'association'. Emotional reactions seemed dissociated from cognitive processes; irrelevant ideas disturbed the course of thinking and were given unwarranted importance, whereas truly related concepts were perceived as disjointed; speech was frequently incomprehensible, bizarre and oftentimes interrupted to take a wholly different course; the meaning of words and sentences was emptied or arbitrarily altered; and opposite concepts were maintained in a state of inner conflict. In short, the plight of these patients was a severe impairment in logical thinking and common sense. As

[1] It is commonplace in discussions of schizophrenia to hastily point out that the disorder has nothing to do with the notion of 'split-personality' as portrayed in Hollywood's shock movies and horror novels. However, as it turns out this caveat is not entirely warranted: the confusion is not originally issued from media and lay misinformation, but had actually been orchestrated by Bleuler himself, his translator, and the psychological profession at large [11].

a consequence, their personality and behavior seemed disunited and unpredictable, and they developed elaborate delusions, states of confusion, and unsettling affective changes. Moreover, these patients were disconnected from their own thought processes and had a hard time disentangling reality from fantasy, leading to hallucinations in the auditory and visual modalities, and eventually to a loss of contact with reality. Motor processes were also affected, including stereotypical behaviors, mannerisms, lack of initiative, disordered actions and agitation, resistance to external stimulations, or even complete stupor and catatonia. Contrary to Kraepelin, Bleuler noted that apart from the defective process of association, cognitive, memory, and perceptive processes were often quite remarkably preserved in his patients. The deterioration was not global, it often concerned rather specific areas of mental life leaving the others unaffected. Furthermore, although he thought that schizophrenia was incurable, he pointed out that the disturbances could remain quite stable over time and did not necessarily lead to a general deterioration. Importantly, Bleuler also highlighted the role of the environment as a powerful modulating factor in the course of schizophrenia. Obviously, such disturbances led to many problems in daily life, and these social consequences in turn influenced the nature, severity, and course of the condition.

In the intervening years, many theories and complements have been adduced to Bleuler's description of schizophrenia [12], but to this day the general idea has survived and continues to be used by professionals and researchers (see table 1 for a summary of Bleuler's concept of schizophrenia and current diagnostic criteria, and table 2 for alternative approaches to schizophrenia). Before Bleuler, however, this picture had never been systematized and existed only, at best, in scattered fragments of the psychiatric literature.

### *Has There Always Been Schizophrenic Patients?*

Bleuler's coinage and systematization of the concept of schizophrenia – following Kraepelin's attempt to classify rationally the different types of mental disorders – has of course been hugely influential in helping identify and categorize a wide group of patients previously thought to be unrelated to each other or suffering from different ailments altogether. Previous to the advent of such modern descriptions and classifications, 'madness' was conceived in very general terms, such as 'possession', 'melancholia', 'vesania', 'furor', 'dementia', and later somewhat more precisely as 'monomania' and 'psychosis'. This makes it difficult to retrospectively examine the existence or prevalence of the disease – as understood in its current acceptation – in older times, and even more so to track down the earliest reports of the condition.

Nevertheless, on the grounds that schizophrenia is fairly recognizable and a rather striking disorder, authors have argued that it must have been reported long before the modern diagnosis had been established. The implication being, rather provocatively, that if no such reports can be found, then schizophrenia must be a new disease. Hare [20] defended precisely this hypothesis, arguing that the scarcity of reports previous

**Table 1.** Schizophrenia: Bleuler's approach and abridged criteria from DSM-IV-TR (American Psychiatric Association, 2000)

| | |
|---|---|
| *Eugen Bleuler's concept of schizophrenia (1911)* | |
| | Against Kraepelin's dementia praecox: deterioration not ineluctable; impairment not global; onset not restricted to the youth; analogy with senile dementia misleading |
| | The syndrome is characterized by a number of cardinal symptoms, always present in all patients: (1) autism (i.e. motor inhibition, social retreat, inwardness in a fantasy world); (2) loosening of associations (i.e. thought disturbances, disorganized speech and ideas, irrational reasoning, loss of the meaning of words and things); (3) inappropriate affects and ambivalence (i.e. felt and expressed emotions are incongruent with current circumstances, attitudes, and intentions, and appear ambiguous, irrational, and unpredictable to others) |
| | As a reaction to the cardinal symptoms, a number of secondary symptoms may or may not appear: hallucinations, delusions, stereotypies, catatonia, mannerisms, and resistance to external stimulations |
| | The concept of dissociation: as expressed by the coinage 'schizophrenia' (literally 'split mind'), the central feature of the disease is not a deterioration but rather a dissociation of otherwise preserved functions |
| | Organic basis: an underlying organic disturbance leads to dissociation, which itself explains all the cardinal symptoms; the secondary symptoms are based on different mechanisms and can be influenced by a number of external factors; Bleuler provides an analogy to osteomalacia, but does not speculate further about the causes of schizophrenia |
| *Diagnostic criteria in DSM-IV-TR, 2000* | |
| A | At least two (or only one if particularly striking or bizarre) of the following characteristic symptoms, present for most of a 1-month duration without treatment:<br>Delusions<br>Hallucinations<br>Disorganized speech and thought disorder<br>Grossly disorganized or catatonic behavior<br>Negative symptoms (e.g. blunted affect, reduced speech, and lack of motivation) |
| B | Substantial social or occupational dysfunction since the onset of disturbance, as compared to the level achieved prior to onset |
| C | The disturbance persists for of at least 6 months (duration), including at least 1 month of symptoms |
| D–F | Exclusion of a direct influence of mood disorders, substance abuse, or a pervasive developmental disorder |

to 1800 indeed leads to the conclusion that schizophrenia is a recent disease, and therefore that it must have been triggered by a specific event around 1800.

Now the hypothesis raises a number of practical problems. As we have said above, the very introduction of a new diagnosis and particular criteria makes it difficult to accurately judge cases prior to these novelties. Information deemed relevant and important at one time might have been entirely neglected in previous times; however, that does not mean that the information did not exist. Moreover, cultural and historical factors might shape the perception of disease and even alter the presentation of syndromes themselves. Likewise, evolving methods of assessment, different beliefs about etiology, persisting traditions for certain treatments, changes in terminology,

**Table 2.** Concepts and interpretations of schizophrenia

| | |
|---|---|
| Phenomenology | Schizophrenia can only be understood by a careful and empathetic examination of the patient's personality and life history. This background check can help understand the patient's belief system and otherwise meaningless symptoms [13]. |
| Schneider's first-rank symptoms | Schizophrenia can best be detected and diagnosed by focusing on a number of symptoms that are specific to the condition. Among them, Schneider [14] identified: hearing one's own thoughts; hearing voices commenting on one's actions; feeling influenced by unseen external forces; believing that others can see one's thoughts; feeling that one's actions are caused by someone else; deriving wild and irrational conclusions from mundane events. |
| Ego psychopathology | Schizophrenia is a reaction to a perceived threat affecting the integrity of the self (one's sense of existing, identity, agency, consistency, and demarcation from others and the world). The model highlights symptoms as a reaction to the feared disintegration of ego functions, which leads to agitation, stupor, and automatisms [15]. |
| Morbid rationalism | Schizophrenia involves an 'anthithetic attitude' towards reality, whereby rigid, dichotomic, and abstract systems of understanding are devised by the patient. Increasingly, the system leads to 'active egocentrism', namely an inner consolidation of the delusional system of beliefs fostered by a detachment from the others and reality [16]. |
| Loss of self-evidence | Schizophrenia is foremost a loss of the 'commonsense' perception of reality. Because of this subtle anomaly, mundane events that are normally taken for granted suddenly lose their obviousness and become perplexing and troubling. Reality as a whole becomes difficult to process, leading to cognitive, perceptive, motor, and social difficulties and increasing alienation [17]. |
| Cognitive disturbances | Schizophrenia is characterized by a host of cognitive impairments affecting executive functions, memory, attention, social cognition, and motor cognition. Several symptoms appear to be grounded on a deficient online self-monitoring system, whereby self-initiated actions and thoughts are perceived as externally generated, leading to auditory hallucinations, self-other confusions, and delusional beliefs [18]. |
| Two-stage models of monothematic delusions | A twofold process explains delusional beliefs in schizophrenia. A misguided perception of reality is first induced by an underlying neuropsychological impairment affecting perceptual, bodily, motor, or emotional processing. The false belief then becomes a delusion as a second impairment, this time involving higher-level cognitive processes such as reasoning and reality monitoring, fosters its acceptance, and prevents its rejection [19]. |

and issues of translation all converge to cloud the picture and make it very difficult to hit beyond all ambiguity the target one is currently aiming at.

Despite these difficulties, identifying convincing cases of schizophrenia previous to the modern descriptions, or, contrariwise, carefully documenting its historical absence or rarity, is of great theoretical interest.[2] The quest for such a case prior to

[2] See [25] for a related discussion on the nature of dissociative amnesia, and the chapter by Dieguez and Annoni [this vol., pp. 137–168].

1800 has not proven very fruitful, and the remaining controversy only further indicates the weakness of the case (see [21–23]).

Bark [24], for instance, has suggested that a character from the Shakespeare canon could be a 'classic description of chronic schizophrenia'. The character is Poor Mad Tom, who appears in four scenes of *King Lear* (approx. 1603–1606), and is actually the character Edgar in disguise. Bark points out the deterioration in social and economic functioning, the presence of paranoid ideas, loose associations, nonsensical talk, hallucinations, social isolation, bizarre behavior, self-harm, and coprophagia. Altschuler [26] added that Poor Tom also presents the 'redundant clothing sign', a peculiarity supposedly specific to schizophrenia. Now, Poor Mad Tom is really Edgar *acting* like a madman; in other words he is merely feigning insanity. Bark argues, nevertheless, that even to depict a character *imitating* schizophrenia, Shakespeare must still have been inspired by actual schizophrenic patients. In fact, the Bard might even have been inspired by beggars themselves pretending to be mad, which would remove the influence still one step further.

Several authors have accepted Bark's suggestion that Poor Tom is a satisfying portrayal of schizophrenia [20, 27, 28]. However, it appears to us that the 'case' is extremely sketchy and rather in line with many other Shakespearian depictions of lunacy, from which Poor Tom does not so dramatically depart. The purpose of the character is also comedic, and for that reason would need to display an exaggerated scene as well as amusing lines. More importantly, the issue that Edgar is merely *imitating* insanity cannot easily be dismissed. That the layperson's idea of what insanity is should happen to coincide with certain schizophrenic symptoms, rather than, say, obsessive-compulsive disorder or restless legs syndrome, in no way is evidence that such schizophrenic symptoms must exist as a natural phenomenon in the first place and for that reason.

Of course, the existence of old historical (real or fictional) cases still would not say much about the prevalence of the disorder at the time. Some rare and isolated striking cases might have come to prominence and led to further portrayals and discussions, without making the disease frequent or widely known in the least. As it seems that no other fictional character has been adduced to demonstrate the existence of schizophrenia prior to 1800, and as Poor Tom appears at the moment to be the most convincing one despite its limitations, one is left to searching for cases from 1800 onwards.

Altschuler [27] proposed that *Diary of a Madman* (1834–1835), one of Nikolaï Gogol's St Petersburg tales, is 'one the oldest cases of schizophrenia'. The short story tells, as the title implies, the experience of mental illness of a low-rank Ukrainian civil servant, Poprischkin, who keeps track of his descent into madness in his diary. Poprischkin writes about perceiving a conversation between two dogs, intercepting a letter correspondence between the dogs, having increasing difficulties at work, believing that he has become the King of Spain (after reading a news story on the subject), being increasingly absent from work, and behaving erratically and impulsively.

The writing itself soon becomes chaotic, and the date entries increasingly absurd (e.g. '86th Martober'). Altschuler takes the following features as indicative of schizophrenia: progressive worsening, disorganized and bizarre behavior, prodromal period with hallucinations or delusions, increasingly disordered speech, and ideas of reference. He could also probably have added a distorted perception of time and a more specific delusion of grandeur (megalomania).

However, the story takes place in a series of works definitely belonging to the absurdist or grotesque genre. *Diary of a Madman* was published next to *The Overcoat*, *The Nose*, and *The Portrait*, stories that could as well be indicative of diverse types of insanity. Rather than providing a description of a specific type of disease, Poprischkin, just like Edgar in *King Lear*, seems to be performing a certain idea of madness.[3] The 'perception' of a dialogue between dogs and the King of Spain delusion seem in this sense but a crude exaggeration, to farcical effect, of certain features easily labeled as aberrant by a receptive reader.

So the question remains: why is schizophrenia so rare and ambiguous in older texts? It seems that either, for whatever reason, schizophrenia has always existed and been frequent, but was never or rarely reported until the 19th century; or it was a very uncommon or even inexistent disease before 1800. On the first hypothesis, it might be argued that clinicians and medical writers were simply fewer in older times, that beliefs about the supernatural nature of mental illness were prevalent (delusions could simply have been seen as prophecies, and hallucinations as 'veridical' apparitions); or perhaps schizophrenia existed but was simply thought to be something else, took different forms, or was clouded by the factors mentioned above. The second hypothesis naturally raises the question of why a disease such as schizophrenia would suddenly appear out of the blue. Some authors have speculated about the triggering event that could have led to the appearance – or at least a radical increase – of schizophrenia in the early 19th century. Cooper and Sartorius [30] blamed the rise of industrialization, Torrey [31] blamed 'civilization' as a whole, and Hare [20] felt it involved more specifically the role of an unknown infectious agent.

Notwithstanding this debate about recency, it seems that schizophrenia had to wait for Eugen Bleuler and, as we will now see, Honoré de Balzac to be formally observed, described, and identified as a unique entity.

## *Louis Lambert* as a Case Report

### *The Creation of Louis Lambert*

*Louis Lambert*, despite its shortness and rather marginal place in the overall balzacian scheme of things, did not come easily to its otherwise remarkably efficient

[3] For a discussion of Gogol's own alleged mental ailments, and especially how his diagnosis was hotly debated among Russian psychiatrists, see [29].

and productive author. Nevertheless, he clearly saw it as one of his greatest achievements: '*[Louis Lambert]* is a work where I sought to challenge von Goethe and Byron, *Faust* and *Manfred*' (letter to his family, 20th July 1832). Balzac reworked it more than ten times and hesitated a great deal as to the place it should take in *La comédie humaine*. At times he displayed enormous pride, but on other occasions he seemed rather despaired with the work. The story was written in 'thirty days and fifteen nights'. It was first published as part of the 4th volume of *Romans et contes philosophiques (Nouveaux contes philosophiques)* in 1832 under the title *Notice biographique sur Louis Lambert*, and was almost immediately reworked and published in a separate volume as *Histoire intellectuelle de Louis Lambert* in 1833. In 1835, *Louis Lambert* was 'moved' in the *Livre mystique*, a volume comprising *Les proscrits* and *Séraphîta*, and including an author's preface. This preface, as well as one already present in the 1832 version, was be removed from subsequent editions; they strongly highlighted the scientific ambitions of the work, not only concerning the 'philosophical' contents, but also its views on the mind, brain, and pathology. *Louis Lambert* was again reprinted in 1836, in a slightly altered version, as part of the collection *Etudes philosophiques* (volumes XXIII and XXIV), and later in 1846 in a larger edition of the complete *Comédie humaine* (volume XVI, 3rd book of *Etudes philosophiques*). Balzac's intentions in writing this work were manifold. He saw it as a response to those who doubted his sanity and talent: 'I had to respond gloriously to those who say that I am crazy [. . .] my reputation and future are at stake', he wrote to his sister. He also clearly wanted the work to be taken seriously by scholars, including doctors, philosophers, and alienists. To achieve this goal, he knew the message should not be too obvious or direct, but be formatted as a novel just like the many others he published at the time: 'Had I written a purely scholarly work, it would have attracted the attention of thinkers, but they wouldn't have even looked at it. However, if they come across it by chance, then they might talk about it'.

As is customary in Balzac's work, his character's biographical details are extremely realistic and detailed [32]. We know, for instance, that Louis Lambert was born in Montoire in 1797 and died at Villenoix on the September 25, 1824. His 'existence' is acknowledged by characters in other works, and he even makes appearances in *Illusions perdues*, *Les martyrs ignorés*, *Le curé de Tours* (previously *Les célibataires*), *Aventures administratives d'une idée heureuse*, and *Un drame au bord de la mer*. His descent into insanity is sometimes mentioned in these works. There are also some connections between Raphaël, the main character of *La peau de chagrin* (1831) and Louis Lambert, and some have speculated that he appears sometimes under different names [33].

Another interesting protagonist of *Louis Lambert* is the narrator, frequently identified as Balzac himself. Indeed, the book is the only one in Balzac's canon to be written in the first-person, and Louis Lambert is first met at the Collège de Vendôme, the institution at which Balzac himself was schooled from 1807 to 1813 (he entered at 8 years of age).

*Psychiatric Biography of Louis Lambert*

The complexity and ambition of Balzac's literary enterprise makes it unlikely that he would write anything carelessly or with no relevance to his general scheme of things. *Louis Lambert* is certainly no exception. The story was reworked and refined over years, and the result is a dense and carefully constructed biographical account of a brilliant young man ultimately overwhelmed by his exalted thought processes, his abstract beliefs and philosophy, and his emotional upheavals (table 3). The psychiatrists and scholars who have analyzed his case tend to follow the author in dividing the course of the disease in three parts [2, 3]. In what follows, we use the same approach, but proceed in reverse order, starting with the third and last stage of Lambert's decay, and concluding with the first signs of cognitive and affective disturbances in Lambert's youth [5].

*Third Stage: Catatonia*

In this final stage, the narrator meets Louis Lambert after having lost contact for some time. He has just recently learned that Lambert has been insane for the last 2 years and is being cared for by his wife (who married him just after his mental breakdown) at her home, which he never leaves anymore. By then, Lambert has ceased to communicate, hardly moves at all, and seems lost in his thoughts, completely disconnected from the external world:

> At last I could see him, and it was one of those spectacles that are stamped on the memory for ever. He was standing, his elbows resting on the cornice of the low wainscot, which threw his body forward, so that it seemed bowed under the weight of his bent head. His hair was as long as a woman's, falling over his shoulders and hanging about his face, giving him a resemblance to the busts of the great men of the time of Louis XIV. His face was perfectly white. He constantly rubbed one leg against the other, with a mechanical action that nothing could have checked, and the incessant friction of the bones made a doleful sound[4] (fig. 2).

Lambert very rarely lays down to sleep, says his wife, although when he does, he sleeps for several days in a row. In fact, most of his time is spent in the same posture, 'with a fixed gaze, never winking his eyelids'. The signs of premature ageing are frightening: 'Alas! he was wrinkled, white-headed, his eyes dull and lifeless as those of the blind. His features seemed all drawn upwards to the top of his head. I made several attempts to talk to him, but he did not hear me. He was a wreck snatched from the grave, a conquest of life from death – or of death from life!'

Louis Lambert's condition at this stage of the novel represents the most severe type of social withdrawal one can find in mental illness, a state frequently labeled 'autism' in the early uses of the concept of schizophrenia, and referred to by Balzac as catalepsy. This is an extreme manifestation of negative symptoms, encompassing all domains of waking life: reduced activity, overall slowness, decreased blinking,

[4] Throughout this chapter we use the French text in [34]; and Clara Bell and James Waring's English translation is available online at http://www.gutenberg.org/files/1943/1943-h/1943-h.htm.

**Table 3.** Summary and examples of Louis Lambert's schizophrenic symptoms

| | |
|---|---|
| *Stage 1: Unusual childhood* | |
| Unusual interests and preoccupations | Precocious and obsessive appeal for theological, mystical, linguistic, psychological, and philosophical matters far out of his reach. Deep significance found in mundane events or items. |
| Pervasive mental imagery | 'When I read the story of the battle of Austerlitz I saw every incident.' |
| Imagination induces bodily sensations | 'If I think with concentration of the effect that the blade of my penknife would have in piercing my flesh, I feel an acute pain as if I had really cut myself.' |
| Belief of being endowed with precognitive, clairvoyant, and disembodiment capabilities; probable déjà-vu experience. | 'I saw this last night in a dream.' 'If my spirit and my body can be severed during sleep, why should I not insist on their separating in the same way while I am awake?' |
| Morbid rationalism | Elaboration of an all-encompassing, supreme and ultimate theory of cosmic significance (an elusive *Treatise on the Will*). Increasing abstraction and loss of contact with reality, increasing inwardness and social isolation. |
| *Stage 2: Cognitive, emotional, and social disturbances* | |
| Delusions of grandeur | 'My head is too weak, it will burst with the vehemence of my ideas.' |
| Mood swings, emotionality | 'I cry and I laugh – I am possessed! Every joy is an arrow of flame; it pierces and burns me.' |
| Ego disturbances | 'No one in the world can conceive of the terrors my fateful imagination inflicts on me.' |
| Apathy, lack of motivation | 'I feel bereft of all strength. Everything is a burden to me; every fiber of my body is inert, every sense is flaccid, my sight grows dim, my tongue is paralyzed, my imagination is extinct, desire is dead.' |
| Experience of influence, feelings of passivity | 'What name can I give to the power that ties my hands and shuts my mouth, and drags me in a direction opposite to my vocation?' |
| Thought-intrusion and thought broadcasting | 'Did not I know, at once, that your carriage had been overthrown and you were bruised? But on that day I had been with you, I had never left you, I could see you.' |
| Self-other confusion | 'We are not yet completely one in mind. At two leagues' distance or at a thousand I ought to feel your pain and sorrows. I shall not believe that I love you till my life is so bound up with yours that our life is one, till our hearts, our thoughts are one.' |
| Catalepsia | 'He had once remained motionless for fifty-nine hours, his eyes staring, neither speaking nor eating.' |
| *Stage 3: Catatonia* | |
| Immobility and lack of communication | 'Louis stood day and night with a fixed gaze, never winking his eyelids as we do.' |
| Stereotyped movements | 'He constantly rubbed one leg against the other, with a mechanical action that nothing could have checked, and the incessant friction of the bones made a doleful sound.' |
| Sleep disorders | 'He very rarely lies down, but whenever he does, he sleeps for several days.' |

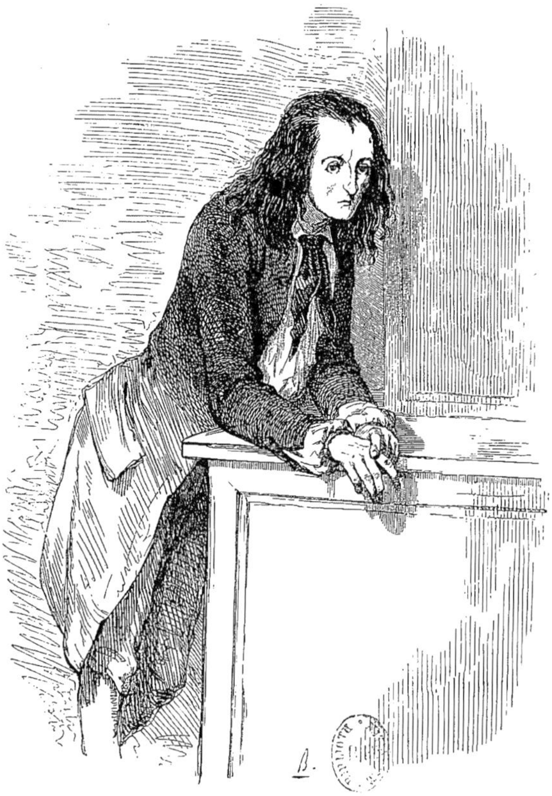
LOUIS LAMBERT.
Il se tenait debout, les deux coudes appuyés sur la saillie formée par la boiserie...

**Fig. 2.** Louis Lambert in the last stage of his disease. Most of his time is spent in this posture. The text reads: 'He was standing, his elbows resting on the cornice of the low wainscot. . .' (from *Oeuvres Illustrées de Balzac*, 1852, Paris: Marescq et Compagnie) [51].

thwarted communication, and unresponsiveness to external stimulation. Lambert also displays sleeping disturbances, as well as motor – and more rarely verbal – stereotypies. These are all classic signs of chronic untreated schizophrenia. But there is much more in Balzac's analysis of the case: the greater share of the book is really devoted to meticulously documenting the steps that progressively led to that final outcome of severe catatonia.

*Second Stage: Cognitive, Emotional, and Social Disturbances*

The second – intermediary – stage of the course of Lambert's illness is provided by his correspondence (namely, the letters recovered by the narrator) and the testimony of his uncle. At this moment of his life Lambert is a young adult trying to make a living, maintain a social life, and progress in his project to write a philosophical work. His ambitions are considerable, but success is not forthcoming. His problem is that he is unable to control and hold together his many ideas and projects, and as a result ends up shutting himself away: 'Compelled to live in himself alone, having no one to share his subtle raptures, he may have hoped to solve the problem of his destiny by a life of ecstasy, adopting an almost vegetative attitude, like an anchorite of the early Church, and abdicating the empire of the intellectual world.' Lambert thinks he has come up with a superior philosophical system that entirely solves the problem of disunity of scholarly knowledge, and will turn him into the guide needed to achieve a new stage of humanity. Yet he feels that his plans are being thwarted by a 'power that ties my hands and shuts my mouth, and drags me in a direction opposite to my vocation'. What is more, he increasingly feels dragged of energy and of the very sense of existence: 'There are moments when the spirit of vitality seems to abandon me. I feel bereft of all strength. Everything is a burden to me; every fiber of my body is inert, every sense is flaccid, my sight grows dim, my tongue is paralyzed, my imagination is extinct, desire is dead'.

Considered in the light of the last stage of the disease and the prodromal signs in his youth (see below), these features are strongly indicative of delusions of grandeur on the one hand and of negative symptoms on the other (apathy, inhibition, disorganization of thought, and loss of motivation), both rather common types of symptoms in schizophrenia. Moreover, the difficulties are attributed to an external source, some 'power', a causal misattribution typical of the early stages of the disease.

Lambert also occasionally displays impulsive behavior. For instance, one evening at the theater he suddenly falls in love with an unknown woman, and is seized by a desire to kill her companion on the spot, 'an effect of animal instinct combining with the almost luminous flashes of a soul crushed under the weight of thought'. Although not explicitly stated, these 'luminous flashes' emerging from the 'weight of thought' are reminiscent of the hallucinated voices that sometimes intimate patients to perform atrocious acts.

The letters provide ample evidence of inner conflict and contradiction, increasing dissociation from reality, as well as a deepening feeling of isolation: 'On all hands we find a precipice! On every side a gulf in which reason is lost [. . .] No one in the world can conceive of the terrors my fateful imagination inflicts on me. It often bears me up to the sky, and suddenly flings me to earth again from prodigious heights.' The handwriting itself displays evidence of a pathological state of mind, as the narrator notices:

> My familiarity with Lambert's writing enabled me in time to decipher the hieroglyphics of this shorthand, the result of impatience and a frenzy of passion. Carried away by his feelings, he had written without being conscious of the irregularity of words too slow to express his thoughts. He must have been compelled to copy these chaotic attempts, for the lines often ran into each other.

There are also hints of ideas of reference, passivity, thought intrusion, telepathic influence and self-other confusion. In the letters to her beloved, for instance, the need for fusion and the feeling of sympathy seem to go well beyond mere lyricism:

> 'At two leagues' distance or at a thousand I ought to feel your pain and sorrows. I shall not believe that I love you till my life is so bound up with yours that our life is one, till our hearts, our thoughts are one. I must be where you are, see what you feel, feel what you feel, be with you in thought. Did not I know, at once, that your carriage had been overthrown and you were bruised?

But on that day I had been with you, I had never left you, I could see you'; and later 'I fancy I could spend whole nights breathing your breath; I would I could steal into every detail of your life, be the very substance of your thoughts – be your very self'.

Anticipating the final catatonic stage, Lambert also suffers the reappearance (see below) of signs of motor inhibition: 'I have sat for hours in a sort of stupor caused by the violence of my passionate yearning, lost in the dream of a caress as though in a bottomless abyss. At such moments my whole vitality, my thoughts and powers, are merged and united in what I must call desire, for lack of a word to express that nameless delirium.' That 'nameless delirium' reaches its full-blown expression a few days before his planned marriage: 'He had once remained motionless for fifty-nine hours, his eyes staring, neither speaking nor eating; a purely nervous affection, to which persons under the influence of violent passion are liable; a rare malady, but perfectly well known to the medical faculty.' As we have seen, he will not recover from that state. What is worse, his very last manifestation of will seemed to have been an attempt at self-castration. His uncle indeed reports having 'found him preparing to perform on himself the operation to which Origen believed he owed his talents.'

It is after this event that Lambert is brought, only once and very shortly, to a doctor. The man is no less than the great Esquirol (a personal acquaintance of Balzac). Unfortunately, he is pronounced 'incurable', and the only medical advice given to his relatives is that he should be 'left in perfect solitude, with nothing to break the silence that was needful for his very improbable recovery.'

This second, intermediary stage of the disease thus works as a subtle transition towards the final – catatonic – outcome. It is marked by a state of inner conflict, grandiose ideas that cannot be reconciled with conflicting 'forces,' and increasing difficulties in controlling his thoughts, emotions, and behavior. This leads to pathological responses, attempts at coping with the situation that will only serve to precipitate his downfall. He first reacts by developing delusions of intellectual superiority (that would explain why he seems to be rejected by society), grandiose ideas and mannerisms, exalted and manic writing (graphomania or hypergraphia), acceleration and flight of thoughts, loosening of associations, and abrupt changes of topic and attitude, as well as unrest, anxiety, impulsivity, and intermittent self-depreciation (perhaps suggestive of auditory hallucinations).

Ultimately, these positive symptoms lead to a general state of indecision and confusion – with a very well-depicted partial lack of insight unto the condition – and progressively to feelings of being trapped and imprisoned inside of himself, culminating in complete withdrawal. In the process, Balzac introduces two additional remarkable features. The first one is the feeling of complete mental fusion with someone else, including fantasies of thought intrusion and telepathic communication. This is now recognized among the most striking early manifestations of schizophrenia (for an early report see [35]). The second one is the attempt at self-castration. Male genital self-mutilation, although infrequent, has since been found to be quite specific to schizophrenia, especially in the presence of delusions of a religious nature [36, 37], which certainly applies to Lambert's mystical obsessions (see below).

Absent any evidence for substance abuse, organic damage, epileptic seizures, or malingering, these detailed manifestations, especially in light of the preceding and following features, can only apply to schizophrenia as we know it nowadays. We also note that Balzac carefully places all these symptoms in the broader context of Lambert's social environment (as well as his childhood and adolescent years). Early onset-schizophrenia must always be examined in this light, as it is well known that particular events and lifestyles can modulate the presentation of the syndrome. In Louis Lambert's case, social isolation, financial problems, thwarted intellectual ambitions, and especially the emotional upheavals introduced by the discovery of passionate love definitely count for much in the emergence and precipitated worsening of his symptoms. Yet some observations from his early years clearly suggest a strong predisposition to develop the disease.

*First Stage: An Unusual Boy*

The 'data' from Lambert's school and adolescent years were obtained by direct and sustained observation by the narrator (Balzac?), his closest friend at the time. As we will see, a number of red flags are suggestive of incipient schizophrenia.

Louis Lambert entered the Collège de Vendôme at 13, on the enthusiastic recommendation of Madame de Staël. The celebrity had met the young boy by chance, as she found him one day reading *Heaven and Hell*, a book by Swedish mystic Emanuel Swedenborg, and was immediately impressed by the youth's vivid intelligence. She saw in him 'a real seer', and took it upon herself that he receive a strong education in the best of schools (after which, 'she probably forgot him' notes the narrator). Lambert was certainly a precocious child. He is said to have read the Bible at age 5, and from then on showed a remarkable interest in matters of religion, science, linguistics, history, and psychology.

Very soon, he develops an intense inner life, fostered by remarkable powers of memory and visualization:

> His memory was prodigious. He remembered with equal exactitude the ideas he had derived from reading, and those that had occurred to him in the course of meditation or conversation. Indeed, he had every form of memory – for places, for names, for words, things, and faces. He not only recalled any object at will, but he saw them in his mind, situated, lighted, and colored as he had originally seen them [. . .] He could remember, as he said, not merely the position of a sentence in the book where he had met with it, but the frame of mind he had been in at remote dates [. . .] His brain, accustomed in early youth to the mysterious mechanism by which human faculties are concentrated, drew from this rich treasury endless images full of life and freshness, on which he fed his spirit during those lucid spells of contemplation.

As Lambert explains, his mental life actually seems to him more vivid than the real world: 'I can draw a veil over my eyes. Then I suddenly see within me a *camera obscura*, where natural objects are reproduced in purer forms than those under which they first appeared to my external sense.' As an example of his peculiar powers of imagination, Lambert tells the following anecdote:

> When I read the story of the battle of Austerlitz [. . .] I saw every incident. The roar of the cannon, the cries of the fighting men rang in my ears, and made my inmost self quiver; I could smell the powder; I heard the clatter of horses and the voices of men; I looked down on the plain where armed nations were in collision, just as if I had been on the heights of Santon.

At times, however, this tendency to inwardness disconnects him completely from the external world: 'On the occasions when he brought all his powers into play, and in some degree lost consciousness of his physical existence, and lived on only by the remarkable energy of his mental powers, whose sphere was enormously expanded, he left space behind him, to use his own words'. Even worse, the imagination sometimes replaces reality altogether, as when self-suggestion induces actual bodily sensations:

> Do you ever feel [. . .] as though imagined suffering affected you in spite of yourself? If, for instance, I think with concentration of the effect that the blade of my penknife would have in piercing my flesh, I feel an acute pain as if I had really cut myself; only the blood is wanting. But the pain comes suddenly, and startles me like a sharp noise breaking profound silence.

Despite these remarkable capacities and Madame de Staël's great expectations, young Louis is not very successful at school. The professors are disappointed by his poor results, he does not make friends (other than the narrator), the vitiated school atmosphere makes him sick, and he seems to live in a perpetual dreamy state. As a result, 'he took refuge in heaven, which lay open to his mind' and increasingly indulged in reading mystical literature and developing ambitious schemes about the universe and the human mind. These 'theories' actually form the background of the entire novel. Balzac himself saw some significance in the works of Swedenborg and other mystics, and he cleverly used *Louis Lambert* as a way to present his own thinking in spiritual matters and the supernatural, while at the same time distancing himself from the most overblown ideas by putting them in the mouth of a disturbed character. Indeed, the narrator is not entirely impressed by Lambert's doctrines, which he describes as 'swathed in the wrappings of the phraseology affected by mystical writers [mystographes]: an obscure language full of abstractions, and taking such effect on the brain, that [. . .] they give rise to phantasies as various as the dreams of the opium-eater'.

As such, of course, an interest in mysticism and grandiose theories is not necessarily indicative of insanity. Yet such a connection cannot be mere coincidence in Louis Lambert's case: the ideas that the human mind is capable of supernatural feats, that will and consciousness are transcendental forces reaching beyond the material world, and that everything in the universe has a hidden relatedness and purpose, cannot but conjure up some cardinal features of schizophrenic cognition. Moreover, far from mere whim or healthy curiosity, Lambert's belief system is strongly reminiscent of what Eugène Minkowski [16] later called 'morbid rationalism'. This refers to the

**Table 4.** Examples of Louis Lambert's philosophical system. The appearance of systematization and rationality is suggestive of Minkowski's concept of 'morbid rationalism'. The original text displays an elaborate and confused use of typographical variations

| |
|---|
| The brain is the alembic to which the 'animal' conveys what each of its organizations, in proportion to the strength of that vessel, can absorb of that 'substance', which returns it transformed into 'will'. The 'will' is a fluid inherent in every creature endowed with motion. Hence the innumerable forms assumed by the 'animal', the results of its combinations with that 'substance'. The animal's instincts are the product of the coercion of the environment in which it develops. Hence its variety. |
| Though space exists, certain faculties have the power of traversing it with such rapidity that their effects are equivalent to its abolishment. From your own bed to the frontiers of the universe there are but two steps: *will—faith*! |
| There are three worlds – the 'natural', the 'spiritual', and the 'divine'. Humanity passes through the 'natural world', which is not fixed either in its essence and unfixed in its faculties. The 'spiritual world' is fixed in its essence and unfixed in its faculties. The 'divine world' is necessarily a 'material worship', a 'spiritual worship', and a 'divine worship': three forms expressed in 'action', 'speech', and 'prayer', or, in other words, in 'deed', 'understanding', and 'love'. |
| 'Three' and 'seven' are the two chief 'spiritual' numbers. |

tendency to categorize reality into discrete and rigid categories, to elaborate complex hierarchical systems of relationships and causality, and to see everything through the lenses of a unique doctrine. Further, such doctrines become increasingly abstract and disconnected from reality, which consolidates their perceived inner 'consistency' and makes them all the more resistant to counterevidence. Minkowski's coinage would certainly apply to Louis Lambert, who even attempted to compose a *Treatise on the Will* (Traité de la volonté), a far-reaching project encompassing all of human knowledge and explaining pretty much everything (table 4).

In retrospect, the first years of Louis Lambert's 'intellectual history' can be seen as early predictors of his forthcoming psychosis. His childhood psychological profile is certainly unusual, and includes, among others, striking signs of precociousness, social isolation, unusual interests, inner withdrawal, trance-like attitudes, loss of contact with reality, confusion of imagination and reality, occult beliefs, extreme emotionality, and 'morbid rationalism'. Moreover, Lambert's occult beliefs – such as precognition, clairvoyance, astral journeying, and telepathy – can retrospectively be interpreted as indicative of loose associations, delusional thinking, and perceptual abnormalities.

## Genius, Mysticism, and Insanity

Having presented at some length Louis Lambert's case history, some further notes can be adduced to put into perspective Balzac's schizophrenic character in the years following its publication. First, we touch on Balzac's interest in mysticism, and note that

*Louis Lambert* was one of the first works in the long tradition of associating mysticism and the occult with madness. We then turn to Balzac's personal relationship with insanity and his – as well as his character's – strange fate in the psychiatric literature.

*Balzac, Lambert, and Mysticism*

Balzac's depiction of mystical and occult themes in *Louis Lambert* is hardly unique. His interest for these topics can be found in numerous other works, including *La peau de chagrin*, *Le cousin Pons, Ursule Mirouët,* and *La recherche de l'absolu*. His personal position on such matters, however, is not easy to pin down (witness the many conflicting attempts to do so, e.g. [38–41]).

Balzac apparently thought of himself as a moderate 'swedenborgist', in the sense that he accepted some ideas of the Swedish mystic, but added a mix of his own Christianity, skepticism, and materialism. In other words, Balzac had no clearly identifiable belief system and was rather open to many different ideas and approaches. Whereas he certainly was interested in occult topics, and especially in the then rising craze for animal magnetism (i.e. Mesmerism), his love for the natural sciences and friendship with the great scientists of his time were probably much stronger. In any case, he used both registers as suited him best [33]. What is more, there is no reason to exaggerate his interest for Swedenborg or mysticism in general: it has indeed been demonstrated that most of his knowledge in this domain, including all the references made in *Louis Lambert*, can be traced back to a single source, *Abrégé des ouvrages d'Emanuel Swedenborg*, a digest published anonymously in 1788 [42]. Likewise, the 'genius' attributed to Lambert should not be overestimated either. Balzac's portrait certainly alludes to the tired trope of the genius-madness analogy, but everything in *Louis Lambert* points against the notion that Lambert is *truly* a superior mind. Rather, the *appearance* of profundity, wisdom and exceptionality are themselves indicative of the aberrant thought processes and behavior that underlie it, a phenomenon Sperber [43] has dubbed 'the guru effect'. Incomprehensible and illogical speech, or even plain mental illness, can indeed under the right circumstances be mistaken for genius. The *Treatise on the Will*, or rather the extracts unearthed by the narrator, would be a good example. A charitable, naïve or particularly well-inclined reader might perhaps see some value in those mysterious and far-reaching aphorisms, but clinicians will see in them clear evidence of a disorganized and deeply disturbed mind (e.g. [4]). Indeed, to *not* read *Louis Lambert* as an early report of schizophrenia, one would have to take his 'theories' (i.e. his symptoms) at face value and thus conclude that Lambert *actually* had reached a superior state of genius and ended up his life as a disembodied spirit in some higher plane of existence.

Around the 1850s it became customary in the neuropsychiatric literature to associate spiritualism, mysticism, and the occult in general with mental pathology. Psychics, seers, ecstatics, spiritualist, table-turners, somnambulists, mystics, and self-appointed prophets were all at some point placed under the watchful and scathing eyes of skeptical doctors [44]. Some examples, it should be pointed out, bear striking resemblances to Louis Lambert's profile, and here again Balzac's work can be seen as pioneering. Perhaps the most striking real-life embodiment of Louis Lambert has been Alexis Didier (1826–1886), a 'magnetic somnambulist' who appeared on the public scene in 1846 (i.e. 14 years after *Louis Lambert* was first published) [45, pp 235–242]. Alexis was purportedly gifted with extraordinary psychic abilities, which were eerily similar to those of Lambert (regardless of whether these 'powers' should be taken as 'real', merely imagined, delusional, or faked somehow). Didier most likely did not suffer from schizophrenia, but his health was fragile and he had epileptic seizures as a child. Moreover, if real, his clairvoyant and other psychic abilities would vindicate Lambert's 'philosophical system' (and thus support the Lambert-as-genius reading of the novel), which raises the intriguing possibility that Alexis Didier in fact had read *Louis Lambert* and set out to launch a career based on incarnating, as it were, Balzac's character [45].

Later, as schizophrenia and related psychoses became fairly well established clinical phenomena, the observation that such patients tended to hold irrational beliefs strongly related to occultist, religious, and conspiracy themes became commonplace. The best-known example of such a patient can probably be found in Daniel Paul Schreber's first-person account of his delusions [46].

*Balzac and Insanity*

Whereas some authors have assumed that Balzac really had known someone who would later become the model for his Louis Lambert, others have surmised that the character might rather be a projection of the author himself (e.g. [6, 33]). Could it be that Balzac experienced symptoms similar to those of Lambert? We have seen that they at least shared some common philosophical interests. We also know that Balzac at some early point had a project similar to Lambert's *Treatise on the Will*, and of course the spectacular scope of *La comédie humaine*, a project aimed at embracing the totality of human behavior, is reminiscent of Lambert's inordinate ambitions as a polymath. At 14, Balzac suffered for some months from a kind of stupor, apparently caused by an excess of reading. This can also be compared to Lambert's sickness during his stay at the Collège de Vendôme, and more generally to the dangers of an unrestrained intellectual life. Balzac was indeed well aware of such dangers and suffered chronically from ailments due to excessive work. In a letter from 1843, after an appointment with Dr. Nacquart, he wrote: 'I have arachnitis, namely a permanent inflammation of the arachnoid or the network of nerves which serve as a membrane to the brain [. . .] The doctor says that this is due to the extreme contrarieties and sensations that follow my excessive working' (quoted in [7, p 477]).

Thus, like Baudelaire, Balzac may have felt several times 'the winds of the wing of foolishness' pass over him, and the writing of *Louis Lambert* seemed to have caused him a great deal of worry [47]. The very act of writing, for him, sometimes involved getting immersed in a trance-like state – involving the consumption of an extraordinary amount of coffee – in which reality and imagination became blurred [6]. It should also be added that Balzac strived to build his own legend as a visionary verging on the brink of madness, which would explain the strange recycling that his persona and his character underwent in the medical literature following *Louis Lambert's* publication.

Indeed, Lambert came to be presented as a 'real' medical case in psychiatric textbooks in the mid-19th century [7, 48]. For instance, Bénédict Augustin Morel, in his *Etudes cliniques* (1852), and Brierre de Boismont, in the third edition of *Des hallucinations* (1862) used Louis Lambert as an example of 'hyperesthesia of sensibility'. Balzac himself was also cited as a good illustration of 'eccentricity' in Moreau de Tours' *La psychologie morbide* (1859). There was even a psychiatric tradition to quote an anecdote involving both Balzac and Esquirol, the great psychiatrist who examined Louis Lambert – and not only failed to help him but let slip the opportunity to isolate schizophrenia as a new medical diagnosis (according, of course, to retrospective readings of this probably fictive meeting; see [7] for a critical analysis of such approaches). The anecdote has it that Esquirol liked to display his novelist friend together with a mentally ill patient, and ask his students which was the madman [48]. Now, with such a background, it is hardly surprising that ill, disturbed, and insane characters, as well as doctors, should be so prominent in *La comédie humaine* (e.g. *Adieu* and *Ursule Mirouët;* see [1, this vol., pp. 225–235]).

## Conclusion: Is Louis Lambert Schizophrenia's Princeps Case?

To date, medical readings of *Louis Lambert* have applied a wide range of diagnostic criteria for schizophrenia, with slight changes in terminology and emphasis, from 1927 to 1950 [2–4]. Other authors have essentially picked up these works and put them into perspective, sometimes adding new clinical details and commenting on various aspects [1, 5, 6], or critically examining their claims using literary and historical analysis [7, 48]. Should we take over and apply today's criteria and nomenclature of schizophrenia to Louis Lambert? Can we pinpoint one specific type of schizophrenia for this patient, rule out all the exclusive criteria and prescribe a course of treatment? We do not think that such an approach is relevant for our purposes here or even that it would be profitable in the long run. First, as we already pointed out, views on schizophrenia have varied considerably ever since – and indeed, even before – the word was coined by Bleuler. The concept is currently under revision, and its definition, etiology, features, underlying mechanisms, and even its very usefulness continue to be hotly debated (e.g. [49, 50]). Second, it should be reminded that Louis Lambert is a fictional character. Despite short appearances in other works, the set of available information has been pinned down forever by the author, Balzac. Finally, the recent refined criteria, descriptions, and terminology for schizophrenia do not bear on the question of Louis Lambert's priority as the first case of schizophrenia. Indeed, it is unlikely that making diagnostic criteria sharper and more stringent could help unearth cases prior to Louis Lambert.

What matters, and is at the moment undisputed, is that *Louis Lambert* indeed offers a striking portrayal of an evolving schizophrenia. The details are numerous and cover virtually all the domains classically affected by schizophrenia, including personality, cognition, emotions, social life, beliefs, and the motor system. It almost seems that Balzac can only be blamed for not having provided the causal origin of the disorder, a disclosure that would arguably have been of some help to contemporary scientists. Still, Balzac vaguely postulated some type of brain damage or dysfunction, and suggested an influence of arousal and stressful events, which is about as much as is known with any certainty about the disorder, as of today.

Balzac could have been informed by extensive medical documentation and personal observations [2, 7] – including perhaps a visit to a mental asylum [47] – and by his careful self-examination [6]. The favored hypothesis, however, is that he knew someone like Louis Lambert, perhaps even met this person during his stay at the Collège de Vendôme, and later reported his observations in a fictional format. The psychiatrists Henri Claude and Joseph Levy-Valensi [3, p 590] wrote:

> There is no question that Balzac has seen a schizophrenic, that he followed his evolution from schizoidy to schizophrenia through all the cyclothymic, and perhaps schizomaniac, manifestations. Before Chaslin, Stranski, Bleuler and ourselves, he sensed the notion of dissociation, before Bleuler and Minkowski, he magnificently described the autistic component, the loss of contact with reality.

Likewise, 'Such precision and perfect truthfulness cannot be the result of imagination, and we have no doubt that Balzac has himself seen the evolution of a dementia praecox [. . .] [B]efore him no one had provided a description [. . .] the novelist had seen what the doctors would not watch' [4, p 310] (see also [2, 6, 7, 48]). There will probably never be a definitive answer as to Balzac's influences in creating (or reporting) Louis Lambert's case. But, for the time being, there does not seem to be any earlier character in literature – nor for that matter any description in the medical literature – providing such a lengthy, organized, and detailed account of what Kraepelin would later call dementia praecox, and Bleuler – still later – schizophrenia. Therefore, it is fair to consider Louis Lambert the princeps case of schizophrenia.

Of course, the case is not 'perfect'. Perhaps if Balzac had provided a full list of schneiderian first-rank symptoms, or a full DSM-IV check-list, then the issue would have been settled a long time ago. Yet, again, one should not forget that we are dealing with a novel. We are left with the possibility that Balzac used the story to introduce a full description of a condition that he found intriguing and interesting, or that he knew much more about schizophrenia than the text shows, but chose to include only the elements that suited his narrative purposes best. In either case, it remains that although there have been countless other examples of mental illness and insanity in literature, none come even close to the level of detail adduced by Balzac in *Louis Lambert*. Gogol's *Diary of a Madman* or Shakespeare's Poor Mad

Tom in *King Lear* are very far from the semeiological richness of Balzac's portrayal of the disease. Balzac goes well beyond a description of raving lunacy or general inadequacy. Louis Lambert is not playing the fool, his decay is not meant for comic relief, and his portrayal is not an allegory. Rather, *Louis Lambert* is plainly what it appears to be: not a caricature of insanity, not some kind of eulogy for otherness and difference, and not a supernatural adventure, but the story of a young man struck by a severely disabling mental illness, laid out in meticulous and carefully structured detail.

In fact, *Louis Lambert* might even favor the recency hypothesis of schizophrenia. The idea that schizophrenia was something new at the time would certainly be supported by the fact that a writer like Balzac, widely held as one of the most penetrating and consummate observers of the emergence of modernity in all of its details, would choose to devote a small part of his monumental project to a clinical case. Indeed, if schizophrenia had been around and well known for centuries, there is no obvious reason why Balzac would waste his ink writing about something unremarkable. Furthermore, Balzac had a large number of very worthy predecessors in his own domain, and it is not unreasonable to think that if he could, and would bother to provide such a striking description of schizophrenia, then others could also have done so earlier. After all, hallucinations, delusions, disorganized speech, apathy, catatonia, bizarre behavior, and early-onset mental disorders have been reported throughout history (one need only think of Cervantes' *Don Quixote*, Molière's *Imaginary Invalid*, Shakespeare's *Hamlet*, Burton's *Anatomy of Melancholy*, or Erasmus' *Praise of Folly*). Yet no one before Balzac provided a complete, course-length, and coherent picture of what came to be known as schizophrenia. If schizophrenia had always existed, this fact, on the face of it, indeed is quite surprising [20].

As such, one final question, perhaps the most important, remains open. If it is true that no one described schizophrenia before Balzac, could it be the case that he was the actual instigator of the very idea of schizophrenia as it came to be known in psychiatry? Could it be that Kraepelin and Bleuler (like perhaps the psychic Alexis Didier) read *Louis Lambert* and exploited this new knowledge in their own practice and theories? As far as we know, this hypothesis has not been thoroughly examined. Rigoli [7] provided ample evidence of cross-readings and borrowings within psychiatric literature and between doctors and novelists in 19th century France, but a balzacian trail in German-speaking psychiatry remains to be investigated. Such an approach might also be applied to the emergence of medical views about occult beliefs, mystical experiences, and spiritual practices. Could Balzac's *Louis Lambert* have influenced the development of pathological discourses for marginal, deviant, and unusual ideas and beliefs? And if so, was this turn of events in line with his own beliefs and desires?

## References


1 Borel J: Médecine et psychiatrie balzaciennes: la science dans le roman. Paris, José Corti, 1971.

2 Abely P: En relisant Balzac, psychiatre occasionnel. Ann Méd-Psychol 1958;116:751–761.

3 Claude H, Lévy-Valensi J: Un schizophrène dans la La comédie humaine. Le Progrès Médical 1934;14: 587–590.

4 Devic A, Morin G: A propos de la démence précoce: Balzac précurseur de Bleuler. Lyon Médical 1927;39: 305–311.

5 Dieguez S: Un héros balzacien schizophrène avant l'heure. Cerveau Psycho 2011;48:80–86.

6 Evans H: La pathologie de Louis Lambert: Balzac aliéniste. Revue d'histoire littéraire de la France 1950;2:249–255.

7 Rigoli J: Lire le délire: aliénisme, rhétorique et littérature en France au XIXe siècle. Paris, Fayard, 2001, pp 477–517.

8 Bleuler E: Die Prognose der Dementia Praecox (Schizophreniegruppe). Allgemeine Zeitschrift Psychiatrie Psychischgerichtliche Medizin 1908;65: 436–464.

9 Bentall RP: Madness Explained: Psychosis and Human Nature. London, Penguin, 2004.

10 Quétel C: Histoire de la folie de l'antiquité à nos jours. Paris, Tallandier, 2009.

11 Mcnally K: Schizophrenia as split-personality/Jekyll and Hyde: the origins of the informal usage in the English language. J Hist Behav Sci 2007;43:69–79.

12 Tandon R, Nasrallah HA, Keshavan MS: Schizophrenia, 'just the facts' 4. Clinical features and conceptualization. Schizophr Res 2009;110:1–23.

13 Jaspers K: Allgemeine Psychopathologie, ed 7. Berlin, Springer, 1959.

14 Schneider K: Clinical Psychopathology. New York, Grune & Stratton, 1959.

15 Scharfetter C: Ego-psychopathology: the concept and its empirical evaluation. Psychol Med 1981;11: 273–280.

16 Minkowski E: Contribution à l'étude de la pensée et de l'attitude autistes (le rationalisme morbide), 1923; reprinted in Minkowski E: Au-delà du rationalisme morbide. Paris, L'Harmattan, 1997, pp 21–33.

17 Blankenburg W: La Perte de l'évidence naturelle: une contribution à la psychopathologie des schizophrénies pauci-symptomatiques. Paris, P.U.F., 1991/1971.

18 Frith CD: The Cognitive Neuropsychology of Schizophrenia. Hove, Lawrence Erlbaum Associates Ltd., 1992.

19 Coltheart M, Langdon R, McKay R: Delusional belief. Annu Rev Psychol 2010;62:271–298.

20 Hare EH: Schizophrenia as a recent disease. Br J Psychiatry 1988;153:521–531.

21 Ellard J: Did schizophrenia exist before the eighteenth Century? Aust NZ J Psychiatry 1987;21:306–314.

22 Hare EH: Schizophrenia before 1800? The case of Revd George Trosse. Psychol Med 1988;18:279–285.

23 Jeste DV, Carman R, Lohr JB, Wyatt RJ: Did schizophrenia exist before the eighteenth century? Compr Psychiatry 1985;26:493–503.

24 Bark NM: Did Shakespeare know schizophrenia? The case of Poor Mad Tom in King Lear. Br J Psychiatry 1985;146:436–438.

25 Pope HG Jr, Poliakoff MB, Parker MP, Boynes M, Hudson JI: Is dissociative amnesia a culture-bound syndrome? Findings from a survey of historical literature. Psychol Med 2007;37:225–233.

26 Altschuler E: Shakespeare knew the layered clothing sign of schizophrenia. BMJ 1999;319:520–521.

27 Altschuler E: One of the oldest cases of schizophrenia in Gogol's Diary of a Madman. BMJ 2001;323: 1475–1477.

28 Andreasen NJ: The artist as scientist: psychiatric diagnosis in Shakespeare's tragedies. JAMA 1976;235:1868–1872.

29 Sirotkina I: Gogol, moralists, and nineteenth-century psychiatry; in Sirotkina I (ed): Diagnosing Literary Genius: A Cultural History of Psychiatry in Russia, 1880–1930. Baltimore, Johns Hopkins University Press, 2002, pp 14–44.

30 Cooper JE, Sartorius N: Cultural and temporal variations in schizophrenia: a speculation on the importance of industrialisation. Br J Psychiatry 1977;130;50–55.

31 Torrey EF: Schizophrenia and Civilization. London, Aronson, 1980.

32 Lotte F: Dictionnaire biographique des personnages fictifs de *La comédie humaine*. Paris, José Corti, 1952.

33 Le Yaouanc M: Autour de 'Louis Lambert'. Revue d'Histoire Littéraire de la France 1956;4:516–534.

34 Balzac H: Louis Lambert; Les proscrits; Jésus-Christ en Flandre. Paris, Gallimard (folio classique), 1980/1832.

35 Starobinski A: Un cas de délire télépathique. Ann Méd-Psychol 1921;2:219–224.

36 Greilsheimer H, Groves JE: Male genital self-mutilation. Arch Gen Psychiatry 1979;36:441–446.

37 Ozan E, Deveci E, Oral M, Yazici E, Kirpinar I: Male genital self-mutilation as a psychotic solution. Isr J Psychiatry Relat Sci 2010;47:297–303.

38 Amblard MC : L'œuvre fantastique de Balzac : sources et philosophie. Paris, Didier, 1972.

39 Ambrière M: Balzac et la recherche de l'absolu. Paris, P.U.F. (Quadrige), 1999.
40 Gauthier H: L'image de l'homme intérieur chez Balzac. Genève, Librairie Droz, 1984.
41 Nykrog P: La Pensée de Balzac dans La comédie humaine. Copenhague, Munksgaard, 1965.
42 Sjödén KE: Balzac et Swedenborg. Cahier de l'Association internationale des etudes françaises 1962;15:295–307.
43 Sperber D: L'effet gourou. L'autre côté 2009;1:17–23.
44 Le Maléfan P: Folie et spiritisme: Histoire du discours psychopathologique sur la pratique du spiritisme, ses abords et ses avatars. Paris, L'Harmattan, 1999.
45 Méheust B: Un voyant prodigieux: Alexis Didier (1826–1886). Paris, Les Empêcheurs de penser en rond, 2003.
46 Schreber DP: Mémoires d'un névropathe. Paris, Seuil, 1975/1903.
47 Pommier J: Genèse du premier *Louis Lambert*. Revue d'Histoire Littéraire de la France 1953;4:484–495.
48 Rigoli J: 'Ce que les médecins n'avaient pas su regarder': prodiges et mirages de la psychiatrie balzacienne. L'Ecrit 2002;48:5–18.
49 Tandon R: The nosology of schizophrenia: toward DSM-5 and ICD-11. Psychiatr Clin North Am 2012;35:557–569.
50 van Os J, Kapur S: Schizophrenia. Lancet 2009;374:635–645.
51 Oeuvres illustrées de Balzac. Paris, Marescq et Compagnie, 1852.

Sebastian Dieguez, PhD
Laboratory for Cognitive and Neurological Sciences, Unité de Neurologie
Département de Médecine, Université de Fribourg
PER 09 (salle 2.106), 5 chemin du Musée, CH–1700 Fribourg (Switzerland)
E-Mail sebastian.dieguez@unifr.ch

Bogousslavsky J, Dieguez S (eds): Literary Medicine: Brain Disease and Doctors in Novels, Theater, and Film.
Front Neurol Neurosci. Basel, Karger, 2013, vol 31, pp 35–43 (DOI: 10.1159/000343250)

# Hysteria in Fin de Siècle French Novels

Olivier Walusinski

Family Physician, Brou, France

**Abstract**
During the second half of the 19th century, sociopolitical conditions and society's interest in psychological questions transformed the millennial concept of hysteria into a sociocultural representation of the female condition and sexuality. Influenced by the public demonstrations of Jean-Martin Charcot at La Salpêtrière, many writers attempted to magnify this neurologist's work in their novels. In this chapter, we will analyze several representative passages written by Jules Clarétie, Camille Lemonnier, Jules Lermina, Octave Mirbeau, Joris-Karl Huysmans, and Gustave Flaubert, bearing in mind the scientific, progressive, and anticlerical ideas of the time.



In 1928, Louis Aragon (1897–1982) and André Breton (1896–1966) published a manifesto entitled *The 50th Anniversary of Hysteria* and concluded: 'Hysteria is not a pathological phenomenon and may be considered a supreme means of expression' [1].

Why 1878–1928? Hysteria is a word forged in ancient times and thus was not new when it appeared in 1878. Georges Gilles de la Tourette (1857–1904) and Paul Richer (1849–1933) noted: 'In 1878, these memorable conferences began at La Salpêtrière, renewing interest in hypnotic studies.' This was the year Jean-Martin Charcot (1825–1893), admitting that his anatomoclinical method had failed to find a brain lesion, postulated a psychic cause and used hypnosis for the first time as a new scientific means for studying behavior [2].

'Supreme means of expression' – here is a source of inspiration for writers. In 1858, Jules Michelet gave us the key for understanding how an illness can become this source of inspiration. 'Each century has its major illness: leprosy in the 13th century, the black plague in the 14th century and syphilis in the 16th century. The 19th century was affected at the two extremes of nervous functioning: thought and love.' These two terms can be used to define hysteria and explain why it became the illness of the century at the end of the 1800s [3].

All translations provided by the author.

The slow transformation of postrevolutionary French society gave rise to a new vision of mental illnesses, following the work of Antoine-Laurent Bayle (1799–1858) describing general paralysis, and that of Philippe Pinel (1745–1826) and Jean-Etienne Esquirol (1772–1840) who 'liberated lunatics from their chains'. The illnesses of the psyche began to be viewed as arising from critical situations in one's personal life or in the collective sociopolitical life. Against this backdrop, medicine was confronted with an increasing number of cases of hysteria, which acquired a sociocultural dimension. The transformation of relations between men and women was still undefined. Women retained their ancestral role as mothers and spouses. Men played a dominant role in society as well as in the family. Misogyny reached its apogee during this time, and women were oppressed and scarcely visible. Women's attempts to throw off these oppressive shackles were either in vain or a source of scandal. Hysteria, a form of rebellion against the familial or social mentalities of the time, became a symbolic means of expression that inevitably led to a rich novelistic output [4].

As shown by Victor Segalen (1878–1919) in his 1902 thesis entitled *Literary Clinicians*, narrative was the most appropriate method for representing psychological phenomena. Shifting from philosophical and religious authorities to the physiologist and clinician, literature in the second half of the 19th century transmitted the words of the learned man, his experience with living organisms, and his ability to shed light on moral and social problems. Was it possible for literature to function on the same level as the laboratory? Honoré de Balzac (1799–1850) paved the way through character development with a strong medical influence. He drew on Hippocratism mixed with phrenology; temperament and constitution marked his characters' faces with passions associated with visceral reactions. The body was subjected to the implacable determinism of heredity and social class, as taught in lessons given by renowned physicians in French hospitals [5].

The lessons of Armand Trousseau (1801–1867) at Hôtel Dieu Hospital, and especially the lessons of Charcot at La Salpêtrière, publically revealed the hereditary and personal antecedents, as well as symptoms manifested spontaneously or those revealed by a methodical examination. These lessons became theater in and of themselves, generating a novelistic narrative for disturbances of body and mind. Charcot provided the image, and Freud would provide the words, as Léon Daudet (1867–1942) might have said. In 1922, Daudet described the painting by André Brouillet (1857–1904), *Une leçon clinique à la Salpêtrière*:

> A famous painting made these sessions at La Salpêtrière widely known. Thirty-five years ago, everyone in Paris was talking about them. In addition to physicians, writers, artists and politicians were in attendance; hysteria and cerebral localisations were part of the secular and republican agenda [6].

Charcot, who embodied the triumphs of medicine and the rise of positivism, addressed his audiences at the confluence of disease and literature (fig. 1). Jules Clarétie (1840–1913) attended Charcot's lessons and was fascinated by the 'Napoleon

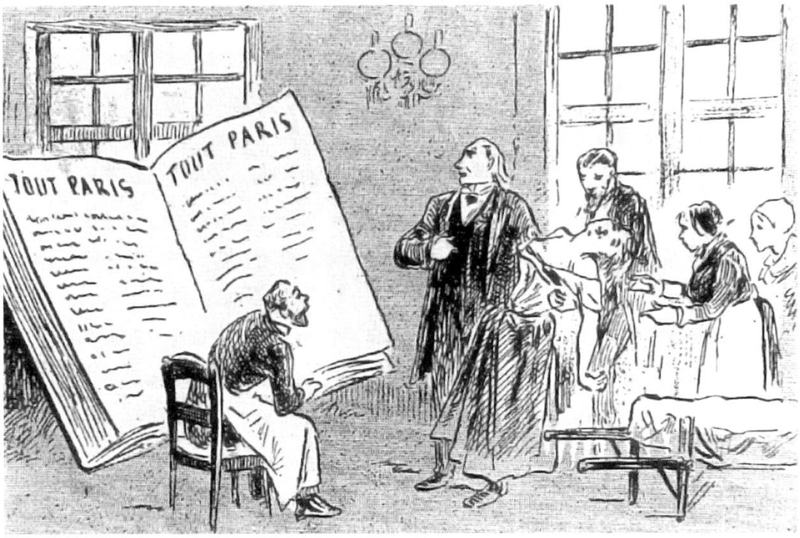


**Fig. 1.** Anonymous caricature of André Brouillet's painting *Une leçon clinique à La Salpêtrière*. Gilles de la Tourette on the left wearing an apron, Charcot, Babinski supporting Blanche Wittman in front of nurses Marguerite Bottard, and Mademoiselle Ecary (private collection of the author).

of neurosis'. He incorporated him into one of his novels, *Les amours d'un interne*, which idealizes the care provided by the doctor [7]. The nurse with whom he is in love questions him: 'Please tell me, if you would, what it is you mean by hysteria.' He replies:

> Definitions are always devilishly difficult. I can tell you what hysteria is not. It is not what people generally believe it to be. For the common man, hysteria entails sensual imbalance, as Monsieur Joseph Prudhomme would say. But this is not at all true. Hysteria is instead a general disturbance of the nervous system. It can take any form – erotic (conforming with popular beliefs), dark, mystical, religious – any form at all. It is, if you will, the exaggeration of anything. The hysteric eats too much or nothing at all, sleeps too much or not enough. She is either absorbed like an idiot or exalted like a maniac. She likes noise, harsh colours, novelistic invention. She wants to be noticed, then left alone. She is not commonplace and her world is the demi-monde, the theatre and the salons of Paris. In fact the city is full of hysterics whose perfectly characterized illness would benefit from Doctor Charcot's care [7].

This definition should be compared to the 1952 definition by Henry Ey (1900–1977): 'Hysteria is a neurosis characterised by somatic hyperexpressivity of unconscious ideas, images and affects' [8]. The DSM-IV uses the Freudian term 'conversion', limiting hysteria to symptoms such as mutism, sensory loss, or motor paralysis by which the conflicts of the psyche are transformed into physical symptoms. This term does not allude to theatrical changes in behavior, which strongly inspired novelists.

Here is how Clarétie transposed the symptoms presented by the mother of the heroine in his moralistic novel:

'The disease', the doctor told Jeanne, 'is not so much madness as a sort of hystero-epilepsy. And if the fits reoccur, I would advise you to take the patient either to Monsieur Charcot, who is an eminent specialist and unrivalled in this area, or to Monsieur Fargeas. Both of them have a department at La Salpêtrière.' Hearing this lugubrious name, La Salpêtrière, for the first time was like hearing a bell toll. Jeanne suddenly had visions of a place of torture, Dantesque with its distraught faces and its sinister cries and grimaces of madwomen. La Salpêtrière! The Bicêtre lunatic asylum for women! Oh, thank God no, we had not yet reached that point! [. . .] A new phase in the disease was beginning and from this day forward, the poor woman's fits became epileptoid. They were perhaps more frightening for Jeanne, who watched as her mother, this good woman transformed into a poor, exquisite creature, was beset with atrocious convulsions and hellish torsions [7].

Joris-Karl Huysmans (1848–1907), another regular at the Tuesday lessons, published *A rebours* in 1884 in an attempt to break with the naturalistic aesthetic in the works of Emile Zola (1840–1902), which he had greatly admired and defended. His 30-year-old hero, Jean Floressas des Esseintes, is an eccentric dandy and a capricious aesthete. He suffers from 'hystero-neurasthenia, a vague disease involving a unique form of atavism characterized by the predominance of lymph in the blood'.

During this singular disease that ravaged families, slowly bleeding its victims, attacks were suddenly followed by calm periods. [. . .] Like all neurotics, he could not stand the heat. [. . .] His ennui became boundless, and his brain was haunted by a confused mixture of libertine and mystical obsessions. He emerged from these reveries annihilated, broken, almost moribund [9].

The medical descriptions of 'digestive hysteria' by Paul Briquet (1796–1881) or Gilles de la Tourette cannot rival with Huysmans' writings: 'The deficiencies of his stomach made it impossible for him to consume varied and heavy dishes. His pains ranged from a bloated, hardened belly to the feeling of an iron poker running through his entrails, to useless and urgent efforts. . . Finally, his appetite disappeared, and his stomach was plagued by a gassy, warm sourness and by dry fires. After any attempt at a meal, he became bloated and gasped for breath, unable to tolerate having his breeches buttoned or a tight vest.' His hero required years of special care and a particular diet. Once 'his digestive functions had been treated, it was time to attack the neurosis' and 'obligate him to interact with other people' [9].

Octave Mirbeau (1848–1917) was one of the zealous propagandists of Charcot's work. Mirbeau was a journalist for the newspaper *L'évènement* (under the pseudonym 'Diable' or 'Devil'). He saw in Charcot the incarnation of 'triumphant medicine'. His description of the hysterical fit was in all points similar to 'major hysteria' [10–12] (fig. 2):

All of a sudden, the patient's vision deteriorates and the eyes take on an expression of anguish. The limbs contract in all directions. Then large movements and convulsions bend the body along the circumference of a circle. This is followed by strange dramatic or comic attitudes. The patient is frightened and sees ghosts or people who want to take her away. Then suddenly, these entities become angels or laughing figures, and she smiles at them. Her state becomes ecstatic. She murmurs

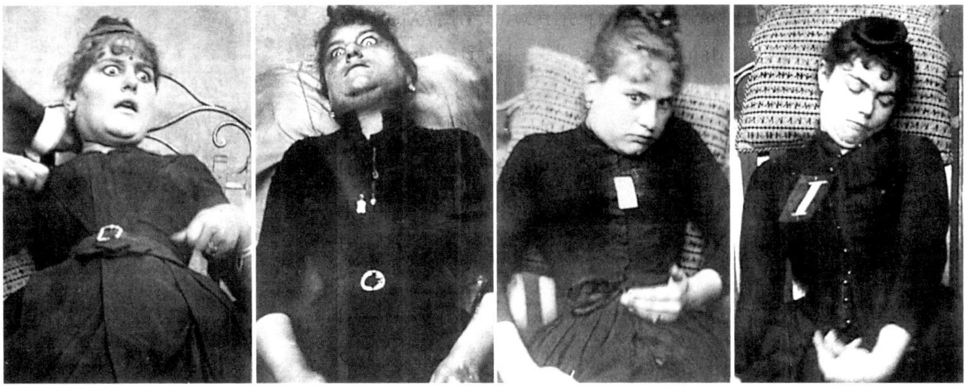

**Fig. 2.** 'Esther' in the clown phase of hysteria major. Esther was one of the hysterics studied by Jules Luys (1828–1897) at Hôpital de la Charité in 1886. Prints of photographs from the period (private collection of the author).

words senselessly. Sometimes she holds an imaginary being in her arms. Finally, she becomes dejected, exhausted, profoundly melancholic [10, 11] (fig. 2).

Strangely, Mirbeau never used the word 'hysteric' to qualify the characters in his novels. For example, the red-haired Clara in *Jardin des supplices* is described as a 'femme fatale' but with unpredictable behavior, suffering from unnamed attacks that are nonetheless characteristic of hysteria [10, 13]:

> She was extraordinarily pale and her body trembled, shaken by nervous spasms. [. . .] Her eyelids were frighteningly open and her eyes were rolled back, so that only the whites were visible. [. . .] All of a sudden, she cried out; the muscles of her face tensed, and nervous twitches shook her chest, arms and legs. [. . .] Then Clara began to thrash. All her muscles stood out, horribly raised and contracted. . . her joints cracked, as if she were a boat tossed about by a storm.

Jules Lermina (1839–1915), a journalist who attacked the empire in numerous pieces, wrote (in prison and later on) social adventure novels which were often pastiches, such as *Le fils de Monte-Cristo, Les mystères de New York,* and *Les hystériques de Paris* (fig. 3). In the third book, he portrayed a demoniacal, vampirish, and manipulative 'femme fatale' who drove her lovers to commit murder:

> But by her monstrously depraved nature, this woman, who was driven by her ardent thirst for riches and grandeur alone, had pushed back the limits of perversity to achieve her purpose. She had no passions other than her immense egoism and an insatiable appetite for pleasure, which were fed by her prodigious character. She was a hysteric in all her terrible and dangerous excitability [13].

One can imagine Lermina's pleasure in naming the police commissioner Bernheim and the judge Tourette, an allusion to the famous dispute between the Nancy and La Salpêtrière schools during the Gouffé-Bompard case, concerning criminal

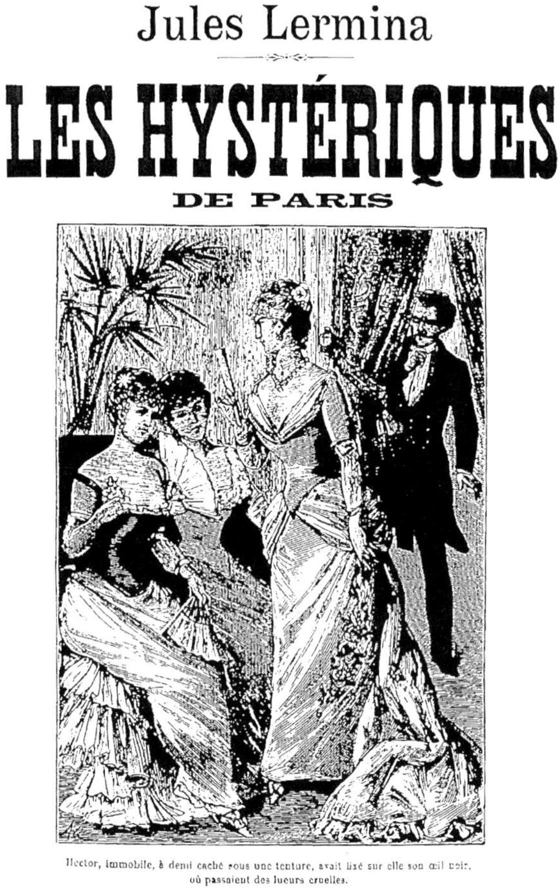


**Fig. 3.** Cover of Jules Lermina's 1885 book (private collection of the author).

responsibility for acts supposedly committed under hypnosis [14]. Lermina's novel portrayed feminine sexuality as threatening and misunderstood by men, as his character was the antithesis of the fragile, submissive woman. As for the myth of the submissive woman, it can be found in *L'hystérique* by Camille Lemonnier (1844–1913). This Belgian author based his book on the case of Louise Lateau, related in 1873 by Désiré-Magloire Bourneville (1840–1909) [15] (fig. 4). The novel is naturalistic and ferociously anticlerical. It portrays the young nun Humilité. This pious and ignorant woman is raped by the abbot Orléa. After 'her ecstatic state', which was most probably hypnosis:

'she recovered from the violence of her attack in a languid depression, as if her blood, which had stood stagnant during her long cataleptic immobility, was slow to begin circulating again. [. . .] She then thanked him with her pale smile, explaining that she felt nothing but a heavy weariness. She had never experienced as much joy during mortification of the flesh: she had perceived Jesus entering her in the form of a great light'. Not only did Lemonnier illustrate the 'duplicity that the Church instills in its servants and forces them to abide by';

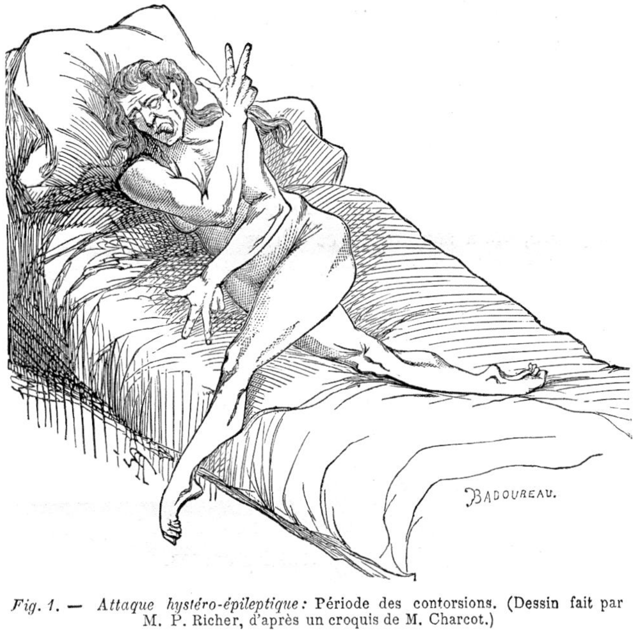
BADOUREAU.
Fig. 1. — Attaque hystéro-épileptique: Période des contorsions. (Dessin fait par M. P. Richer, d'après un croquis de M. Charcot.)

**Fig. 4.** Engraving of Louise Lateau in Désiré Magloire Bourneville's book (private collection of the author).

he portrayed the final phase of hysteria major with special emphasis, in the Charcot tradition. Lemonnier implicitly associated this phase with the millennial myth of menstrual influences:

> Sister Humilité's illness had long been irregular and chaotic; it came to manifest itself as periodical phenomena. Starting Wednesday of each week, slight tumefaction swelled her hands and feet as well as her side. By Thursday, the blisters had popped, releasing a mist of blood that, like red dewdrops, trickled along the flesh. Then on Friday, around noon, the final attack was signalled by the prodromes of ecstasy. The ecstatic state lasted around three hours. Suddenly a bloodcurdling cry rang out, expressing both terror and supplication. Humilité fell face-first to the ground, arms open on either side of her body, in the posture of the Lord crucified [16].

Emile Zola was faithful to the ideas of Charcot in *La foi qui guérit*. In *Lourdes* (1894), he examined how 'miracles (referring only to a recovery outside the realm of curative medicine) make up a category of acts that are not exempt from the natural order of things' [17]. Marie, the heroine, is stricken by a mysterious disease that leaves her immobilized, and for this reason makes the journey to Lourdes. She is afflicted by classic uterine suffocation:

> 'The weight in my left side, which had made it difficult to breathe, moved up,' revealed Marie, 'and the pain was so intense I thought I would die. But it passed up through my chest, then up through my throat. It was then in my mouth, and I spit it out violently. . . It was over, I was no longer sick. My illness had flown away'.

Convinced she has been cured, Marie is 'ecstatic and radiant. She seemed ignorant of all that was going on around her, waiting in rapture for the miraculous to occur'. The hysterical paralysis disappears at the same time femininity is renewed, in keeping with Charcot's staging:

> As she felt the source of her blood flow forth in her, the source of her life as a woman, wife and mother, she had a final fit of anguish, and an enormous weight rose from her belly into her throat. Only this time, it did not stop, it did not suffocate her. Instead it burst out of her open mouth and flew off with a cry of sublime joy: I'm cured, I'm cured! [18].

Zola used the novel to paint a portrait similar to the one Charcot and Richer depicted in *Les démoniaques dans l'art* in 1887 [19].

As emphasized by Charles Richet (1850–1935), 'of all the hysterics found in novels, the most vibrant, the truest and the most passionate is Madame Bovary' [20]. The novel by the same name, the masterpiece of Gustave Flaubert (1821–1880), was published in 1857. Paradoxically, its content rather than its style made it a success – and a scandal. The novel's theme is feminine passion that far exceeds the accepted custom and habit of the times, and thus goes against religious teachings and social rules. There is detailed description of daydreaming, double adultery, irresolvable debt, the heroine's suicide, the bourgeoisie's mediocrity, and the banality of life in the French provinces.

Written well before Charcot's work, *Madame Bovary* describes Emma's melancholy ('mournful day – dark atmosphere') and without ever using the word 'hysteria', it relates a phenomenology of 'nervous irritation and excitation': 'suffocation, swelling, dizziness, a strong arterial pulse and teeth grinding'. In his correspondence with his mistress Louise Collet (1810–1876), Flaubert mentioned a 'nervous fit' suffered by Emma Bovary, which in the book was replaced by 'nervous upset' (an implicit reference to his own attacks of temporal lobe epilepsy) [21]. Emma confused the 'sensuality of luxury with the joys of the heart, and elegant habits with refined sentiment.' Flaubert's aesthetic intention was to describe hysteria without naming it. This disease of hypersensitivity could even involve nervous fits, when the unsatisfied desire for love reached its height:

> 'She would at last possess the joys of love, this feverish happiness she had given up on attaining. She was entering into a marvellous realm where everything would be passion, ecstasy and frenzy.' Her moods were an enigma for her naive husband, representing medicine: 'Charles sank into his chair, overcome. He tried to figure out what could be wrong with her, imagining a nervous illness and shedding a few tears. He had the vague impression of something disastrous and incomprehensible surrounding him.'

Flaubert laid the groundwork for his reader to attribute the behavioral problems to the contrast between the hopes for an intellectually, emotionally, and sexually satisfying life, and the narrow reality imposed by society's moral order. This contrast leads to psychic disorders and suicide [4, 22]. All of these narratives draw on hysterical psychology to illustrate the analogy between ecstasy and possession. They strike a balance between moral interpretation and drama, as does Charcot's iconography, colored by Bourneville's anticlerical progressivism. Although it is impossible here to analyze the entire literary output from the period, it is clear that hysteria acted as a stage for showcasing the female body, where the backdrop of the female condition revealed itself. Hysteria bears witness to the era in which it arose, when the millennial representation of female submission was giving way and a new, independent woman was emerging, a forerunner to 20th century feminists.

## References


1 Aragon L, Breton A: Le cinquantenaire de l'hystérie (1878–1928). La Révolution Surréaliste 1928;11: 20–22.
2 Gilles de la Tourette G, Richer P: Hypnotisme; in Dechambre A (ed): Dictionnaire encyclopédique des sciences médicales. Paris, Masson & Asselin, 1887, 4è série (F-K), pp 67–132.
3 Michelet J: L'Amour. Paris, Louis Hachette, 1858.
4 Marquer B: Les 'romans' de la Salpêtrière. Réception d'une scénographie clinique: Jean-Martin Charcot dans l'imaginaire fin-de-siècle. Genève, Droz, 2008.
5 Segalen V: Les cliniciens ès-lettres. Thèse. Bordeaux, Imprimerie Yves Cadoret, 1902.
6 Daudet L: Les œuvres dans les hommes. Paris, Nouvelle librairie nationale, 1922.
7 Clarétie J: Les amours d'un interne. Paris, E. Dentu, 1881.
8 Ey H: Entretiens psychiatriques. Paris, Privat – PUF, 1952.
9 Huysmans J-K: A rebours. Paris, G. Charpentier, 1884.
10 Mirbeau O: Le jardin des supplices (Vingt compositions originales de Auguste Rodin). Paris, A. Vollard, 1902.
11 Cornille C-E: Sur quelques dégénérés dans les œuvres d'Octave Mirbeau. Thèse Médecine. Lille, Imprimerie coopérative 'La Gutenberg', 1920.
12 Michel P: Mirbeau et Charcot: la vision du 'Diable'. Cahiers Octave Mirbeau 2004;44:53–67.
13 Lermina J: Les hystériques de Paris. Sceaux, Imprimerie de Charaire et fils, 1885.
14 Bogousslavsky J, Walusinski O: Gilles de la Tourette's criminal women: the many faces of fin de siècle hypnotism. Clin Neurol Neurosurg 2010;112: 549–551.
15 Bourneville DM: Louise Lateau ou la stigmatisée belge. Collection Science et Miracle. Paris, Aux bureaux du Progrès Médical, 1873.
16 Lemonnier C: L'hystérique. Paris, G. Charpentier, 1885.
17 Charcot JM: La foi qui guérit. Revue Hebdomadaire (Paris, Plon-Nourrit) 1892;1:112–132.
18 Zola E: Les trois villes: Lourdes. Paris, G. Charpentier and E. Fasquelle, 1894.
19 Charcot JM, Richer P: Les démoniaques dans l'art. Paris, Delahaye et Lecrosnier, 1887.
20 Richet C: Les démoniaques d'aujourd'hui. Etude de psychologie pathologique. Revue des Deux Mondes (Paris) 1880;37:340–372.
21 Jallon P, Jallon H: Gustave Flaubert's hidden sickness; in Bogousslavsky J, Boller F (eds): Neurological Disorders in Famous Artists. Front Neurol Neurosci. Basel, Karger, 2005, vol 19, pp 46–56.
22 Beizer J: Ventriloquized Bodies: Narratives of Hysteria in Nineteenth-Century France. Itaca, Cornell University Press, 1994.



Olivier Walusinski
Family physician, private practice
20 rue de Chartres
FR–28160 Brou (France)
E-Mail walusinski@baillement.com

Bogousslavsky J, Dieguez S (eds): Literary Medicine: Brain Disease and Doctors in Novels, Theater, and Film.
Front Neurol Neurosci. Basel, Karger, 2013, vol 31, pp 44–51 (DOI: 10.1159/000343234)

# The Nadja Case

Julien Bogousslavsky

Center for Brain and Nervous System Diseases, GSMN Neurocenter, Clinique Valmont,
Glion/Montreux, Switzerland

**Abstract**

On October 4, 1926, a young woman who seemed lost in the street met one of the most important writers of the century, André Breton, who had just published the *First Manifesto of Surrealism* two years before. The young woman was named Léona Delcourt, but one used to call her Nadja. She fell in love with Breton, but he remained more interested in her poetic strangeness, which expressed itself in her conversation, drawings, and letters. Their intimate relationship lasted only ten days, but correspondence continued until March 1927, when she developed acute psychosis and was interned in psychiatric wards for the rest of her life. A few months later, Breton published *Nadja*, one of the most famous novels of the twentieth century. He had intentionally written it as a clinical report (though violently criticizing psychiatry and psychiatrists) lacking emotional features, and it was partly influenced by his own neuropsychiatric experience during the war as a medical student working with Raoul Leroy and Joseph Babinski. Breton's apparent coldness associated with the dramatic fate of Nadja has often been interpreted unfavorably, as he supposedly missed a diagnosis of paranoid schizophrenia in her. However, a careful look at Nadja's letters to Breton suggests that hallucinations and delirium were absent before the March 1927 decompensation, and her behavior may be one of the best available examples of the fascinating poetic instability which may precede acute psychosis.



Published in 1928, *Nadja* [1] is the most famous novel by André Breton (1896–1966), the leading figure of the surrealist movement. It reports in a 'clinical way' (as mentioned by Breton himself in the second edition in 1963) the meeting between Breton and Nadja, a young woman who seemed to wander freely in Paris with no personal roots. The relationship lasts for about ten days, during which the couple visits places in the capital, before the novel ends stating the 'madness' of Nadja and her disappearance in the French psychiatric asylum system, contrasting with the surge of Breton's exalted love for another woman called 'X' (Suzanne Muzard, who would finally marry the writer Emmanuel Berl, after a prolonged struggle between him and

Breton). For Breton, this new relationship was prepared by the poetry and mystery of his meeting with Nadja, and the book concludes with the famous phrase, 'beauty will be convulsive or will not be at all'. In part because Breton decided to eliminate emotional feelings from his text and because it appears that Nadja was in love with him, contrary to his feelings toward her, the reader typically develops a strong empathy for Nadja along with a significant rejection of the narrator, who is felt to be egoistic and cold.

**André Breton as a Neuropsychiatrist**

While objectively the story reported by Breton leaves little doubt about some kind of mental disorder in Nadja, subsequent studies on the work have emphasized the poetic magic of the young woman rather than a psychiatric condition. A legend even developed around Nadja's figure, and people began to doubt that she really existed. Some speculated that she was a famous person of the time, such as Blanche Derval, the actress of the 1921 scandalous (a child was killed by lesbians) play *Les détraquées* [2] by Pierre Palau and a certain 'Olaf', in fact the neurologist Joseph Babinski, who had attended the premiere with a fake beard [3]! While this assumption on the identity of Nadja was wrong, the hypothesis was interesting because Breton, who had started medical studies in 1913, indeed had worked during the war under Babinski for several months in 1917 in his service at La Pitié. The legend developed to such a point, that a couple of decades later, fake Nadjas (including one from Norway, who was quite insisting) announced themselves to Breton or institutions in Paris [4]!

Nadja's legend was certainly supported, though probably involuntarily, by Breton's attitude; he set up much secrecy around her, even mistaking her own real name in his own research to have news from her over three decades later [4]! Moreover, in the novel, Breton gives obvious clues for a mental condition in Nadja, but he also strongly criticizes psychiatry and psychiatrists, even publishing a photograph of Professor Henri Claude, Chairman of Psychiatry at the University of Paris and head of Hôpital Sainte-Anne, with the comment: 'his low and stubborn forehead'. Here and in the following years, Breton assumed a position clearly foreshadowing the antipsychiatry current which developed in the 1960s and 1970s. This attitude is particularly striking since in 1916 Breton had envisioned to become a psychiatrist during his war service at the military neuropsychiatric center of Saint-Dizier with Dr. Raoul Leroy [5]. Leroy was chief alienist at Ville-Evrard, and he introduced Breton to war psychiatry, encouraging him to read many textbooks by Charcot, Magnan, Régis, and Ballet, and having him examine patients as a resident, although he was not even 'médecin auxiliaire' in the medical-military hierarchy. Breton learned current issues on hysteria, including psychoanalytic concepts which were summarized in the monograph by Régis and Hesnard [6], the first book to introduce Freud's theories in the French language. On the other hand, Leroy joked about hysteria, even suggesting that he had intimate relationships with Charcot's famous patients when he was studying at La Salpêtrière. In his correspondence to his friend Théodore Fraenkel, Breton states that he was helpful to Leroy in making several good diagnoses where others had failed, including Dr. Cruchet, who would later report epidemic encephalitis, a condition which bears his name with von Economo [7]. Breton even became rather exalted by psychiatry, emphasizing its hazy boundaries with poetry and creativity in statements such as: 'Oh German poetry, Freud, Kraepelin!' [5]. He wrote up several case reports for Leroy, although none was published with their names. In particular, he was impressed by a patient who denied that there was a war, and subsequently quoted him in his own poetic production [8]. It is striking that Breton often quoted medical issues from that time in his later literary work, including echolalia and Ganser syndrome (taken form Costanza Pascal's book on dementia praecox) [9] in the *First Manifesto of Surrealism* (1924), or lilliputian hallucinations (in fact, first reported by Leroy in 1909 [10]) in *L'air de l'eau* (1934).

However, Breton was also negatively impressed by primitive, gross features in many patients, who were not really 'poets', and he also became disappointed with psychiatrists, whom he compared with plant engineers [5]. He switched his admiration towards Joseph Babinski, of whom he had acquired the *Titres et travaux* volume of 1913, which he subsequently kept all his life in his private library, with his ex-libris designed by Salvador Dali. After Saint-Dizier and a time as stretcher bearer on the front near Verdun, he spent several weeks in Babinski's service in 1917, where he admired his skills in exploring the clinical examination of patients, something he remembered well several decades later [7]. However, Babinski was not at all interested in psychiatry and he denied emotional-psychological factors in hysteria, which he considered as 'auto-suggestion', with unclear boundaries with simulation, and completely at odds with his master Charcot [11]. It is likely that along with a re-immersion into the Parisian literary world and Babinski's attitude showing Breton that medicine was not what he had expected, contributed to his decision to discontinue his medical studies [7] shortly after he was appointed 'médecin auxiliaire' on July 1, 1919, roughly seven years before he met Nadja.

## Léona Delcourt

Nadja's real name was Léona Delcourt (1902–1941), but this remained unknown to the public until the 2002 exhibit 'La révolution surréaliste' at the Centre Pompidou in Paris, where a hotel receipt in her name at the time she was seeing Breton in November 1926, also with notes signed 'Nadja', was displayed [12]. More recently, a Dutch journalist made a thorough inquiry and discovered documents in the family and institutions, which shed light on the life of this woman [13]. Originally from Lille in northern France, she became pregnant at 16 years of age during the war, presumably from a British officer, before she went to Paris under the care of a 'protector'. In Paris, Delcourt had several 'friends' and probably prostituted herself from time to time; she was even arrested for a small cocaine business. It is not clear why she called herself Nadja, but this may have been with reference to the pseudonym (Nadja) of the American actress Beatrice Wanger. Breton, however, stated that it corresponded to the first part of the Russian word for 'hope' [4]. In the novel, Breton reports how he met Nadja in the street on October 4, 1926, and the rest of the story focuses on the following ten days, when Breton and Nadja wander around Paris. After a night they spent together in a hotel, the relationship changed and became mainly epistolar until Nadja developed acute hallucinations and delirium in Hôtel Becquerel on March 21, 1927, and had to be interned at the Infirmerie Spéciale du Dépôt de la Préfecture de Police, from where she was transferred the same day to the Hôpital Sainte-Anne. Three days later, she was referred to the Perray-Vaucluse asylum in the vicinity of Paris, before her parents obtained her transfer to the Bailleul asylum close to Lille on May 14, 1928, where she died on January 15, 1941, without having ever left psychiatric wards.

## In the Labyrinth of Asylums

During her way through the psychiatric institutions, she was first examined by Dr. Benjamin Logre and his chief at the Infirmerie Spéciale, Dr. Gaëtan Gatian de Clérambault [4], who became famous for his theory of mental automatism in psychosis. This is a fascinating coincidence since Breton's first surrealist experiments dealt with automatic writing with Philippe Soupault in the book *Les champs magnétiques* in 1920; Breton introduced the term 'automatism' in his very definition of surrealism (psychic automatism reflecting the real functioning of thinking) [14]. De Clérambault was fascinated by young women with delirium and required that all of them be presented to him. In his own annotated copy of the monograph by Sérieux and Capgras on psychosis, he wrote down the names of several patients he had seen over the years with his associates, along with the exact type of delirium according to the Sérieux and Capgras classification, and it is fascinating to discover the name 'L. Delcourt', corresponding to 'persecution delirium' [4] (fig. 1).

In Logre's report at the Infirmerie Spéciale, one reads:

> Polymorphous psychic disorders. Depression, sadness, anxiety. Anxiety phase with fear. Begs to be killed immediately. At other times, wants to dance, she sings, manierism, ideas of influence. One acts upon her from a distance, one speaks to her, one guesses her thoughts, one sends odors to her, one works in her body with electricity. She is a medium. She has been prevented to eat for 3 days. Ideas of negation. She has no more saliva. Manierism. Bizarre speech. Inappropriate sudden gestures. Sees individuals on the roofs of her house. Wants help. Scandal. Apparently she has been disturbed for a few weeks only. General fatigue. Thinness. Inanition. Pulse: 130.

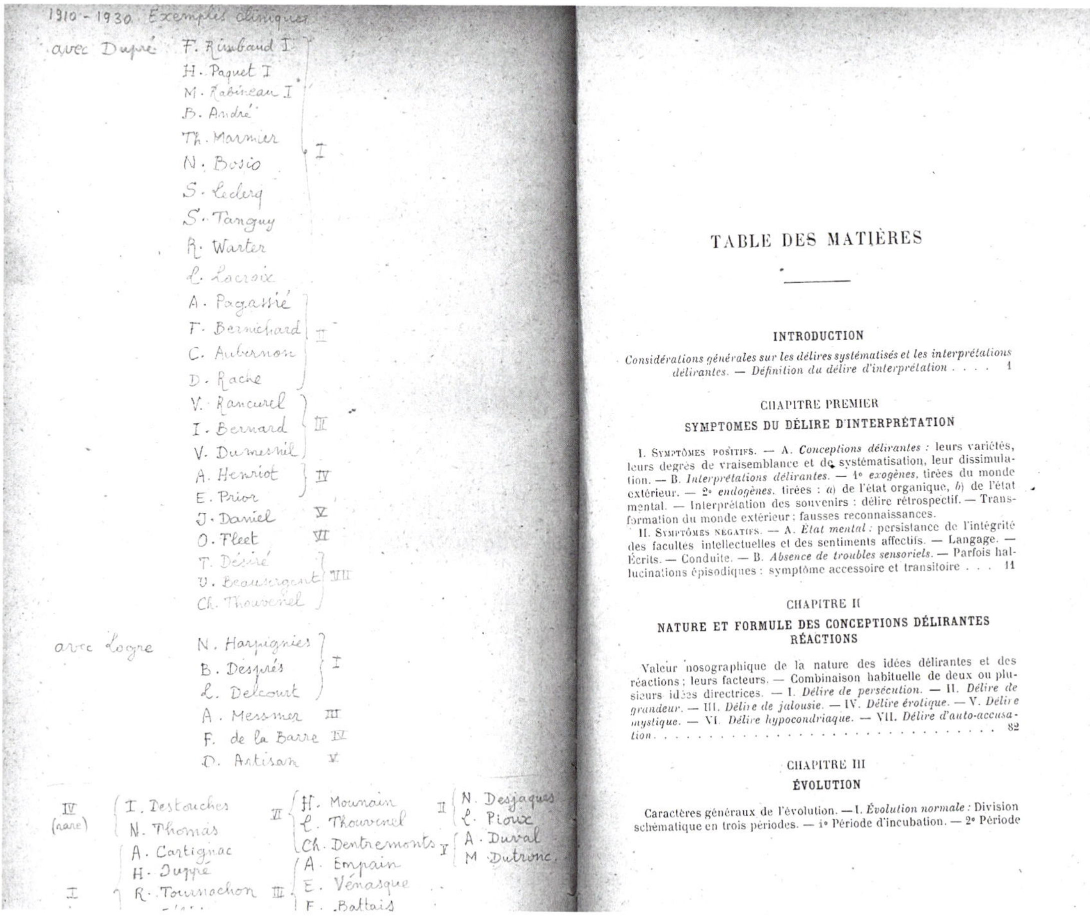


TABLE DES MATIÈRES

INTRODUCTION

*Considérations générales sur les délires systématisés et les interprétations délirantes. — Définition du délire d'interprétation* . . . . 1

CHAPITRE PREMIER

SYMPTOMES DU DÉLIRE D'INTERPRÉTATION

I. Symptômes positifs. — A. *Conceptions délirantes :* leurs variétés, leurs degrés de vraisemblance et de systématisation, leur dissimulation. — B. *Interprétations délirantes.* — 1° *exogènes*, tirées du monde extérieur. — 2° *endogènes*, tirées : *a*) de l'état organique, *b*) de l'état mental. — Interprétation des souvenirs : délire rétrospectif. — Transformation du monde extérieur ; fausses reconnaissances.
II. Symptômes négatifs. — A. *État mental :* persistance de l'intégrité des facultés intellectuelles et des sentiments affectifs. — Langage. — Écrits. — Conduite. — B. *Absence de troubles sensoriels.* — Parfois hallucinations épisodiques : symptôme accessoire et transitoire . . . 11

CHAPITRE II

NATURE ET FORMULE DES CONCEPTIONS DÉLIRANTES
RÉACTIONS

Valeur nosographique de la nature des idées délirantes et des réactions ; leurs facteurs. — Combinaison habituelle de deux ou plusieurs idées directrices. — I. *Délire de persécution.* — II. *Délire de grandeur.* — III. *Délire de jalousie.* — IV. *Délire érotique.* — V. *Délire mystique.* — VI. *Délire hypocondriaque.* — VII. *Délire d'auto-accusation* . . . . . . . . . . . . . . . . . . . . . . . . . . . 82

CHAPITRE III

ÉVOLUTION

Caractères généraux de l'évolution. — I. *Évolution normale :* Division schématique en trois périodes. — 1° Période d'incubation. — 2° Période

**Fig. 1.** List of patients examined by de Clérambault in Gaëtan Gatian de Clérambault's personal copy of the book by P. Sérieux and J. Capgras, *Les folies raisonnantes* [17]. The name of Léona Delcourt appears in the series of patients examined with Benjamin Logre at the Infirmerie Spéciale. She has been included in category I of Sérieux and Capgras, i.e. persecution delirium (private library, Switzerland).

After her referral to Sainte-Anne, she was not admitted to the wards, but remained at the admissions, where she was examined by Dr. Auguste Marie, who wrote: 'State of anxious agitation. She fights for the Right, for the Good, for freedom, one has hypnotized her, but she is a medium, she is attacked by electricity and 'gagoméphitiques' [sic, a neologism]'. Auguste Marie was one of the first psychiatrists to be interested in painting and graphic productions by mental patients, even building up a famous collection, which mysteriously disappeared after it was exhibited in Sainte-Anne in the 1950s. However, there is no indication that he knew that Nadja indeed produced drawings, in particular the famous design, *La fleur des amants* (The Lovers' Flower; fig. 2), an activity which had been encouraged

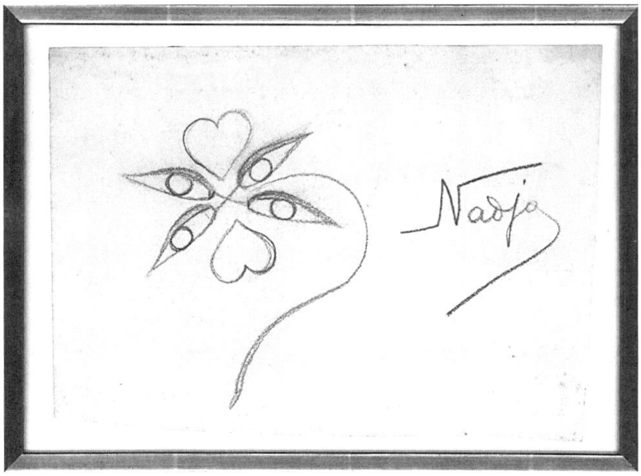

**Fig. 2.** *La fleur des amants* (The Lovers' Flower), original drawing by Nadja, end of 1926 (private library, Switzerland).

and supported by Breton during their relationship. Three days later, on March 24, she was transferred to the asylum of Perray-Vaucluse under the care of Dr. Paul Courbon, the son-in-law of Paul Sollier, the famous pupil of Jean-Martin Charcot, who had followed Marcel Proust during his 1905–1906 'cure' [15]. Courbon wrote: 'Manierism and mutism syndrome with alteranting anxious vs. incoherent mimickry. Meagerness, poor general state.' During the following weeks and months, the patient's state did not evolve much, as reported in the chart, which shows mainly: 'same', or 'nervous agitation'. The only people who were allowed to see her were her parents; the surrealists Paul Éluard and Louis Aragon were not given permission to visit her. It remains uncertain whether Breton went and tried to see her, but unpublished documents from the Delcourt family now in a private collection clearly show that Breton did write to her after her internment. Unfortunately, all Breton's letters to her were burned by her family shortly after she died, along with her own letters to her daughter. When she was finally transferred to the Bailleul asylum one year later, Courbon's diagnosis was unequivocal: 'dementia praecox with intellectual incoherence and impulsiveness'. Three nurses were necessary to proceed with the journey in safe conditions. In Bailleul, the psychiatrists who attended her until her death in 1941 were Dr. Maupaté and Dr. Briche, who did not alter the diagnosis of 'dementia praecox', 'schizophrenic state', and 'paranoid dementia'. A few notes by the nursing staff emphasize 'singing, dancing, hitting, hallucinations, undressing with self-exhibition, impulsive, violent, noisy (even at night under her ideas of influence), shouts, destroys, gesticulates and speaks alone [. . .] believes to see Englishmen and Americans who come to torture her, to possess her, to take out the white of her eyes.'

## Did André Breton Miss the Diagnosis?

One of the question marks which remains in the Breton-Nadja story is the apparent lack of recognition by Breton of a mental disorder during his relationship and his correspondence with her [4]. While he later (in particular in the novel) quoted clues which suggested a mental disorder, he also seemed to minimize the situation, even complaining to his wife that the instability and 'folly' of his mistress Suzanne Muzard ('X' at the end of the novel) was much worse than that of Nadja [Breton A: Letter to his wife Simone, October 8, 1928]. It has been suggested that at the time, Breton may have forgotten much of his neuropsychiatric training, or that he was so fascinated by Nadja and her poetic aspects and productions that he missed the signs [5]. Elements of these factors may well have played a role, but I think that the most likely explanation why Breton did not recognize the severe psychosis of Leona Delcourt during the 'Nadja episode' is that it was absent. Indeed, in the novel, Breton carefully noted features which a posteriori suggest elements easy to integrate into a diagnosis of a psychotic pathology after the development of the decompensation with hallucinations and delirium which led to internment. However, during their relationship, only Nadja's strangeness was really obvious, and it could easily be seen through the periscope of poetic features, which Breton was looking for. Psychotic traits are not synonymous with clinical psychosis, and in a way, accusing Breton of having missed (and exploited, as a writer) a distressing psychiatric condition looks like a trial where sentencing would precede the exposure of the facts [4]. Moreover, it has been shown that Breton tried to help Nadja, including with rather large amounts of money which he himself did not have much of at the time. Already at the time of the publication of the novel, it was clear that he had no doubt about the true diagnosis of his former friend, as shown by his inscription in Valentine Hugo's copy of the book: 'I barely dare to offer this doll of the paranoid dementia' [Breton A. Dedication in Valentine Hugo's copy of *Nadja*, 1928–1929]. In the novel itself, Breton concludes that he has no illusion of the fact that people will elaborate on his own responsibility in the development of Nadja's delirious ideas and her subsequent fate, but he replies that he prefers to ignore these 'cretins' and 'leave them in peace', preferring to attack violently psychiatry and psychiatrists. However, people often regret that Breton never expressed specific regrets on the way his relationship with Nadja evolved, and this lack of perceived guilt is well exemplified in Suzanne Muzard's remark that Breton's only excuse was that he was not in love with Nadja [16].

Along with the extraordinary description of this ten-day relationship in the novel, the Nadja's letters to Breton (now in the Bibliothèque Littéraire Jacques Doucet in Paris and in a few private collections) indeed represent one of the best available and most moving reports of the strikingly unstable mental and affective situation of someone just before acute psychotic decompensation. Léona Delcourt developed acute psychosis, but in fact there was no 'Nadja case'. The story of Nadja shows how strangeness and its potentially artistic consequences finally evolved towards a clinical psychiatric disorder in this young woman, but without altering the poetic features of her letters to the man she loved, to whom she wrote [4]:

*I am afraid of myself* (October 22, 1926).
*Man of stone, understand me* (November 11, 1926).
*And so I will be nice – like a quiet toy* (December 1, 1926).
*Outside I am automatically the sidewalks which leads to the grave* (December 2, 1926).
*Perhaps my survival from this great mystery will sort out to be powerful and happy* (January 15, 1927).

*It still rains*
*My room is dark*
*The heart in an abyss*
*My reason dies*
(January 25, 1927).

## References


1 Breton A: Nadja. Paris, Gallimard, 1928.
2 Article about the performance at the Théâtre des Deux-Masques of the play by Pierre Palau and Olaff [Joseph Babinski] Les détraquées. Comoedia, Paris, February 16, 1921.
3 Philippon J, Poirier J: Joseph Babinski. Oxford, OUP, 2009.
4 Bogousslavsky J: Nadja et Breton: Un amour juste avant la folie. Paris, L'Esprit du Temps, 2012.
5 Bonnet M: André Breton, naissance de l'aventure surréaliste. Paris, José Corti, 1988.
6 Régis E, Hesnard A: La psychanalyse. Paris, Alcan, 1914.
7 Haan J, Koehler P, Bogousslavsky J: Neurology and surrealism: André Breton and Joseph Babinski. Brain 2012, E-pub ahead of print.
8 Breton A: Sujet. Nord-Sud, No 14, April 1918.
9 Pascal C: La démence précoce. Paris, Alcan, 1911.
10 Leroy R: Les hallucinations lilliputiennes. Ann Méd Psychol 1909:279–289
11 Bogousslavsky J: Hysteria after Charcot: back to the future; in Bogousslavsky J, (ed): Following Charcot. A Forgotten History of Neurology and Psychiatry. Karger, Basel, 2010.
12 La révolution surréaliste. Exhibition at the Centre Pompidou. MNAM, Paris 2002.
13 Albach H: Léona, héroïne du surréalisme. Paris, Actes Sud, 2009.
14 Breton A: Manifeste du surréalisme. Paris, Sagittaire, 1924.
15 Walusinski O, Bogousslavsky J: À la recherche du neuropsychiatre perdu: Paul Sollier (1861–1933). Rev Neurol 2008;164:239–247.
16 Muzard S: Les confidences inachevées de Suzanne Muzard; in Sebbag G (ed): André Breton, l'amour-folie. Paris, Jean-Michel Place, 2004.
17 Sérieux P, Capgras J: Le délire d'interprétation. Paris, Alcan, 1909.



Julien Bogousslavsky, MD
Center for Brain and Nervous System Diseases
GSMN Neurocenter, Clinique Valmont
CH–1823 Glion/Montreux (Switzerland)
E-Mail jbogousslavsky@cliniquevalmont.ch

Bogousslavsky J, Dieguez S (eds): Literary Medicine: Brain Disease and Doctors in Novels, Theater, and Film.
Front Neurol Neurosci. Basel, Karger, 2013, vol 31, pp 52–59 (DOI: 10.1159/000343253)

# *The Great Neurosis* of Dr. Joseph Gerard

Jean-Jacques Lefrère[a] · Frédéric Rouillon[b]

[a]Institut National de la Transfusion Sanguine, [b]Hôpital Saint-Anne, Paris, France

**Abstract**

*The Great Neurosis*, of Dr. Joseph Gerard, was published in 1889 in Paris. The book, intended for the general public, shows the different varieties of neuroses through picturesque and instructive examples. Its scientific and medical value is poor, but provides us with the various meanings of the word 'neurosis' in the late nineteenth century.


*The Great Neurosis*, a book of 518 pages, was published in 1889 in Paris. As explained by its author, Dr. Joseph Gerard, in his 'Exposition of the principles', the book has no scientific ambition: it is didactic and, devoid of any medical-scientific jargon, is aimed at a broad audience: 'We have tried to popularize science under the most attractive form and best suited to our temperament: *entertain while teaching*.' To this end, Gerard embellished his chapters with anecdotes and case reports written in the tone of the moment, which are not always high-end, but dramatic and inspiring. His stories could have been used as a canvas by a tired Maupassant – a very tired Maupassant – because you cannot argue that the vigorous style of the writer of *Bel-Ami* is up-to-date. A few pages would not discredit an anthology of stupidity. Two centuries later, the website of the 'Internationale Crétiniste' cites this sentence from the book: 'The drunkard is always a former drinker of water, even, for that to go back to the time of its withdrawal.'

Joseph Gerard was born in Pont-à-Mousson, March 17, 1834. Son of policeman, he started a career in the military at a very young age. At 17, he was admitted to the Cavalry School of Saumur, joined the Sixth Cavalry and saw action in the Crimean campaign. When peace returned, he was chosen to be part of the 'Cent-Gardes', an elite troop of the Second Empire. During the Italian campaign, he was awarded the Military Medal on the battlefield of Solferino and was promoted to lieutenant in the campaign against Prussia in 1870, where he was wounded in the Battle of Sedan, and for which the deposed emperor personally awarded him the Legion of Honor.

In 1871, Gerard returned to civilian life and enrolled at the School of Medicine in Paris, where he obtained the title of Officer of Health. Then he signed on as a physician on a transatlantic boat, went to America, and successfully passed his doctor's examinations at the University of Livingstone. Back in Paris in 1875, he opened a consulting office. Soon after, tired of the lack of trust in foreign diplomas, he began, though already somewhat mature, to get the French equivalents: he did a baccalaureate degree in literature and sciences, and completed his medical studies in 1885. His thesis on artificial insemination caused an outcry at his jury, which rejected it: the fact being very rare, the author will draw, if not some glory, at least wide publicity. The following year, Gerard created the prototype of the 'SOS médecins', a public service 'medical phone' to accelerate rescue in emergencies. He also became famous as a 'curative hypnotist', publishing in 1866 a monograph in which he mocks the scholars who deny the value of this new science (*Magnetism Looking for a Social Position,* with a preface by *Victor Hugo*). After experimenting with various genres in his early years, composing a *Treaty of Failures*, a drama, and a comic opera libretto, he published several works; however, he did not always win the approval and esteem of his peers. Some of his works even caused some controversy in the medical world, such as *Practical Treatise on Diseases of the Genital Tract of Women* (1877), *Boards of Hygiene and Nutrition for All Stages of Life, Summarized in Three Thousand Aphorisms* (1880), *Contribution to the History of Artificial Insemination* (1885, the thesis rejected by the Faculty), *Book for Mothers* (1886), *New Causes of Infertility in Both Sexes* (1888), *Guide of Hypnotist* (1891), and *The Doctor of Madam or Odyssey of a Chaste, Professional Novel* (1893). Gerard also led an ephemeral weekly, *Medicine Illustrated*, published between November 1887 and January 1889. He died in 1898.

In the first part of *The Great Neurosis*, entitled 'Pieces of the trial', the author describes the central nervous system as being composed of 'cells and tubes housed in a box' (the skull and spine) and considers the brain, the most protected organ, as being primordial for the human body. He cites its role in the will and judgment in order to establish his hypothesis of a dual function – induction and deduction – as well as its importance in the memory of instincts, 'the phenomena of intelligence and all psychic transactions that make us be an individual [. . .] sometimes reasonable.' The brain is thus compared to a 'deus ex machina', to an army general, and to a just and honest government, which lowers the heart – this 'convict sentenced to beat all his life' – to the rank of a 'viscera that would be nothing without nerve impulses'. This superior function draws its energy from the electric force stored in the cerebral ventricles: the right lobe for the positive pole, the left one for the negative. Obviously aware that this comparison to 'a battery' is as simplistic as fanciful, Gerard handles this by saying: 'We do not care, this is a problem of physics that will one day find its solution.' He hastens, furthermore, to add that he is 'a semi-scholar and a semi-literate who wishes to link the point of views of anatomists and physiologists on the one hand and of novelists and moralists of the other one on disorders of the mind.'

If such considerations fail to recall the dichotomy (always real today) between neuroscientific and philosophical points of view on psychopathology, they cannot excuse the conceptual fragility of the explanations given by Gerard on the sources of life, vital economy, and transformation of forces. Today, they no longer have any medical and scientific basis, nor on the history of ideas, nor on the physiology of the central nervous system. The most that can be retained is the emphasis put on the influence of the environment, considered as crucial, even more than the innate ('some native qualities [. . .] but nothing compared to the qualities acquired through education'). We can also underline the emerging concept of the unconscious of 'brain intermediaries', as compared to intermediate administrative bodies, which recognizes unconscious acts and automatisms such as those of a piano player. However, as there is also question of automatic actions and functions such as walking or breathing, we are far from Freud's notion of the unconscious.

In another chapter, entitled 'Way of life', Gerard rejects the idea that religion is founded on miracles and that diseases are to be blamed on evil or divine causes. Advocating a scientific approach, he extols the experimental method ('the Deacon Paris will now be called Charcot, Luys, or Liebant Bernheim, and the exorcist will be replaced by hypnotist'), but advocates not straying from the ideological position of 'enjoying life and not live to enjoy' and prohibiting excess so as not to 'burn and die early'. In the neuroses, Gerard sees 'a product of refined civilizations', and his book seeks to demonstrate 'that anyone [who] wants to get out of his social sphere without having the right stuff in him, loses his vital balance and becomes fatally dark in the turmoil of a storm skull.' The chapter entitled 'Countryside calm' holds the cities responsible for the tension of the nerves, which he likens to tightly strung violin which would almost be destroyed by the high-pitched sounds these strings would make. This view is not unlike that of Beard, who, in the late nineteenth century, blamed modern and urban life in the genesis of the American disease that he called neurasthenia. In describing the city as a 'hundred-headed Minotaur which devours its victims,' Gerard foreshadows the Yuppie syndrome ('young urban professionals'): dynamic executives stressed by overwork and an exhausting lifestyle. He then develops an analogy with the war economy, responsible for excessive spending, and with conscription, which induces a forced displacement of men from the countryside to the barracks of the cities, where they take 'leisurely strolls' and later refuse to devote themselves to field work. 'In time of peace, standing armies devour the nutritious juices of the Nation' concludes our good doctor in an antimilitarist flight that must have seemed out of place to many readers warmed by the 'spirit of revenge'.

In the second part of the book, which is devoted to portraits of neurotics, Gerard suggests a definition of neurosis quite consistent with that of his time:

> . . .a condition that seems to have its seat exclusively in the nervous system; it is always without fever and without lesion, even at autopsy. [. . .] The neurosis appears mostly intermittently by simple malaises – headaches, neuralgia – but also sometimes by serious disorders and even frightening, that can achieve separately, simultaneously or successively parts of the nervous system devoted to the feeling, to the intelligence.

Gerard individualizes two subtypes. The 'little neurosis', the most common, which is characterized by:

> . . .a special state of the feeling touching on the general constitution and inducing a temperament said *nervous*, mainly consisting in an excess of impressionability causing one to feel very intensely certain sounds that are not felt by those whose nerves are calm: scratching of nails on a stove pipe, grinding of glass using a knife, cork cut with a razor, violent ringing of the bell, etc.'

He indicates, however, that while the number of people affected by 'little neurosis' is considerable, it is not a real disease, but a simple 'nervous constitution' without consequences 'in well-educated people who know how to understand each other'. This does not apply to the 'great neurosis', 'the only, the true', which is a pathology having its evolutionary phases and affecting sensitivity, emotivity, senses, or intellectual centers. Its consequences are terrible when it affects 'the senses or intellectual centers' because it then leads to 'real storms of the soul' and 'most terrifyingly morbid manifestations of thought, leading to senseless and most disordered acts'. Therefore, the 'great neurosis' appears as a nosological entity with no identifiable cause. Here we find the dichotomy between pathological personality and characteristic disturbance, and this dichotomy is still present in modern nosography, such as that of the *Diagnostic and Statistical Manual* or that of the *American Association of Psychiatry*.

In this 'great neurosis', Gerard distinguishes three levels. The first level is marked by a 'vague sadness' and by a 'pain starting from the pit of the stomach then radiating to the chest and flanks', the subjects have manifestations of anxiety and 'spasmodic and constricting pangs of all the motor nerves', their voice is altered, their throat is constricted, and tears come easily to their eyes. Such a condition leads to the spleen, to hypochondria and to a 'gloomy obsession with the idea of suicide', but without acting on it. Everything still works inside ('the disease is snoring, but the pistons are at rest'). The second level, 'progressive development of the first', is manifested by vapors, a 'tremor', and nervous breakdowns, while 'the soul gets involved and becomes ill.' Then 'weird conceptions of the mind' and 'aberrations of thought' occur, 'the moral sense is obliterated, the passions become perverted and normal reason collapses in the most lamentable mess'. The third level is characterized by a crisis 'of unprecedented violence, but of which the individual has no more responsibility this time' (he 'suddenly fell with a cry, he rolls on the floor, his chest gasping the swollen neck, with a grimacing face'). At this point, neurosis has become hysteria or epilepsy, requiring an urgent internment to protect society. In fact, 'the latent epilepsy may manifest as a criminal act,' attests Gerard, citing the Legrand du Saulle. This description evokes the lessons of Charcot on hysteria at Salpêtrière Hospital of Paris.

The book then introduces no less than fourteen clinical cases intended to illustrate the psychopathological variants of the great neurosis: 'essential neurosis', 'neurosis by failure', 'neurosis by training', 'occupational neurosis', 'neurosis of idleness' and that of 'burnout', 'neurosis of ambition', 'vicarious' neurosis, 'religious' neurosis, 'protean' neurosis, 'mystical' neurosis, 'conjugal' neurosis, 'literary' neurosis, neurosis 'of outward show', and even neurosis 'of a people' (by the contagiousness of symptoms). As fun as some of these 'clinical' descriptions are, they make little account of those already formulated by psychiatrists at the time of Gerard. Similarly, the 'neuroses of internal origin', which the chapter 'Third party' details, are inspired more by psychopathology than by medicine, whether it is the neurosis of the stomach (with his 'bad digestion which focuses on the brain'), alcoholic neurosis, skin neurosis, respiratory neurosis, genital neurosis, senile neurosis, neurosis of the player, congenital or diathesis neurosis, ordinary neurosis, or hypnotic neurosis, which gives Gerard an occasion to glorify the magnetism developed by Mesmer more than a century earlier.

The final section summarizes the treatments of the time. Gerard considers that 'hygiene plays a huge role' and that hydrotherapy is a valuable treatment: 'All types of hydrotherapy are good, since the simple general lotion made using a sponge, to the wet sheet, to the watering of the garden and finally to the shower that our *hydrothéropates* [sic] execute so successfully.' The author also advocates trips to the countryside and, a pioneer of light therapy, emphasizes the importance of exposure to light. The book ends with some medications used in the treatment of neurosis (polybromide, bromide of camphor, gold bromide) and stating the need to divert the individual from his pathogenic environment – the only measure that appears to retain its relevance today.

What to think of such a book today? Indeed the concept of neurosis has always been unclear. In 1900, on the topic of neuropathic disorders, Pierre Janet said that while it is 'difficult to analyze one in particular', it is still 'more delicate and more vague to formulate a general conception about all these diseases, which everyone talks about without much understanding, but which one summarizes under the term *neurosis*'. The term was proposed in 1769 by William Cullen of Scotland in his *Synopsis Nosologiae Methodicae* to designate a whole variety of nerve diseases – the comas, the spasms, the insanities – as well as other general diseases, such as fevers or cachexias, as opposed to local diseases. With Pinel, however, neuroses were called 'diseases without injury' and attributable to moral causes. This negative conception inspired Georget who, in his *Dictionary of Medicine* (1840), considered them as turmoil 'chronic, non-hazardous, intermittent, without fever, in appearance, capable of ringing on suffering such that the subject feels very sick.' The neuroses summarize 'periodic headaches, hypochondria, catalepsy, chorea, hysteria, asthma, nervous palpitations, stomach ache with or without vomiting, and neuralgia.' We find here the heterogeneity of the inventory established by Gerard in his book.

In the late nineteenth century, one witnesses a divergence of neurological concepts because of the influence of Charcot, inspired by Babinski, or by that of Beard, who attributes the 'neurasthenia' to spinal exhaustion. It is also the time of the psychodynamic approaches of Janet and Freud. Alienists and psychiatrists stay

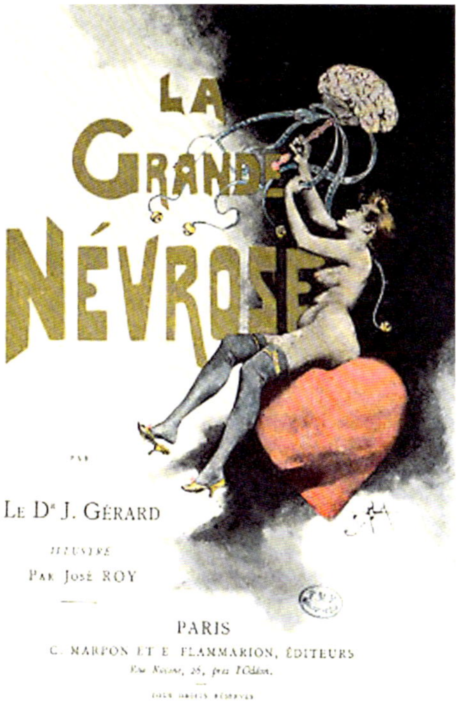


**Fig. 1.** Front cover of *The Great Neurosis*, Marpon et Flammarion, Paris,1889.

out of the way, however, with Kraepelin (Germany) devoting only a few dozen pages to the psychogenic neuroses in his voluminous treatise, and Gilbert Ballet (France) citing only phobias and obsessions in his monumental opus. Ultimately, though, neuroses will be rehabilitated, in psychiatric classifications, in the middle of the twentieth century. Then the term 'neurosis' itself, too inaccurate and tainted by ideology, will disappear from psychiatric science after two centuries of mixed fortunes.

Finally, a few words need to be said about the 230 illustrations that José Roy, an illustrator who then enjoyed some reputation, produced for *The Great Neurosis*. Participating in the overt intention of Gerard to 'learn in fun', they always 'stick' to the text, of which they highlight a simple sentence, phrase, or word. With a gently ironic good humor, they often play on contrast and antinomy, lightening up a work which is primarily professorial. Some are 'pornographic' as one said at the time (this adjective has subsequently acquired a much sharper sense). In 1890, the cover picture – a naked woman sitting on a heart and grasping the stem of a brain floating in the air like an octopus in his element (fig. 1) – and Roy's illustrations for Gerard's *The Artificial Fertilization* brought him condemnation for offending public decency from the Criminal Chamber of the Court of Appeals of Paris. Roy, whose real name was Joseph-Marie Roy, illustrated many other books that had this

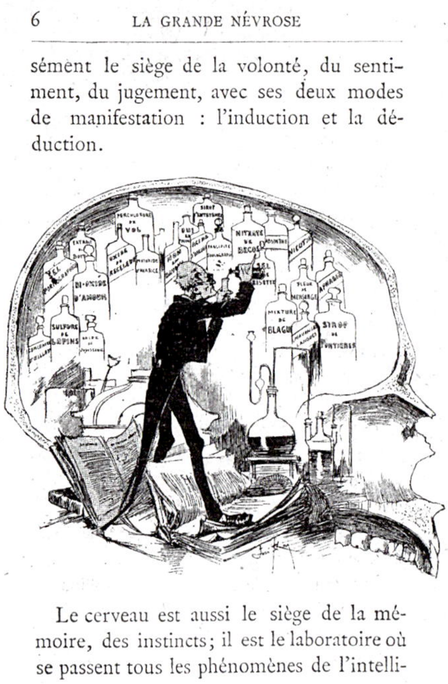
6 LA GRANDE NÉVROSE

sément le siège de la volonté, du sentiment, du jugement, avec ses deux modes de manifestation : l'induction et la déduction.

Le cerveau est aussi le siège de la mémoire, des instincts; il est le laboratoire où se passent tous les phénomènes de l'intelli-

2

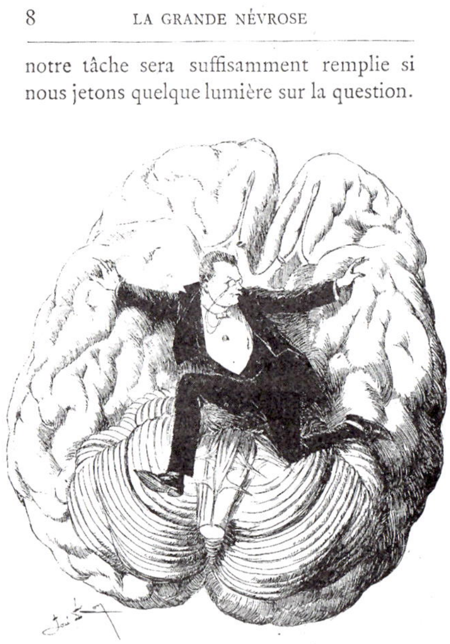
8 LA GRANDE NÉVROSE

notre tâche sera suffisamment remplie si nous jetons quelque lumière sur la question.

3

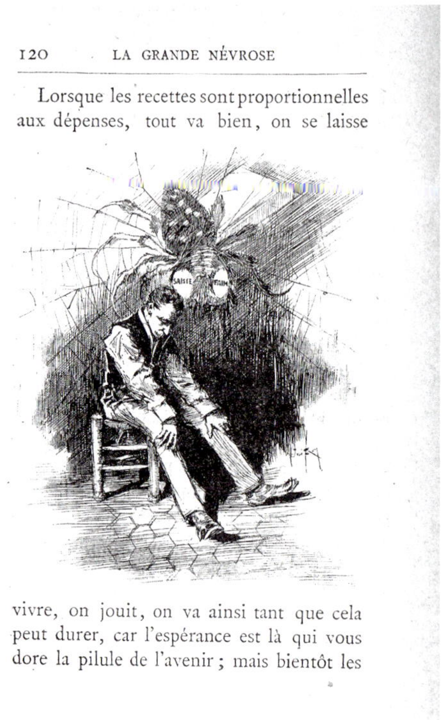
120 LA GRANDE NÉVROSE

Lorsque les recettes sont proportionnelles aux dépenses, tout va bien, on se laisse vivre, on jouit, on va ainsi tant que cela peut durer, car l'espérance est là qui vous dore la pilule de l'avenir; mais bientôt les

4

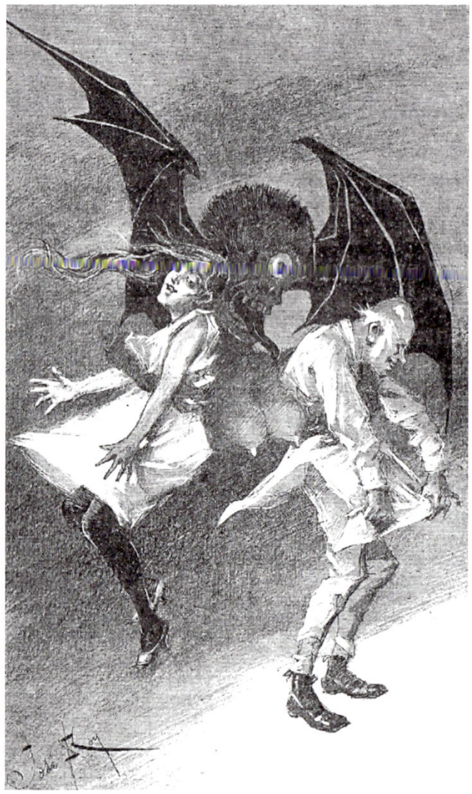

5

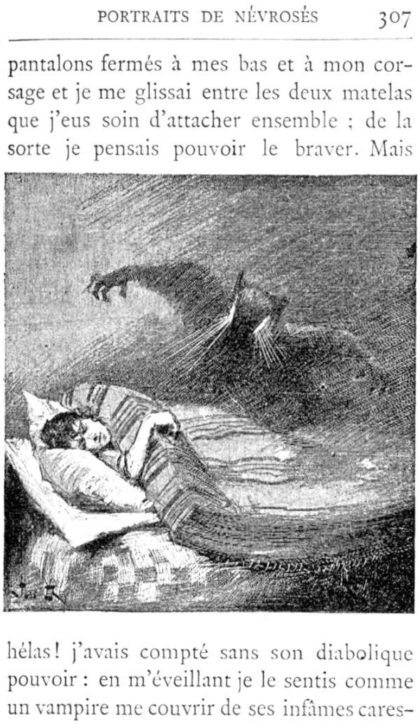

PORTRAITS DE NÉVROSÉS 307

pantalons fermés à mes bas et à mon corsage et je me glissai entre les deux matelas que j'eus soin d'attacher ensemble ; de la sorte je pensais pouvoir le braver. Mais

hélas ! j'avais compté sans son diabolique pouvoir : en m'éveillant je le sentis comme un vampire me couvrir de ses infâmes cares-

6

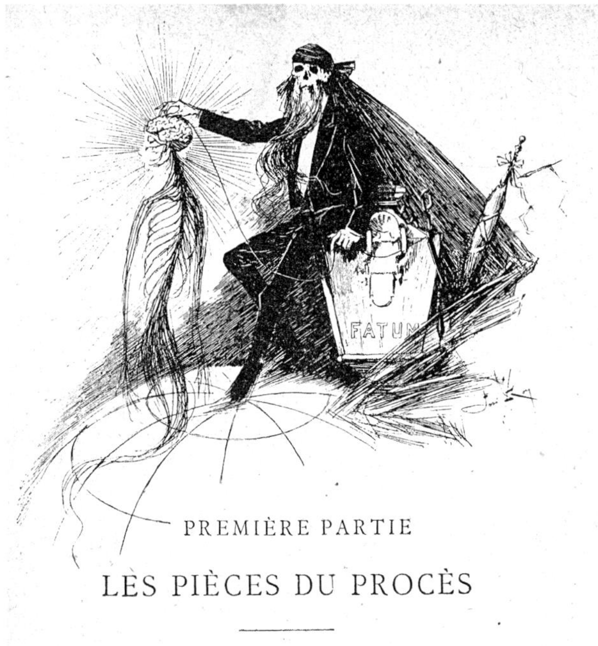

PREMIÈRE PARTIE

LES PIÈCES DU PROCÈS

7

**Figs. 2–7.** Illustrations from *The Great Neurosis*, Marpon et Flammarion, Paris,1889.

type of 'corrupting' nature, such as *Robe montante* by Catulle Mendès, *Jambes folles* by Emile Testard, or *La Charmeuse d'hommes* of Jules de Gastyne. Some pictures in *The Great Neurosis* bring out morbid fantasy, of which this turn-of-the-century period was particularly fond (fig. 2–7). They are an opportunity to recall that José Roy was also the first illustrator of the *Chants de Maldoror*, with the frontispiece he gave to the Genonceaux edition in 1890. The first in the chronology, the last by the genius. . .

Dr. Jean-Jacques Lefrère
Institut National de la Transfusion Sanguine
6 rue Alexandre-Cabanel
FR–75015 Paris (France)
E-Mail jeanjacqueslefrere@orange.fr

Bogousslavsky J, Dieguez S (eds): Literary Medicine: Brain Disease and Doctors in Novels, Theater, and Film.
Front Neurol Neurosci. Basel, Karger, 2013, vol 31, pp 60–68 (DOI: 10.1159/000345058)

# Psychopathic Characters in Fiction

Bartlomiej Piechowski-Jozwiak[a,b] · Julien Bogousslavsky[c]

[a]Department of Neurology, Princess Royal University Hospital, Farnborough Common, Orpington, and [b]King's College Hospital, London, UK; [c]Center for Brain and Nervous System Disease, GSMN Neurocenter, Clinique Valmont, Glion/Montreux, Switzerland

**Abstract**

The theme of psychopathy has fascinated artists and the general public for centuries. The first concepts on psychopathy came from the parasciences, such as phrenology where anatomical features were linked to certain psychopathic/immoral behaviors. The concept of psychopathy was recognized by forensic psychiatry a few decades ago and this official recognition was followed by the emergence of scientific and clinical guidelines for the diagnosis and prognosis of psychopaths. These modern tools can also be used for historical purposes by allowing us to look back on fictional works and identify psychopaths in literature. Interpretation of fictitious psychopaths needs to be related to the historical situation in which the novels were written; such investigations can be both enriching and thrilling.


The theme of psychopathy has fascinated artists and the general public for centuries. It has been at the heart of orally transmitted and written stories on mad emperors, kings, and wizards. An early interest in psychopaths can already be seen in ancient Persian literature in *The Book of One Thousand and One Nights*. The theme recurs in Medieval and Renaissance literature and in works influenced by Romanticism, Realism, and Naturalism as the whirlpool of psychopathy gained momentum. In the 20th and 21st centuries, there has been a huge growth in the genre of 'thriller' or 'horror' fiction, a particularly fertile ground for psychopathic characters. The fictional psychopathic character is usually created by the writer as part of 'ars poetica' and does not necessarily follow known and accepted clinical scenarios – hence the need for subtle and critical interpretations of psychopathic behavior in literary fiction.

## Theory of Psychopathy

The first concept of psychopathy was described by the French psychiatrist Philippe Pinel at the beginning of the 19th century as a partial defect of mental function with affective insanity without a positive, i.e. delusional, component (known as 'Manie sans délire') [1]. Affected individuals present with defective morality and problems with emotional and behavioral control, but at the same time their intellectual function is preserved. However, it appears that mania without delirium may not have a moral inclination and, thus, moral insanity would be a form of mania leading to furious instinctive behaviors ('instincte fureur') [2].

English physician and ethnologist James Cowles Prichard in his *Treatise on Insanity and Other Disorders Affecting the Mind* described moral insanity as a 'morbid perversion of the natural feelings, affections, inclinations, temper, habits, moral dispositions, and natural impulses, without any remarkable disorder or defect of the interest or knowing and reasoning faculties, and particularly without any insane illusion or hallucinations' [3]. In other words the intellect of the morally insane is unaffected, but their feelings and habits are profoundly aberrant.

This concept was developed further by Hervey Cleckley, an American psychiatrist [4]. According to Cleckley, psychopathy should be perceived as a constellation of affective, behavioral, and interpersonal features. The affected individuals have a mask of sanity with preserved intelligence and a surface demeanor that disguises severe underlying abnormalities such as selfishness and impulsivity, a lack of empathy and remorse, and a desire to dominate. Hence, psychopathy may be described as a disconnection between affect and cognition. Psychopaths have diminished capacity for remorse and insufficient behavioral controls.

In contemporary clinical practice, the Psychopathy Checklist, Revised (PCL-R) is a widely accepted tool for assessment of psychopathy [5]. It was developed by Robert Hare, a Canadian criminal psychologist, and is based on Cleckley's criteria. This is a clinical rating scale used to predict the odds for reoffending criminal behavior and to assess the probability of rehabilitation. The scale is based on two pillars. First is emotional detachment, including core personality traits of psychopathy such as callousness, manipulativeness, and lack of remorse. The second pillar focuses on antisocial behavior and the assessment of the type of violent and impulsive acts that are often associated with psychopathy [6].

Psychopathy may also be viewed as the overlap of personality disorders, including antisocial personality disorders and dissocial behavior as defined by the DSM-IV criteria [7]. Emotional impairment in the form of lack of guilt is also part of the criteria. Only one third of individuals with an antisocial personality disorder meet the criteria of psychopathy [8].

Psychopathy may be divided into two groups: developmental psychopathy and acquired sociopathy [6]. The latter form may follow brain injury, especially of the frontal lobes. In these cases the impulsive aggression and antisocial behavior is triggered by external factors and may be the leading presentation, while in developmental psychopathy the process may be more multilevel, including goal-orientated actions aimed at financial and sexual gain and increased status. In addition, these individuals may have problems dealing with feelings of fear and a sense of isolation from other people whose emotions they find difficult to comprehend [8]. It seems that developmental psychopaths demonstrate both core personality traits of psychopathy and antisocial behavior on the PCL-R scale while acquired sociopaths score higher in antisocial behavior on the PCL-R scale [6].

## Brain Abnormalities in Psychopaths

The first concept of anatomical differences in psychopaths was proposed by the Swiss physiognomist and poet, Johann Caspar Lavater, at the end of the 18th century in *Physiognomische Fragmente zur Beförderung der Menschenkenntnis und Menschenliebe* [9]. He suggested a link between facial features and crime. Later Franz Joseph Gall, a German neuroanatomist, founded phrenology, which is currently considered a pseudoscience. Gall originally developed cranioscopy to try and determine an individual's mental and moral properties based on the anatomy of the skull [10]. Cesare Lombroso, an Italian physician and criminologist, introduced the concept of a 'naturally born criminal' ('reo nato'). According to Lombroso, psychopathy with criminal behavior was inherited and could be identified based on anatomical features that revealed atavistic properties. He described a regression of human features in criminals that made them resemble the lower primates more closely and marked them out as not fitting into the civilized world. Lombroso conducted multiple post mortems in a quest for physical stigmata to prove his theories. He identified several features that he associated with 'criminal types', including the shape of the forehead and ears, cranial malformations, facial asymmetry with prognathism, long arms, etc. [11]. The results of his studies were widely disproved and scientifically discredited, but they did create interest in the idea of investigating the concept of a criminal mind.

The case of Phineas P. Gage provided a basis for linking focal brain damage with personality changes and development of socially unacceptable behavior. Mr. Gage was a railway worker who had never had any problems fitting well into society. However, he then suffered a severe brain injury when a heavy metal rod pierced his left eye, penetrating his skull, damaging his frontal lobe, and exiting at the top of his head [12, 13]. Physically, Gage made a good recovery from this accident. He had no weakness and no cognitive impairment with preservation of perception, memory, cognition, and speech. However, he was 'no longer Gage', presenting with an unstable affect and a lack of patience and respect for others. He found decision-making difficult and his social functioning became aberrant. In short, Gage's behavior became psychopathic due to an acquired condition [13].

## Frontal Lobe

Following the Phineas Gage case, the frontal cortex became the primary topic of research in the field of psychopathy. There were numerous reports linking acquired sociopathy with damage to the orbitofrontal cortex and decreased volume of the prefrontal area in the dominant hemisphere, as confirmed with magnetic resonance imaging of the brain. There is data on the significant loss of prefrontal gray matter in people with antisocial personality disorder. The reduction of cortical volume was linked to impaired decision-making and learning problems [6]. When comparing psychopaths who were not caught following their crimes ('successful') to those convicted ('unsuccessful'), Yang et al. [14] found a significant reduction in the prefrontal gray matter in the latter group. Individuals with prefrontal cortex damage present with disinhibition and impulsivity, distractibility, and impairment of decision-making. This constellation of symptoms is also known as the 'frontal lobe personality' trait and is quite often seen in acquired psychopaths (pseudopsychopathic behavior) [6]. However, the role of frontal lobe dysfunction and the occurrence of violence in individuals with psychopathy have been a matter of debate among scientists [8].

## Temporal Lobe

The other group of symptoms associated with psychopathy such as lack of empathy and disturbed reactions to fearful and sad facial expressions may lead to difficult interpersonal relationships and targeted aggression. The anatomical substrate for these traits lies in the temporal lobe and in the amygdala [8]. The amygdala plays a crucial role in aggressive behavioral patterns. Data from neuroimaging studies show an association between amygdala dysfunction and occurrence of psychopathy. It was found that violent offenders had smaller volumes of amygdala as confirmed by volumetric magnetic resonance imaging. In patients with temporal lobe epilepsy and aggression, the volume of amygdala was found to be decreased as well [8]. Functional magnetic resonance studies also confirmed reduced amygdala function in individuals with high scores on the PCL-R scale during processing of negative valence words [8].

The results of a study on 372 male individuals in a maximum security mental hospital showed that 20% of the patients from the most violent group had focal temporal electrical abnormalities on EEG in the form of slowing and/or sharp waves, and 41% had either dilated temporal horns or reduced size of the temporal lobe as demonstrated with computed tomography of the brain. In the least violent group, the results were 2.4 and 6.7%, respectively [15]. In addition, posterior hippocampal volume loss was demonstrated to be significant in incarcerated violent offenders [16]. An exaggerated anterior hippocampal structural asymmetry (right volume greater than left) was shown in unsuccessful (convicted) when compared to successful (unconvicted) psychopaths and healthy controls [17]. This anatomical difference may be responsible for disruption of hippocampal-prefrontal connections which consequently may lead to dysregulation of affect, poor contextual fear conditioning, and lack of ability to interpret cues [6].

The link between organic disorders of both frontal and temporal lobes in the occurrence of antisocial, aggressive, and disruptive behaviors was demonstrated in patients following herpetic encephalitis and in those with frontotemporal dementia [6]. In a very recent paper, Gregory et al. [18] demonstrated that violent offenders with antisocial personality disorder and psychopathy had significant reduction of gray matter in the anterior rostral prefrontal cortex (Brodmann 10) and temporal poles (Brodmann 20/38) when compared to offenders without a psychopathic syndrome. These structures are involved in empathic processing and moral reasoning as well as in guilt and embarrassment functions. All of these attributes are impaired in psychopaths.

## Corpus callosum

The neuroanatomical basis of psychopathy is complex. As brain function requires the interconnection of many important centers, any disconnection of these may lead to certain abnormalities, including psychopathy. There are reports of increased callosal volume, increased callosal length, and decreased callosal thickness in psychopaths with antisocial personality disorder when compared to healthy controls. The importance of callosal function is backed by the findings of abnormalities in interhemispheric processing in psychopathy, such as reduced evoked potentials amplitudes [6].

## Psychopaths in Thrillers – From Antiquity to the Third Millenium

In contrast to forensic psychiatry, the profiles of psychopaths in literature are fictionalized for the sake of scene setting and storyline. They do not necessarily match the PCL-R criteria of psychopathy. The main features of fictitious psychopaths are high intelligence, goal orientation (for financial and sexual gain and societal status), deceptiveness, and impulsive often violent behavior. These traits are accompanied by mercilessness, lack of empathy, and an inability to feel guilt or remorse – in sum all the characteristics society associates with malevolence. Retrospective analysis using modern psychological tools may lead us to consider some historical figures such as the classic 'mad emperors' Caligula and Nero as psychopaths. We should remember though that 'bad' characters in fiction may have been invented, at least in part, to represent those features that were most unwanted and socially disapproved of at the time of writing. Hence the importance of interpreting psychopathic characters in the context of the societies in which they lived. The modern study of psychopathy in both fact and fiction began during the 18th century as part of Romanticism and the

Enlightenment. Developments in the field have been stimulated by medical science but also by parasciences like phrenology. This rich, complex and often interwoven genealogy has led to a parallel blossoming of knowledge and prejudice, understanding, and stigmatization.

Thrillers are by definition designed to provide readers with a sort of fearful excitement. The narrative gradually builds up a feeling of suspense and unease, often heightened by a surprise in the denouement, the classic 'twist in the tale' [19]. Using this definition we can take a literary trip back in time to search out those villains/bad characters who have thrilled the readers through the centuries.

One of the first fictitious psychopathic characters in literature is the Pardoner in *The Canterbury Tales* (Chaucer). He does not want to work or beg, but he longs for money, wool, cheese, and wheat, and enjoys drinking liquor and ale. He wants to take advantage of the vulnerable – poor widows, servant boys, etc. He preaches moral tales purely for his own profit and admits to being a vicious person. Perhaps most shockingly, at least in the eyes of his contemporaries, the Pardoner says he does not want to follow the apostles, which in the late 14th century would have been considered rebellious and seditious. Analyzing his behavior retrospectively with PCL-R, we can state that the Pardoner lacked remorse and empathy, was manipulative, and lied. His lifestyle was parasitic and he lacked realistic long-term goals, giving him both PCL-R factors 1 and 2.

Barabas, from '*The Jew of Malta*' (Christopher Marlowe, 1589) is another fictitious psychopathic character. A wealthy Jewish merchant who loses his fortune when the Turks demand tribute from the Maltese, Barabas plots against the Governor of Malta whom he blames for his bankruptcy. He uses his own daughter Abigail to turn the Governor's son against his father, a ruse that ultimately leads to the death of both men in a duel. After realizing the role she played in her father's plot, Abigail joins a nunnery, only to be poisoned by her father for becoming a Christian. Finally, Barabas turns to the Turks – the catalyst for the whole tragedy in the first place – helping them to invade Malta and becoming Governor himself. In the case of Barabas we can see a whole variety of psychopathic features such as manipulativeness, lack of guilt, egocentrism, and focusing on wealth and social status above all else.

Shylock from *The Merchant of Venice* (Shakespeare, 1596–1598) is another wealthy Jewish merchant presented as a psychopathic character. He agrees to lend money without charging interest to Antonio, a prosperous – and anti-Semitic – Venetian entrepreneur. As an act of revenge provoked by Antonio's prejudice, Shylock attaches one very specific condition to the loan, if Antonio does not pay the money back on time, he will have to give up a pound of his flesh. This condition meets with some surprise, but Shylock's proposal is considered as a sign of generosity rather than a vicious plan. Unfortunately, Antonio's business plans fail when his fleet is lost at sea, and he cannot repay the loan. Shylock refuses an offer from Antonio's friend to repay double the sum and demands one pound of the debtor's flesh. However, Antonio's ally discovers that as stated in the contract Shylock can take just flesh but not blood, exactly one pound, no more no less, as otherwise according to Venetian law his goods would be confiscated. Based on these revelations Shylock agrees to be paid three times the owed amount, but this is rejected. The Duke of Venice decides that because Shylock is Jewish, and thus an 'alien', he must give his fortune to the state and Antonio. By the end of the play Shylock is forced to convert to Christianity as well as give away his fortune. As we can see in this story, Shylock assumed that he might be in the position to ask Antonio for a pound of his flesh without asking for a high return rate for the loan. He simply puts money above human values. He agrees to lend the money without charging interest, but then adds the sadistic pound of flesh business to the agreement. Such behavior shows an all too human desire for revenge against prejudice and social ostracism rather an obsession with money. Shylock wants to cause pain and humiliation, even if only metaphorically, in vengeance for the slights and cruelty which are meted out to him as a Jew, an alien, and outsider. This looks like a meticulous calculation, exploiting an opportunity to exact revenge and show no mercy.

A real encyclopedia of psychopathic behavior was presented in '*Les 120 journées de Sodome*' (Marquis de Sade, 1785). De Sade takes the reader through the story of four wealthy men who seal themselves up in the medieval castle of Saint-Martin-de-Belleville, together with a group of young men and women. The four men are the Duc de Blangis, known to have amassed his fortune by poisoning his mother and sister; the Bishop, Blangis' brother and an enthusiastic sodomite; the President de Curval, a judge who enjoys sentencing innocent people to death, and Durcet, a banker. These four men embark on a 4-month orgy of sexual, emotional, and physical abuse, with their victims even including their own daughters. Female brothel keepers are invited to the castle, together with eight studs renowned for the length of their penises. Stimulated by stories told by the veteran prostitutes, the four men engage in a variety of abuses that are divided into four categories – simple passions (no actual sexual penetration, pedophile acts, coprophagia), complex passions (pedophile acts with flagellation, blasphemous activities, deflowering children), criminal passions (sodomizing children, inflicting physical injury), and murderous passions (skinning children, disemboweling a pregnant women, killing newborns). In this novel we can see all aspects of psychopathy represented by four libertines who let nothing restrain them from their desire to experiment with extreme and perverted forms of sexual behavior.

Fyodor Dostoyevsky in his novel *Crime and Punishment (Преступлéние и Наказáние)* published in 1866 provides a thorough dissection of a psychopathic profile with his portrayal of Rodion Raskolnikov, who plans to kill a verminous pawnbroker for her money. Raskolnikov tries to find a rationale for this murder by emphasizing the good use he will make of the pawnbroker's money; he attempts to turn a terrible act into something that is not only positive but also somehow inevitable – an expression of 'natural justice'. Eventually Raskolnikov manages to kill the pawnbroker and, by accident, her sister as well. After this botched assault he steals just a small amount of money. The double murder remains undetected for some time, but Raskolnikov is obsessed by his violent crime. At one point he becomes delirious and wanders the streets of Saint Petersburg, behaving in a manner that suggests he is trying subconsciously to own up to the crime he has committed. Raskolnikov meets a constable named Porfiry and confides in him. As Porfiry listens to his outpourings, he begins to suspect that Raskolnikov killed the pawnbroker and her sister. Tormented by guilt, Raskolnikov eventually confesses to the murder and is sentenced to penal servitude in Siberia. The case of Raskolnikov is fascinating as it lets us see clearly the story of an intelligent man who succumbs to an urge to use violent and predatory behavior to try and gain the social and financial advantages he thinks he deserves. However, unlike many other characters with psychopathic traits, Raskolnikov is eaten up by guilt and remorse following his crime.

Moving on to 20th century literature, *The Silence of the Lambs* and *Hannibal* by Thomas Harris need to be mentioned. In both novels the dark character is represented by Dr. Hannibal Lecter, a gifted forensic psychiatrist, serial murderer, and cannibal. *The Silence of the Lambs* features another villain, Buffalo Bill, whose signature crime involves flaying overweight women to make aprons of their skin in a form of twisted 'haute couture'. Bill honed his sewing skills in a center for vocational rehabilitation where he was sent at the age of 12, having been abandoned by his mother and adopted by his grandparents whom he then killed. When hunting for his victims, Bill's technique was to pretend to be vulnerable and ask for help. Any kindhearted, overweight woman who took pity on him was attacked, kidnapped, and starved until her skin was loose enough for 'harvesting'. By wearing a woman's skin and hiding his genitals Buffalo Bill believes he can become a woman, attaining not only sexual and physical transformation, but also acquiring the power and potential of giving birth.

In *Hannibal,* Dr. Lecter is being chased by his former patient, Verger, a sadistic pedophile who seeks revenge for being mutilated during a therapeutic session. He wants to feed Lecter to wild boars but is outwitted by the doctor who convinces Verger's sister to kill him because she was abused by her brother when she was a child. Lecter then drugs an FBI officer, Starling, with mind-altering medications in order to transform her into a stand-in for his dead sister. He invites her for a dinner where they both eat human brain taken from a living victim and the evening culminates with them having sexual intercourse. In both of these novels we can see a prismatic reflection of De Sade's sadistic libertine practices together with perversion of the sexual drive and a striving for domination, control, and supremacy. Lecter shows a clearly grandiose sense of self-worth and he corrupts the values of the medical profession which has given him the knowledge and skill to indulge his taste for cannibalism. Both Buffalo Bill and Lecter are role models for psychopaths.

The quest for psychopaths in literature is never-ending. Creative fiction writing coupled with rapid changes in social and moral values and in the global economy mean we can expect that the concept of psychopathy both in forensic psychiatry and literature will continue to evolve. Tracking these developments can be a thrilling experience.

## References


1 Tuke DH (ed): A Dictionary of Psychological Medicine. London, J. & A. Churchill, 1892, vol 2, p 813.
2 Verplaetse J: Chapter 7: Moral insanity as a disorder of the moral sense; in Localising the Moral Brain: Neuroscience and the Search for the Cerebral Seat of Morality, 1800–1930. Berlin, Springer, 2009, p 195.
3 Prichard JC: Treatise on Insanity and Other Disorders Affecting the Mind. London, Sherwood, Gilbert, and Piper, 1835, p 92.
4 Cleckley H: The Mask of Sanity. St. Louis, Mosby, 1976.
5 Hare RD, Neumann CN: The PCL-R Assessment of Psychopathy: Development, Structural Properties, and New Directions; in Patrick C (ed): Handbook of Psychopathy. New York, Guilford, 2006, pp 58–88.
6 Weber S, Habel U, Amunts K, Schneider F: Structural brain abnormalities in psychopaths – a review. Behav Sci Law 2008;26:7–28.
7 Herpertz SC, Sass H: Emotional deficiency and psychopathy. Behav Sci Law 2000;18:567–580.
8 Blair R: Neurobiological basis of psychopathy. Br J Psych 2003:5–7.
9 Shookman E (ed): The Faces of Physiognomy: Interdisciplinary Approaches to Johann Caspar Lavater. Columbia, Camden House, 1993.
10 Simpson D: Phrenology and the neurosciences: contributions of F. J. Gall and J. G. Spurzheim. ANZ J Surg 2005;75:475.
11 Lombroso C: Le crime, causes et remèdes. Librairie C. Reinwald. Paris, Schleicher Frères, 1899.
12 Campbell HF: Injuries of the cranium – trepanning. Ohio Med Surg J 1851;4:31–35.
13 Damasio AR, Everitt BJ, Bishop D: The somatic marker hypothesis and the possible functions of the prefrontal cortex. Philo Trans R Soc London B Biol Sci 1996;351:1413–1420.
14 Yang Y, Raine A, Lencz T, Bihrle S, LaCasse L, Colletti P: Volume reduction in prefrontal grey matter in unsuccessful criminal psychopaths. Biol Psychiatry 2005;57:1103–1108.
15 Wong MT, Lumsden J, Fenton GW, Fenwick PB: Electroencephalography, computed tomography and violence ratings of male patients in a maximum-security mental hospital. Acta Psychiatr Scand 1994;2:97–101.
16 Laakso MP, Vaurio O, Koivisto E, Savolainen L, Eronen M, Aronen HJ, Hakola P, Repo E, Soininen H, Tiihonen J: Psychopathy and the posterior hippocampus. Behav Brain Res 2001;118:187–193.
17 Raine A, Ishikawa SS, Arce E, Lencz T, Knuth KH, Bihrle S, LaCasse L, Colletti P: Hippocampal structural asymmetry in unsuccessful psychopaths. Biol Psychiatry 2004;55:185–191.
18 Gregory S, Ffytche D, Simmons A, Kumari V, Howard M, Hodgins S, Blackwood N: The antisocial brain: psychopathy matters: a structural MRI investigation of antisocial male violent offenders. Arch Gen Psychiatry 2012;69:962–972.
19 Patterson J (ed): Thriller. Ontario, MIRA Books, 2006, p iii.



Bartlomiej Piechowski-Jozwiak, MD
Consultant Stroke Neurologist, Clinical Lead for Stroke, Department of Neurology
Princess Royal University Hospital, Farnborough Common
BR6 8ND Orpington, Kent (UK)
E-Mail bpiechowski@gazeta.pl

Bogousslavsky J, Dieguez S (eds): Literary Medicine: Brain Disease and Doctors in Novels, Theater, and Film.
Front Neurol Neurosci. Basel, Karger, 2013, vol 31, pp 69–76 (DOI: 10.1159/000343256)

# Misidentifications in Pirandello's Plays and Short Stories

Maurizio Paciaroni · Thomas Kilcline

Stroke Unit and Division of Cardiovascular Medicine, Santa Maria della Misericordia Hospital, University of Perugia, Perugia, Italy

**Abstract**

Luigi Pirandello was an Italian playwright, novelist, short story writer, poet, and one of the leading dramatists of the twentieth century. Pirandello used his plays and short stories to express his life philosophy which included the irony and bitterness of self-deception. In his works, his characters possess highly complex personalities, portrayed by ongoing and overlapping conflicts between illusion and reality. These manifestations of double personalities and confusion between imagination and reality are today known as psychopathological phenomena, classified as both delusional misidentification and reduplication syndromes. Here, individuals misidentify and reduplicate places, people, or events. These delusional syndromes (Capgras, Frégoli, intermetamorphosis, syndrome of subjective doubles) occur primarily in psychiatric illnesses (i.e. schizophrenia) and organic illnesses (i.e. right hemispheric stroke). For Pirandello, reality was highly subjective in all humans. However, misidentification and reduplication syndromes can manifest when this subjectivity gets out of control. With his works, Pirandello made philosophical concepts which had previously only been discussed by intellectuals available to a much larger audience. Pirandello continued to elaborate upon this concept of mutable ego, established by Blaise Pascal in the 1600s and carried on by the French psychologist Alfred Binet.


## Luigi Pirandello (1867–1937)

Luigi Pirandello (fig. 1) was an Italian playwright, novelist, short story writer, poet, and one of the leading dramatists of the twentieth century. Born in Girgenti (now Agrigento), Sicily, on June 28, 1867, his father was the owner of a rich sulfur mine and played an important role in the industrial and commercial life of Girgenti and Porto Empedocle. Coming from a well-to-do family permitted him a comfortable childhood and adolescence. Pirandello began his studies at home with private tutors, then went on to attend a technical institute, and later changed his course of study to humanities where he excelled in oratory and literature. Pirandello attended the universities of Palermo, Rome, and Bonn. During this university period, he wrote and

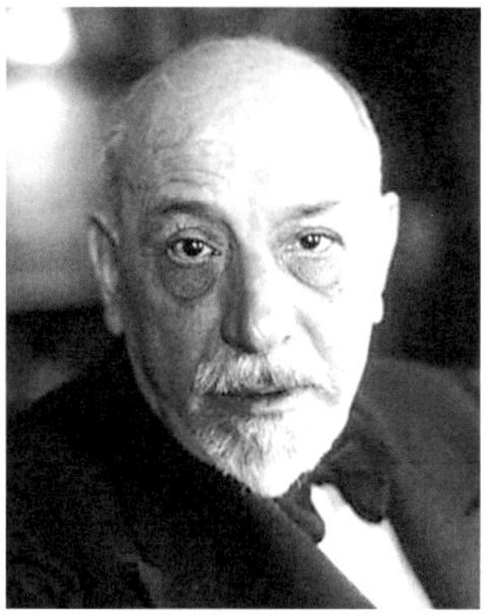

**Fig. 1.** Luigi Pirandello (1867–1937). Source: Agence Meurisse.

published two volumes of poetry. Although his father wanted him to follow a career in business, Pirandello had no desire in fulfilling his father's request.

Pirandello earned his doctorate in philology with a thesis on the dialect of his native Girgenti before setting off for Rome to teach and write in 1893. In 1894, a series of melancholy events that were to becloud his entire life began. Specifically, his father arranged his marriage to Antonietta Portulano, the daughter of a wealthy sulfur merchant. She was of a violent and capricious nature, which contrasted sharply with his gentleness and erudition. Nevertheless, the first five years of marriage were relatively untroubled and produced three children: Stefano, Rosalie, and Fausto. In 1903, a landslide shut down the sulfur mine in which the families' capital was invested. As result of this financial disaster, his wife developed frequent hysterical attacks and a persecution mania which manifested itself in a frenzied jealousy of her husband. Pirandello's torment ended with her admittance to a sanatorium in 1919 [1]. This separation from his wife was very difficult for Pirandello, despite her morbid jealousies and hallucinations which caused him great suffering. In fact, still in 1924, he continued to believe that he could take care of his wife at home. Antonietta, however, would never leave the asylum until her death in 1959; she described it as both her prison and her protection against the resurgence of the phantasms overwhelming her.

These bitter experiences determined the themes of his most characteristic works, already perceptible in his early short stories: the exploration of the tightly closed world of the forever changeable human personality. Over his career, Pirandello wrote six novels, some 250 short stories and about 50 plays. It was the novel *Il fu Mattia Pascal* (The Late Mattia Pascal; 1904) that first brought him fame. Of the other five novels, the best known are *I vecchi e i giovani* (The Old and the Young; 1913), *Si gira* (Shoot!; 1916), and *Uno, nessuno, centomila* (One, None, and a Hundred Thousand; 1926). It was not until 1916, however, that he turned his attention to the theater, and only in 1920, when he was past 50, that he seriously began playwriting. His first stage success was a comedy entitled *Liolà* (1917), written in the Agrigento dialect followed by the play entitled *Così e', se vi pare* (Right You Are, If You Think You Are; 1918). He

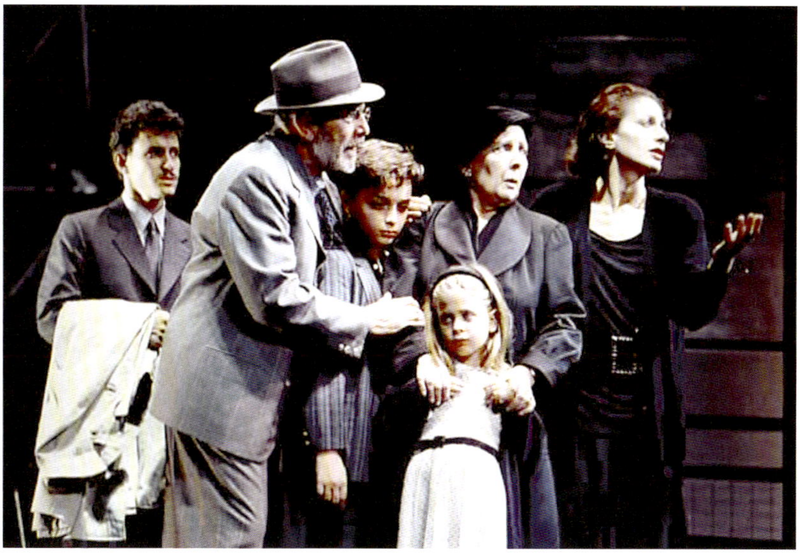

**Fig. 2.** A representation of the play *Sei personaggi in cerca di autore*: from the left Stefano Onofri, Enrico Maria Salerno, Luca Maria Michienzi, Regina Bianchi, Veronica Visentin, Benedetta Buccellato. Archive of E. M. Salerno – Photo Tommaso Le Pera. Debut: Teatro Antico, Taormina, Italy, Summer 1991 (with the permission of Tommaso Le Pera).

wrote a large number of dramas which were published between 1918 and 1935 under the collective title of *Maschere nude* (Naked Masks). In 1921, Pirandello presented his most famous play, *Sei personaggi in cerca di autore* (Six Characters in Search of an Author; fig. 2). It had successful but scandalous openings in Rome and Milan; 1922 saw the successful opening of another play, *Enrico IV* (Henry the Fourth). In 1925, patronized by Benito Mussolini, he founded his own theater in Rome. This venture, while artistically successful, proved financially disastrous. By this time, however, his fame had spread to North and South America, throughout Europe, and as far as Japan, and his works were translated into many languages. It was also in the theater that Pirandello finally found a more understanding relationship with a woman, the actress Marta Abba, for whom he dedicated most of his later plays. In 1934 Luigi Pirandello was awarded the Nobel Prize for Literature. He died in his home in via Bosio, in Rome, on December 10, 1936.

## Pirandello's Philosophy

With the beginning of the 'dramatist phase' of his life, Pirandello used his plays and short stories to express his personal philosophy which included the irony and bitterness of self-deception. Pirandello was always preoccupied with the problem of identity. He was fascinated with the question: 'What are people really like?' According to

Pirandello, the self exists to oneself only in relation to others; it consists of changing facets that hide an inscrutable abyss. Pirandello shared the view that the concept of identity is not unitary. That is, what seems like an irreducible and monolithic nucleus of multiples, is in fact a prism. The projected self does not have the same face as the interior self, it is only a mask that man unconsciously assumes in order to adapt himself to his social context. Every individual has a unique manner in a mobile game. Identity for Pirandello is played within two relatively discreet contexts, the social and the theatrical. Both contexts are explored in his characteristic texts, revealing how the interplay of identity and politics is played out. The theories of role and personality, role and actor, and role and author, all come together in a confrontation between relativism and idealism that distinguishes Pirandello's drama, and condemns the political philosophy that it analogically produces [2]. This duality highly reflects the Sicilian social structure made up of tight-knit family groups where austere Catholicism and rigid code of honor cohabitates with explosive and violent temperaments. Thus, born in a land of contradictions and deceptions, Pirandello knew well of self-deception as he grew up peering behind masks. Pirandello considered this his basis of comedy. His plays are entirely enigmatic, their characters seemingly unpredictable, basically bewildered in the face of life's contradictions and, like life itself, not readily definable [3].

Another concept responsible for spreading distorted self-perception in Pirandello's work is the mirror. In fact, the image of doubleness fools one into believing that appearance is reality. The mirrored image of the body is mostly an external object, like a name or some other trace of the self, which allows self-consciousness to take place within a social field of differences. The mirror in Pirandello's discourse formulates a paradox of semiotic identity but refuses to account for the real breakdown of semiosis, the cases of genuine doubleness and exact resemblance that emphasize the inadequacy of language to name objects absolutely [4].

In his novel, *Il fu Mattia Pascal*, the protagonist, after winning a lot of money at a casino, abandons his wife and family and is taken for dead. His fortune turns into tragedy, however, when after losing all his money and documents, he seeks to return to his previous life. His wife, believing him dead, in the meantime has remarried and Mattia is told by the authorities that he does not exist. When introduced to others, Mattia says 'I'm the late Mattia Pascal'. The core message of this masterpiece strongly evokes Pirandello's philosophy: nothing is sure in our lives, reality is not absolute but relative, and so is man.

In the play *Così e', se vi pare*, the truth is portrayed as being subjectively and fundamentally different for each observer. Here, two of the main protagonists hold contradictory notions about the identity of the third protagonist. In the end, no definitive identity is agreed upon, due to an incapacity on the part of the three to view things in the same manner. For this, we the audience, are persuaded that the truth is not singular.

In *Vestire gli ignudi* (To Clothe the Naked; 1923), the main protagonist tries to establish her individuality by assuming various identities, which are successively stripped from her; she gradually realizes her true position in the social order and in the end dies 'naked' without a social mask, in both her own and her friends' eyes [5].

Similarly in *Enrico IV,* Pirandello's protagonist loses his mind after falling from a horse at the end of a masquerade. After this, the man believes he is a medieval emperor. This illusion is coddled by a wealthy relative who surrounds the delirious man with a grotesque retinue of servants and courtiers. Finally, after twelve years, the injured man recovers his sanity, but continues to feign insanity because he prefers this world of illusions to the painful real world in which he had been abandoned by the woman he loved. When this woman and her lover come to visit, 'Henry IV' is overcome with rage and mortally wounds his rival. Now, for the protagonist it is more imperative than ever that the pretense of madness continues in order to avoid the legal consequences of his actions. He continues in his role as Henry IV for the rest of his life.

The analysis and depiction of self is artfully portrayed in Pirandello's masterpiece *Sei personaggi in cerca di autore* where the stage substitutes reality [5]. In it, a group of actors are preparing to rehearse for a Pirandello play. Shortly after starting the rehearsal, they are interrupted by the arrival of six other characters. The leader of the latter characters, the father, informs the manager that they are looking for an author. He goes on to explain that the author who created them did not finish their story, and that they, therefore, are unrealized characters who have not yet been fully brought to life. The manager tries to throw them out of the theater, but becomes more intrigued when they start to describe their story. After telling their story, the manager agrees to become the author for them. But several artistic difficulties are encountered including that the characters do not like his play as they had opposing perceptions. Fed up with the whole situation, the author calls for an end to the rehearsal [6]. The play exemplifies the Pirandellian philosophy that art, due to its immortality and predictability, is superior over life, which is a continuous succession of mutations and unpredictable events made more difficult by the fact that a convergence regarding perception is for the most part unattainable.

Mahida [6], in analyzing *Sei personaggi in cerca di autore,* states that Pirandello believes that 'life imitates art and art is better than life because it gives us the chance to reflect upon our past and our present experience of life. To this extent, art is superior to life'.

Finally, Pirandello's 1925 novel, *Uno, nessuno, centomila,* recounts the tragedy of a man who struggles to reclaim a coherent identity for himself in the face of an inherently social and multifaceted world. Prompted by an innocuous observation on the part of his wife, the protagonist Vitangelo Moscarda is led to believe that his friends' perceptions of his character are not at all what he imagines. In order to upset their assumptions, he takes on various masks to salvage some sort of stable identity. This continuous and dynamic reworking of his projected profile leads to a blurring of reality and illusion [7].

As suggested by Hochman [3], the Pirandello philosophy can be summarized in three dominant themes: (1) man creates both his personality and his life, ultimately becoming imprisoned by them; (2) reality is relative, changing with the viewer; and (3) art is the ultimate reality, superior to life because of its permanence, and yet inferior to it because of its immobility. Behind all these themes lie several basic conflicts, including those between the primitive life force and life as conceived by man and society, between nature and form, truth and appearance, and face and masks.

### Misidentifications and Duplications in the Works of Pirandello

Pirandello acknowledged the influence of the French psychologist Alfred Binet (1857–1911) on his philosophy. In fact, Binet, in his work of 1892, *Les altérations de la personnalité*, wrote that every man has an ego that crumbles in his lifetime: our personality changes over time. According to Binet, personality is not a fixed entity, permanent and unchangeable: it is a synthesis of phenomena that vary with the elements that compose it. This concept of mutable ego had already been described by the French philosopher Blaise Pascal (1623–1662) in the 1600s. Although Pirandello never allegedly read his works, his philosophy possesses many of the tenets proposed by Sigmund Freud (1856–1939), which were the foundation of modern psychiatry that was responsible for laying the groundwork for the contemporary classification of double personalities and confusion between imagination and reality. Delusional misidentification syndromes are rare and are classified together because they often co-occur and interchange [8]. Although misidentification syndromes have been reported in neurological patients with organic brain disease, especially involving the right hemisphere (i.e. stroke), most cases occur in psychiatric illness (i.e. primary psychotic disorders such as schizophrenia). There are four principle subtypes of misidentification syndrome:

1 Capgras syndrome, which was first described by Capgras and Reboul-Lachaux in 1923 [9], who reported a patient believing that her family and other individuals had been replaced by identical doubles. The syndrome refers to the delusional denial of identification of familiar people and their replacement by doubles who are physically – but not psychologically – identical to the misidentified people [10].

2 Frégoli syndrome, first described by Courbon and Fail in 1927 [11], is characterized by a false identification of a familiar person among strangers. In this case, the patient maintains that the familiar person (who is usually believed to be a persecutor) differs in physical appearance from the stranger but is the same person psychologically [10].

3 Intermetamorphosis syndrome, first described by Courbon and Tusques in 1932 [12], is a variant of Frégoli syndrome. Here, the patient believes he has changed into another person without any change in physical appearance. In reverse intermetamorphosis, however, the patient believes that he is another person and that his physical appearance has also changed [13].

4 The syndrome of subjective doubles, first described by Christodoulou in 1978 [14] is characterized by the delusional conviction that others have taken on the patient's physical appearance [10].

Other misidentification syndromes include: temporal reduplication, autoscopic phenomena, and mirrored-self misidentification. Temporal reduplication leads to ongoing déjà vu phenomena as the affected person believes that present events had already happened in the past. Autoscopic phenomena are similar to Capgras syndrome, where the patient believes he is an imposter. Finally, in mirrored-self misidentification, the patient is unable to recognize his own reflected image. However, the capacity to recognize others in the mirror often remains intact [15].

## Conclusions

In the works of Pirandello, his characters possess highly complex personalities and he was able to communicate this by describing the ongoing conflict between illusion and reality which are overlapping. With his works, Pirandello made philosophical concepts which had previously only been discussed by leading intellectuals available to a much larger audience. Pirandello continued to elaborate upon this concept of mutable ego, established by Blaise Pascal in the 1600s and carried on by the French psychologist Alfred Binet. It was Sigmund Freud, allegedly unknown to Pirandello and vice versa, with the advent of psychoanalysis, who gave rise to contemporary psychiatric care. This is something which Pirandello would have greatly applauded, as this allowed patients to be treated in private practices instead of warehoused in asylums worldwide.

## References


1 Whitfield JH: Luigi Pirandello. 2012. http://www.biography.com/people/luigi-pirandello-9441495.
2 Dombroski RS: Laudisi's laughter and the social dimension of Right You Are (If You Think So). Modern Drama 1973;16:337–346.
3 Hochman S: McGraw-Hill Encyclopedia of World Drama, ed 2. New York, McGraw-Hill, 1984.
4 Quinn ML: Relative identity and ideal art: the Pirandello conflict and its political analogy. J Dramatic Theory Criticism 1989;3:73–85.
5 Luigi Pirandello – Biography. Horst F (ed): Nobel Lectures, Literature 1901–1967. Amsterdam, Elsevier, 1969. Nobelprize.org.11 Feb 2012. http://www.nobelprize.org/nobel_prizes/literature/laureates/1934/pirandello-bio.html.
6 Mahida CA: Exploring difference between 'art' and 'life' in Pirandello's Six Characters in Search of an Author. Review of Research. Int Online Multidisciplinary J 2011;1:1–3.
7 Pepe A, Wolff S, Van Godtsenhoven K: One, none and one hundred thousand profiles: re-imagining the Pirandellian identity dilemma in the era of online social networks (cited as arXiv:1109.3428v1 [cs.SI]). Ithaca, Cornell University Library, 2011.
8 Devinsky O: Delusional misidentifications and duplications. Neurology 2009;72:80–87.
9 Capgras J, Reboul-Lachaux J: L'illusion des socies dans un delire systematise chronique. Bull Soc Clin Med Ment 1923;11:6–16.

10 Christodoulou GN, Margarati M, Kontaxakis VP, Christodoulou NG: The delusional misidentification syndromes: strange, fascinating, and instructive. Curr Psychiatry Rep 2009;11:185–189.
11 Courbon P, Fail G: Illusion de Fregoli. Bull Soc Clin Med Ment 1927;15:121–124.
12 Courbon P, Tusques J: Illusions d'intermetamorfose et de la charme. Ann Med Psychol (Paris) 1932;901: 401–406.
13 Piechowski-Jozwiak B, Bogousslavsky J: Neurobehavioral syndromes; in Paciaroni M, Agnelli G, Caso V, Bogousslavsky J (eds): Manifestations of Stroke. Front Neurol Neurosci. Basel, Karger, 2012, vol 30, pp 57–60.
14 Christodoulou GN: Syndrome of subjective doubles. Am J Psychiatry 1978;135:249–251.
15 Villarejo A, Martin VP, Moreno- Ramos T, Camacho-Salas A, Porta-Etessam J, Bermejo-Pareja F: Mirrored-self misidentification in a patient without dementia: evidence for right hemispheric and bifrontal damage. Neurocase 2011;17:276–284.

Maurizio Paciaroni, MD
Stroke Unit and Division of Cardiovascular Medicine
Santa Maria della Misericordia Hospital
University of Perugia, IT–06126 Perugia (Italy)
E-Mail maurizio.paciaroni@med.unipg.it

Bogousslavsky J, Dieguez S (eds): Literary Medicine: Brain Disease and Doctors in Novels, Theater, and Film.
Front Neurol Neurosci. Basel, Karger, 2013, vol 31, pp 77–115 (DOI: 10.1159/000345912)

# Doubles Everywhere: Literary Contributions to the Study of the Bodily Self[1]

Sebastian Dieguez

Laboratory for Cognitive and Neurological Sciences, Département de Médecine, Hôpital de Fribourg, Université de Fribourg, Fribourg, Switzerland

**Abstract**

The topic of the double is a hallmark of romantic, gothic, and fantastic literature. In the guise of the second self, the alter ego or the doppelgänger, fictional doubles have long fascinated critics, clinicians, and scientists. We review classical approaches to the theme and propose a broad clinical and neurocognitive framework from which to examine major instances of the motif in literature. Based on neurological disorders of the bodily self (including unilateral and whole body illusions and duplications), as well as related experimental approaches, we provide examples of literary depictions of bodily fragmentation and splitting; autoscopic hallucinations; the classical doppelgänger, second self, or heautoscopic double; the feeling of a presence; out-of-body experiences; and so-called near-death experiences. Examples include works from Guy de Maupassant, E.T.A. Hoffman, Edgar Allan Poe, Robert Louis Stevenson, Fyodor Dostoevsky, Rudyard Kipling, and others. We discuss these literary cases of doubles from a neurocognitive perspective, and suggest that common mechanisms of the bodily self are involved in the emergence of pathological illusory doubles, literary creations of the double, as well as widespread cultural and religious beliefs about the existence of doubles and the soul.


Ein Heiliger sagt: Es stirbt, wer Gott erblickt!
Doch auch wer sich selbst schaut, lässt das Leben!
*Franz Werfel* (*Spiegelmensch*, *Magische Trilogie*, 1920)

This chapter provides a wide overview of the literary theme of the double from a neurocognitive point of view. The double in literature is a ubiquitous and age-old motif that became a hallmark of the romantic, gothic, and fantastic genres. In the guise of the second self, the alter ego or the doppelgänger, fictional doubles have

[1] Parts of this chapter have been presented at the 5th International Congress on Spatial Cognition, Rome, September 4–8, 2012.

long fascinated writers and critics [1–6], as well as medical researchers [7–10]. At the same time, researchers and writers interested in the occult and paranormal phenomena have likewise given a fair share of attention to such phenomena, pinning down the double as a cultural phenomenon. A considerable amount of theorizing has been devoted to this topic from a wide range of perspectives, including attempts to relate pathological instances of illusory doubles with their literary counterparts [7–13].

Here we follow a similar approach, providing examples of different types of literary doubles organized under a scientifically informed taxonomy. We also take a step beyond mere illustration by arguing that specific neuropsychological mechanisms underlie all instances of doubles (literary, psychological, cultural, and pathological), providing the background for the human proclivity to see and produce doubles everywhere [14–17]. We will argue that the motif of the double arises from the action of specific neurocognitive mechanisms involved with bodily awareness, spatial cognition, multisensory integration, and self-other discrimination. All these capacities of the human mind, indeed, seem to converge to provide our species with a phantom companion onto which our actions, beliefs, desires, emotions, and needs can be safely projected and which can serve as a sophisticated simulation device for planning, anticipating, comparing, and fantasizing. In that sense, we all carry one or several doubles within us, but only in specific cases can they appear to 'leak' into extrapersonal space (i.e. the real world) and become an illusory autonomous being.

In literature, this idea culminated in the 19th century with the theme of the doppelgänger. Through this literary device, it seems that writers were experimenting with the idea of being located in space and being *oneself,* a single bodily entity endowed with a sense of ownership and a sense of agency, differentiated from the others, seamlessly integrating widely different sensory information into single and meaningful percepts, and grounding higher-level aspects of cognition upon the bodily senses.

Drawing on literary material serves to outline some historical trends. Here as in several other cases in this volume, fictional characters similar to actual clinical descriptions were reported before medical research formally identified such symptoms. In fact, the great popularity of the literary double and the widespread awareness of cultural beliefs in paranormal instances of doubling phenomena might in the present case have encouraged and guided clinical investigations of similar phenomena. But more specifically, the sheer variety and striking profiles of fictional doubles might be treated as raw data to inform systematic taxonomies and distinguish different underlying mechanisms of clinical doubles. Such an approach, for instance, has proven fruitful for the study of self-portraiture in painting. Whereas visual, disembodied, and corporeal types of self-portraits could be related to autoscopic hallucinations, out-of-body experiences and heautoscopy (doppelgänger-type phenomena) and their underlying neurocognitive mechanisms [18], here we describe a broader range of literary and clinical conditions, including the feeling of a presence and so-called near-death experiences. The approach can be said to take place in the broader field of cultural cognition, tackling the idea that cultural phenomena, including literary creations and paranormal beliefs, are 'bounded variations within limits set by human cognitive capacities' [19; see also 15, 20]. Conversely, such an analysis could help explain the wide appeal of stories of the double by showing how they neatly fit and tap into human cognitive architecture and its mechanisms. In this sense, the literary double, together with popular beliefs about paranormal doubles, might be seen as an instance of 'cultural recycling of cortical maps' [21].

In the next sections, we provide an overview of the double in literature, its definition, main features, and origins, as well as several explanations, interpretations, and theories developed over the years. We then review principles of cognitive science and clinical syndromes we think are of the utmost relevance to the literary double, including autoscopic phenomena – those syndromes involving the visual duplication in extrapersonal space of the own body, and related conditions. We then proceed to highlighting key examples of literary doubles, attempting to frame them in terms of spatial cognition and bodily awareness, and emphasizing their similarity to clinical syndromes. We conclude with general comments about how literature might enrich and refine current models of the self by delineating those phenomenological features that are shared with 'real life' cases and argue for a common origin of literary, cultural and clinical doubles.

## The Literary Double, or the Doppelgänger

### *Definition and Taxonomies*

We have already mentioned several times the notion of a 'literary double'. Many readers will have spontaneously conjured up images of split- or double-personalities such as *The Strange Case of Dr. Jekyll and Mr. Hyde* (1886) or Norman Bates, the disturbed motel manager of Hitchcock's *Psycho* (1960). Yet the term 'double' more usually refers to the encounter with a duplicate of oneself. The double is thus an exteriorized self, and as can be imagined its appearance is rarely good news for the original self from which it emanates. Jean Paul Richter is credited for having coined, in a footnote to his novel *Siebenkäs* (1796), the term 'doppelgänger' which he thusly defined: 'So heissen Leute, die sich selber sehen' (this is what people who see themselves are called). A more elaborate definition was provided by Herdman [4]: 'a second self, or alter ego, which appears as a distinct and separate being apprehensible by the physical senses (or at least, by *some* of them), but exists in a dependent relation to the original.'

The heyday of this type of double was undoubtedly the 19th century, with classic stories from E.T.A. Hoffman, Edgar Allan Poe, Fyodor Dostoevsky, and Guy de Maupassant. Yet, although the literary double can be more or less readily distinguished from competing fictional entities such as vampires, ghosts, zombies, fairies, or demons [22, 23], its specific contours and features have proven difficult to pin down.

In fact, there is hardly a single author writing on the topic that has not warned right at the outset of conceptual problems plaguing the issue. The concept of the double has been said to provoke 'confusion' [24], to be 'embarrassingly vague' [25] or 'destined to vagueness' [26], and to suffer from 'lack of any clarification' and being used indiscriminately 'for a case of biological twinship and for a case of psychopathic hallucination, with no apparent realization that the two are entirely different things' [1]. Indeed, too loose a definition would encompass too many cases, if not the entirety of the literary canon. Friends, brothers, enemies, lovers, complementary and antagonistic characters, parallel lives, impostors, disguised characters, good and bad cops, past and future selves – all could under some view be considered instances of the literary double, and this does not even include animals, objects, places, cities, and worlds, all of which have also been 'literary doubles' at some point. As Jourde and Tortonese [27] put it: 'No sooner one starts talking about the double than one sees them everywhere.' Writers of stories of the double themselves have seemed ambivalent about the idea. Dostoevsky's *The Double* (1846/1866), often considered the paradigmatic case of the literary doppelgänger, was really for its author a parody of sorts of what he already saw as an overtired literary motive. And Vladimir Nabokov [28], who also freely played with the romantic and gothic conventions of the genre, threw his arms in the air and famously declared, 'The *Doppelgänger* subject is a frightful bore'.

On the other hand, too narrow an approach would have the unfortunate effect of dismissing cases widely held as belonging to the double motif. *The Strange Case of Dr. Jekyll and Mr. Hyde*, for instance, is strictly speaking a story of metamorphosis from person 1 to person 2, 'there is never more than one mind [. . .] there is never more than one body' [1]. Not only are the characters never directly confronted or copresent[2], they do not even look alike and do not seem to share a strong psychological bond [29]. Under such criteria, then, *The Strange Case of Dr. Jekyll and Mr. Hyde* would not belong to the double theme. Yet, as Vladimir Nabokov pointed out in his lecture on the novel, both characters never operate completely independently from the other. In fact, the entire point of the story is precisely that, contrary to appearances and Victorian conventions, the good doctor and the ugly beast actually have much more in common than they would dare to admit. Otherwise, indeed, the very device of a transformative chemical compound would be ineffective: the dominating and immoral Hyde would see no need to revert to the boring and scrupulous Jekyll, and the conventional Jekyll would never feel the temptation and urge to switch again to the rebellious Hyde [30] (fig. 1).

The sheer diversity of stories including one instance or another of 'double' phenomena has led to attempts to distinguish and classify different types of literary doubles: not only are there doubles everywhere, but there are several kinds of doubles (table 1).

[2] Indeed, one should remember that when the story first appeared, it read at the same time like a mystery and a medical case report: the shocking revelation that Jekyll and Hyde are actually one and the same person would come only near the end of the narrative in Dr. Jekyll's first-person 'statement of the case'.

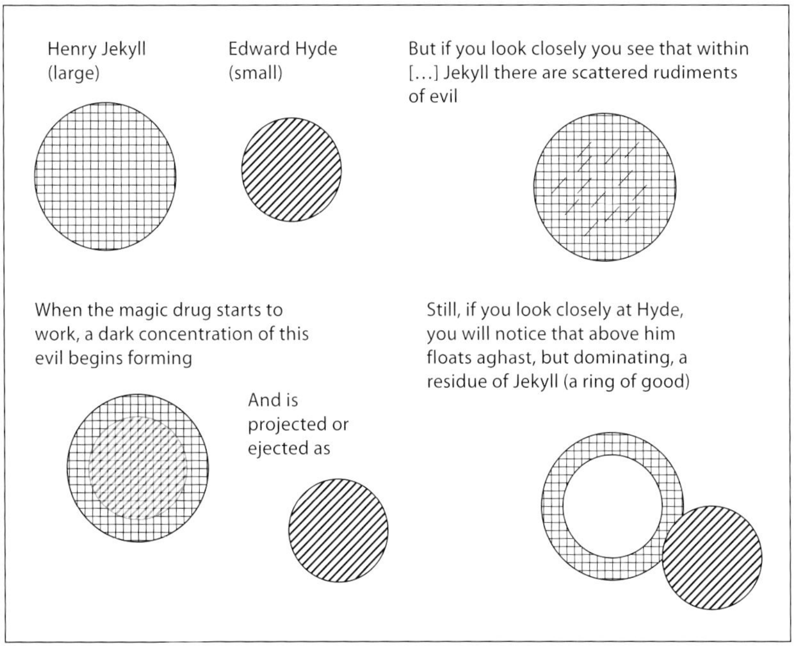


**Fig. 1.** Nabokov's 'model' of *The Strange Case of Dr. Jekyll and Mr. Hyde* (adapted from [159]).

The second self can be real or illusory (i.e. supernatural or psychological), conscious or unconscious, internal or external, physical or mental, divided or duplicated, and so forth. As we will see, this variability of the literary double is reminiscent of the richness of clinical disorders, as well as experimental approaches, of the bodily self and symptoms affecting own body parts or spawning illusory doubles of the whole body. Of course taxonomies of literary doubles and of clinical disorders cannot reasonably be expected to overlap perfectly; however, the similarities are sufficient to suspect a common neurocognitive origin for both.

*Origins of the Literary Double*

The origins of the literary double have often been traced to age-old beliefs about the human soul and the afterlife permeating the human condition across all cultures. The idea of a second self or a phantom double, indeed, is so to speak self-contained in such beliefs: the physical body, and even the material world, was often thought to be reflected by a companion image – a subtle body and otherworld – capable on some occasions of manifesting itself to the living. The power of the imagination, the fascination with dreams, the experience of shadows and reflections, and the existence of twins all point to the inherent duality of the human mind, its ability to fabricate surrogates and fictions, to navigate between real and counterfactual worlds. As Herdman [4] puts it: 'The double as a literary device has its roots in human experience, natural,

**Table 1.** Taxonomies of the literary double

| Author | Types of doubles | Description |
|---|---|---|
| Tymms [2] | Psychological doubles | Doubles born of the unconscious powers of the human imagination. |
| | Trivial/allegorical doubles | Doubles consciously depicting the tug-of-war between good and evil forces. |
| Rogers [24] | Latent doubles<br>Manifest doubles | A Freudian approach exploiting the distinction between the symbolic (manifest) appearance of unconscious processes and their hidden (latent) significance. |
| Herdman [4] | Supernatural doubles<br>Psychological and allegorical doubles | The true double motif should never involve mere hallucinations or insanity, or be merely symbolic (psychological and allegorical doubles). Its deep significance lies in its supernatural origins: the double must be 'real' to fully embody its moral, religious and atonement functions. Along the 19th century, this 'true' double began to 'decline'. |
| Keppler [1] | Second self as twin brother<br>Second self as pursuer<br>Second self as tempter<br>Second self as vision of horror<br>Second self as saviour<br>Second self as the beloved<br>Second self in time | Despite the recurrent motif of the second self as the embodiment of a character's emotional and psychological weaknesses, its many different faces illustrate the complex interplays between the first and second self. In this bidirectional interplay, specific to each different case, lies the importance of the literary second self. |
| Jourde and Tortonese [27] | External subjective doubles<br>Internal subjective doubles<br>Objective doubles | Subjective doubles involve a character (usually the narrator) confronting his own double. They are external in cases of autoscopy or identical doppelgängers, and internal in cases of possession, hauntings or alternating personalities. The double is said to be objective when a character observes doubling phenomena happening to other characters. |
| Bargalló [5] | Doubles by fusion | Two different characters become one and the same. |
| | Doubles by splitting | One individual gives birth to two different characters. |
| | Doubles by metamorphosis | One character progressively, or suddenly, loses his original identity and is replaced by another one. The process can be reversible, or not. |
| Rosset [36] | Doubles by duplication | These doubles copy an original model, which remains unaltered by the process. |
| | Doubles by replacement | Here the double attempts to suppress the original, either by usurping its identity, or by destroying it. |
| Martín López [29] | Same person exists in two or more alternate worlds (i.e. different temporal and/or spatial dimensions)<br>Two persons with different identities, yet equal in some essential and relevant features, coexist in the same world.<br>The character looks at his own dead body. | The taxonomy highlights the subtleties between mechanisms of duplication and splitting. Mirrors, portraits, photographs, shadows, statues, and dolls can serve to implement these mechanisms. |

religious, psychological and parapsychological, and in the reflections of such experience in legend and folklore' (see also [2, 27, 31]).

German romanticism later concentrated its concerns about magic and the occult, the self, psychopathology and psychology, and symbolism into the theme of the double, which was soon followed by similar developments in the Victorian Anglo-Saxon world, France's 'fin-de-siècle', and Russian writers' bent for the absurd. The 19th century, indeed, seemed perfectly appropriate for the emergence of the doppelgänger: scientific discoveries questioned the limits between man and animal, as well as between man and machine; the grip of religion progressively led its place to a secularized and less secure world; boundaries between the occult and the physical sciences were beginning to be traced yet remained quite fuzzy; and neurology, psychology, psychiatry, and philosophy opened the Pandora's box of the unconscious, releasing strange phenomena such as hypnosis, hysteria, and divided consciousness. These developments paved the way for a new understanding of the human condition, questioning the limits of identity and the self, and the public seemed more than ever eager for scary and chilling stories.

This sudden emergence of the modern self also brought its own lot of anxieties. With tensions between older traditions and a newfound excitation for self-discovery, exploration, and individuality, the uneasiness provoked by the idea that we are not quite what we thought we were, the foreboding images of yet so many unknown and shocking news to come, it is no wonder that people felt divided and that writers saw the double motif as the perfect way to express this predicament [32].

*Features and Functions of the Literary Double*

What are the features of this imaginary double, then? And under what circumstances is it said to appear? Webber [33] suggested some criteria. For instance, the second self is visual in nature, not necessarily because the original self can always see it, but mainly because it *demands* to be seen, it is a figure of 'visual compulsion'. The double is also autonomous, which means that it departs in some way from the original self, i.e. it is not an exact replica and has features and a life of its own. Indeed, sometimes it is not explicitly stated that the double is really a duplicate of another self, and one has to read between the lines to detect the special affinities and resemblances that betrays the real identity of the second self. As such, the double is often a symbolic representation of a tug-of-war between conflicting elements present in the original self, the inner fight being externalized and embodied in a separate individual. The second self is also very frequently the product of a male individual, almost always some type of bachelor or lonely gent.

As such, the classical psychoanalytical view that the double represents a projection of the unconscious or the superego, isolating or reificating, as it were, a painful or unacceptable parcel of one's inner conscience that is being either repressed or denied [24, 34], is only one among many. The double can certainly be a representation of narcissism, as in Wilde's *The Picture of Dorian Gray* [35], but more generally it appears in some moment of crisis, being a mixture of ambiguous feelings, paralyzing indecision, unacknowledged self-contempt and guilt, stinging humiliation, loneliness, or failure of self-knowledge. Far from being helpful to the individual, the double more often than not symbolizes a punishment for misguided pride, vanity, envy, ambition, immorality, and depravity. Herdman [4] also highlights that the double is often there to put the individual back on the path to his fate, correcting the course taken by his illusions and conceits, and showing him his true nature.

The emergence of the double can often be cast in psychiatric terms. It appears as a reaction to trends towards depression and self-destruction, it flourishes on states of dissociation, confusion, and depersonalization, and strives on paranoid beliefs. In *A Raw Youth*, Dostoevsky expressed this idea of the double as representing mental illness, or the first stage towards insanity: 'What then precisely is the 'double'? The 'double', at any rate according to a medical work by an expert which I afterwards read for the purpose, is nothing but the first stage in some serious mental derangement which may lead to a pretty bad conclusion.' He added, referring to Versilov, the character displaying the double phenomenon and likely depicting Dostoevsky himself, that the double involved a 'bifurcation' of his feelings and will' (see [9, 31]). As is evident from numerous literary accounts of the double, such as Maupassant's *The Horla* and Poe's *William Wilson*, the entrance in the world of insanity is rarely unrelated to a more general foreboding of death. Rank [34], most notably, has theorized the literary double as a reminder of mortality, a harbinger of death. On this idea, it can also be seen as the opposite, i.e. the pervasive illusion that one is immortal. When the original self is annihilated, the second self takes over, either in this world or in another. This idea, of course, is far from restricted to literature, and indeed has spawned many beliefs and myths about the afterlife, leading philosopher Clément Rosset to declare: 'I therefore denounce the double as a major illusion of the human mind. . .' [36].

## A Toolbox for Applied Studies of the Bodily Self

Before we examine in some detail examples of the literary double, we provide in this section an overview of concepts, methods, and clinical disorders pertaining to the topic of the bodily self. Recent years have indeed witnessed a renewed interest in the bodily self as a topic of empirical and theoretical study. A remarkable range of disciplines and perspectives have contributed theories, methods, studies, and models tackling the underlying mechanisms and the broader implications of the human awareness of having and being a body, situated in space, and distinct from the external world and other bodies. This rapidly burgeoning field is still in need of some systematization, but we suggest here that it already provides a coherent toolbox ready to be applied to specific questions pertaining to other fields, and as such its relevance to the understanding of the literary double should be self-evident.

*Theoretical Concepts for the Bodily Self*

The most frequent representation of the literary double is as a spatially situated and embodied entity. Even in cases where the double is not seen but merely 'sensed,' such as in James' *The Jolly Corner* or Maupassant's *The Horla*, it is still sensed as 'someone out there'. Cognitive neuroscience provides an ample set of concepts, methods, and data pertaining to the perception and awareness of the self, and specifically the bodily self, in peripersonal and extrapersonal space in both healthy and abnormal states.

The idea of a bodily self is derived from related concepts such as body schema, body image, cenesthesia, or corporeal awareness [37]. It refers broadly to the human experience of being, having, and controlling a body. Although this experience is arguably the most mundane and taken for granted that can be imagined (the body is indeed the background scene for *all* that ever happens to us and *everything* we ever do; it is indeed 'always there' as William James put it), scientists and philosophers have progressively been able to deconstruct its mechanisms and inner architecture. 'Ownership', for instance, refers to the specific sense of *owning* our body and its parts; it is the normal experience of ascribing a tag of 'mineness' to that specific body that happens to be mine (as compared to bodies of other persons and external objects) [38, 39]. 'Agency', on the other hand, is thought to involve a separate set of principles, by which we ascribe a tag of 'authorship' to the actions that we voluntarily initiate [40, 41]. There are a number of documented cases where ownership and agency can go wrong, and even in nonpathological states, one can sometimes be unsure about the ownership of one's limbs, for instance if an arm has gone numb or if several hands get mixed together. Likewise, we can perform actions involuntarily, not knowing 'who' exactly 'did it', or feel agency over actions that someone else performed, or that happened by chance [40–42].

These concepts are closely associated to those of 'self-location' and 'visuospatial perspective'. Our awareness of our body is dependent upon the postures we hold, our relationship with gravitational force, our orienting in a stable space, and generally provides a strong spatial overlap of our center of consciousness with our body, indeed within our body. From this place, we perceive the external world from the first-person perspective, yet we are also able to compute spatial contingencies *as if* from someone else's point of view, from the third-person perspective [43–45]. Indeed, we can 'see through the eyes of others' using 'perspective-taking' and 'counterfactual' thinking, simulation abilities that allow us to hold and compare multiple points of view, and further develop fictional scenarios in alternative places and times (e.g. [46]). We can likewise empathize with others by putting ourselves in their shoes. Yet at the same time, we hold strong psychological and physiological imperatives to maintain a robust sense of self-other distinction [47], and this is achieved through a manifold multilevel system, ranging from cellular functions to memory systems, and also including strong cultural influences. More generally, the notion of 'embodied cognition' has been used as an overarching principle according to which many of our cognitive and behavioral faculties are directly derived from, or dependent upon, our conscious or unconscious experience of the body. This includes apparently abstract faculties such as language, numerical cognition, and time perception [48].

A central role has been ascribed to a pre-existing neural representation of the body – a body-template of sorts, possibly innate – for the emergence of the bodily self and its components [49–51], although authors have also highlighted the large flexibility and plasticity of this underlying scaffold (e.g. [52, 53]). Specifically, the principles of *multisensory integration* have been put forward, together with models of action prediction and proprioceptive anticipation, as guiding online modulations of our bodily self [51, 54]. Indeed, too rigid a representation of our body would presumably be ineffective in an ever flexible and unpredictable world. Thus, for instance, by using tools, by wearing clothes, or by cooperating with fellow humans, we *extend* our bodies in a nontrivial sense. Conversely, this ability to project the bodily self beyond its physical limits also involves the *incorporation* of external objects. We feel the page under the tip of our pen, we integrate the boundaries of our car as if it was our own body, and on a good day the saxophonist might experience his instrument as an integral part of himself [55, 56].

This cursory overview of the ongoing theorizing of the bodily self provides some cues as to the relevance of cognitive science to the literary double. However, this will be even more explicit with the following introduction to experimental methods and clinical syndromes, which indeed provide the raw data for the very idea of the bodily self and its mechanisms.

*Experimental Paradigms for the Bodily Self*

In recent years, researchers have devised a number of experimental procedures inducing illusory body experiences, sometimes reminiscent of the disorders described in the next section. Although the specifics differ somewhat between different approaches, it suffices to say that most of these methods are based on the induction of multisensory conflicts. In the 'rubber-hand illusion', for instance, a participant watches as a fake hand lying in front of her is repetitively stroked, while her real hand, lying nearby the fake hand but hidden out of view, is stroked in exactly the same fashion. This usually induces the strong, and somewhat eerie, sensation that the fake hand has become part of one's own body [57, 58]. As a safe and noninvasive manipulation of bodily ownership, this illusion demonstrates the relevance of multisensory integration for the bodily self. Indeed, not only is an external object suddenly part of one's body representation, but it also seems to momentarily replace its physical counterpart, as the latter becomes mislocalized in favor of the fake hand and also seems to manifest sudden changes in autonomic functions [59].

Likewise, the simultaneous stroking of one's own finger together with someone else's finger, when two people press their hands together palm to palm, induces a strange feeling of numbness 'for' the other person's finger [60]. In this case, not only is someone else's body part mistakenly thought to belong to one's own body, but a specific phenomenological sensation other than mere touch is experienced in the process, providing a kind of psychophysiological affinity projected to a foreign body part.

The principle of visuotactile induction of illusory ownership has been subsequently extended to studies of face, multiple limbs, and full body ownership, stretching the limits of the bodily self [51, 61, 62]. Using fake or prosthetic limbs, video projections, simple mirrors, virtual-reality techniques, vestibular stimulations, diverse types of tool-based tasks, and even specific types of drugs, as well as multiple methods of measurement such as subjective questionnaires, accuracy of pointing or reaching towards body parts or objects, distance estimations, differential reaction times to visual or tactile stimuli, diverse physiological modulations, and neural activations and dynamics, scientists have been able to demonstrate the conditions under which the bodily self can extend, incorporate, divide, project, enlarge, transform, and generally be altered in many ways in perfectly healthy participants (see reviews in [62–64]).

### *Altered States of Bodily Consciousness*

Two broad sets of disorders of the bodily self provide a continuous phenomenological landscape that appears strikingly relevant to, and perhaps even foundational for, the literary double. Together with the burgeoning experimental approaches hinted to in the previous section, they represent an outstanding and robust framework for a modern reading of tales of the doppelgänger and related phenomena. Indeed, disorders and illusions ranging from phantom limbs to full-blown projection of illusory bodies form a wide array of neurological manifestations which, were they to appear in a progressive fashion in single individual, would vividly picture a gradually extruding and disowned second self from the physical body[3] [16, 17, 53, 65–71].

#### Lateralized Disorders

The first set of disorders involves lateralized symptoms of the bodily self, or conditions affecting specific body parts. These include the widespread phantom limb experience, which concerns the vast majority of amputation patients. The term 'phantom limb' is strikingly accurate and evocative, as it denotes the vividly felt presence of a nonexisting limb, seemingly replacing its lost physical counterpart, yet frequently differing from it in particular respects, and holding a strong psychological and physical affinity with the patient's self. Phantom limbs can be felt in peculiar postures, they can be painful, they can differ in shape and in location from the original limb – sometimes experienced as detached from the body, floating 'out there' as 'debris of phantoms lost in space', vanishing and reappearing without warning [17, 73]. Moreover, they often are remarkably dependent on psychological, physiological, and environmental factors.

Phantom phenomena of body parts are not restricted to amputees. Just like neural reorganization following the traumatic peripheral insult have gone a long way in explaining the origins of the syndrome [74], disturbances directly affecting the neural

[3] Perhaps not surprisingly, a similar view has lent itself to more esoteric conceptions. E. Bozzano [72], for instance, saw the continuity between phantoms of body parts and full illusory doubles as indicative of the existence of a disembodied soul.

structures underlying the bodily self – due to strokes, epileptic seizures, tumors, migraines, or other etiologies – have been shown to induce phantom experiences of body parts. As such, these particular sensations have been called 'delusional reduplication of body parts' and 'supernumerary phantom limbs', as they involve the vivid experience of a body part in addition to its physical counterpart. In some instances, the illusory limb can even be voluntarily moved, and some patients, not necessarily delusional, have claimed to be able to feel and see it [75]. Tactile sensations projected onto external space are also found in other conditions, and indeed in simple illusions such as the rubber-hand and numbness illusions (see above), and have been grouped under the heading 'exosomesthesia' [76].

Brain damage, of course, can have many other effects on the bodily self. In hemiasomatognosia and anosognosia for hemiplegia, for instance, a specific limb or even an entire half-body can apparently vanish from consciousness, the patient behaving as if these parcels of her own body never existed, not paying attention to them, and oftentimes denying that they suffer from any ailment. In somatoparaphrenia, such attitudes can go a step further as the patient will affirm that her impaired body parts belong to someone else, sometimes mistaking a limb for another person, a piece of a corpse, or an animal, and claiming that a foreign body is sharing their bed [77]. Similar disorders, which can be due to strokes, brain traumas, tumors, epileptic seizures, or migraines, involve conscious feelings that a limb has disappeared, sensations of size alterations restricted to a limb, or even the experience that one's body has split in two separate parts [67, 78].

### Illusory Duplications of the Full Body

These extraordinarily diverse disorders and alterations of the bodily self do not stop at isolated body parts. Another set of clinical symptoms involves misrepresentations and mislocalizations of one's entire body. These disorders are strikingly similar to age-old reports of paranormal phenomena such as apparitions, hauntings, possessions, and otherworld journeys, and indeed their progressive scientific documentation, investigation, and classification can be said to have gone a long way towards their demystification [15, 37, 79–82]. Current taxonomies have been based upon seminal works spanning the 20th century [10, 53, 65, 69–71, 83–86], and encompass a set of conditions called 'autoscopic phenomena' [13, 79, 87, 88] (fig. 2). Etymologically, these conditions generally involve 'looking at oneself' or some disturbance involving the illusory externalization of one's bodily self. The simplest occurrence involves the hallucinatory experience of seeing oneself, usually as if one were looking at one's mirror reflection, yet without a mirror (autoscopic hallucination). In those cases, the experience of a visual double does not directly compromise awareness of the physical body and the self.

Now consider the case of out-of-body experiences, which also frequently involves seeing one's own body in external space. Here the experience of the bodily self is radically altered, as self-location and the visual perspective are seemingly centered

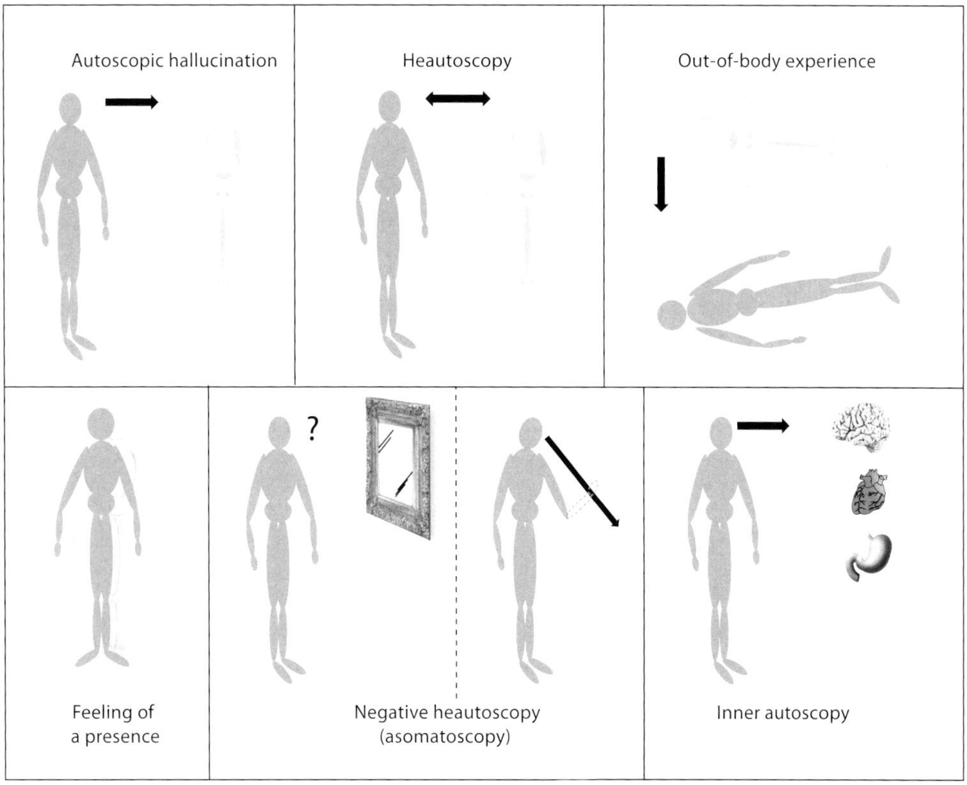


**Fig. 2.** Autoscopic phenomena of neurological and psychiatric origin: phenomenological descriptions. 'Autoscopic hallucination': the visual impression of seeing a double of one's body in extrapersonal space (right figure, light grey), as if reflected in a mirror. The vantage point is centered on the usual egocentric visuospatial perspective, namely the physical body (left figure, dark grey). Self-localization, visuo-spatial perspective and embodiment are normal. 'Heautoscopy': the experience of seeing or feeling a double of one's own body in extrapersonal space, accompanied by strong somesthetic and vestibular sensations in one's own body. The double may not be an exact visual duplicate of the self, yet a strong feeling of psychological sameness and affinity is experienced between both, leading to confusion as to the current localization of the self or the body (alternating or bilocation of self-localization and visuospatial perspective). 'Out-of-body experience': the experience of having left one's body and seeing oneself and the environment from an elevated and disembodied vantage point (top figure, light grey). Visuospatial perspective and self-localization are centered in the 'double', while the physical body (lower figure, dark grey) is often felt as empty and foreign. 'Feeling of a presence': the vivid feeling of a physical presence of another person (or 'shadow') nearby one's body. The sensation is sometimes conceptualized as heautoscopy without the visual element, but the 'presence' is not necessarily recognized as a double of oneself. 'Negative heautoscopy' (also called 'asomatoscopy'): the failure to see one's own body, either when looked at directly (right panel) or via a reflecting surface (left panel). 'Inner autoscopy' (or 'internal heautoscopy'): the hallucinatory perception of one's internal organs (viscera, heart, brain, nerves, or skeleton) as projected in extrapersonal space, mostly known from early reports of patients with hysteria (adapted from [13]).

on the second, externalized, self. The perceived body, thus, is believed by the experient to be that of her original physical body. Moreover, unlike autoscopic hallucinations, the perspective is often that of an elevated position, as if one were floating in the air [88, 89]. Out-of-body experiences sometimes happen during a crisis and life-threatening situations, thus bolstering the vivid impression that one has indeed left one's physical body and entered a different plane of existence, in accordance with widespread cultural and religious beliefs. These specific instances, because of their rich phenomenology and importance for wider anthropological issues, deserve a specific category, and indeed have been the basis of much 'near-death experience' lore [90].

Between autoscopic phenomena and out-of-body experiences, which can be considered as extreme poles of the autoscopic phenomena continuum, clinicians have isolated another syndrome called heautoscopy. This is probably the condition closest to the literary doppelgänger. During heautoscopy – much more so than during other autoscopic phenomena – a strong psychological, affective, and physical affinity is felt between the original and the projected self. Patients report seeing a duplicate of themselves in external space, which can or cannot be physically resembling (and indeed is often visually less sharp than during autoscopic hallucinations and out-of-body experiences), and can either imitate their movements or behave quite independently. Unlike the previous types of autoscopic phenomena, during heautoscopy the location of the bodily self is ambiguous: it can alternate between the physical and the second self, or even be experienced in both simultaneously (i.e. bilocation). Heautoscopy is often accompanied with strong emotional reactions and somesthetic alterations; it can be a very unsettling experience, sometimes leading to self-harming behavior [12].

On clinical, phenomenological, and neuroanatomical grounds, clinicians have also classified the 'feeling of a presence' among autoscopic phenomena, although in these cases the second self is frequently conceived as another person or an indiscriminate 'shadow person', and is not seen directly. Such 'sensed presences' are classically encountered in conditions of isolation or in extreme environments, in which case they have been known as the 'third man factor' [91]. Finally, there are the much less frequent reports of 'internal heautoscopy' and 'negative heautoscopy', whereby patients, respectively, report seeing their internal organs as projected in external space or fail to see their own body, either upon direct examination or through a reflecting surface [13, 83].

Taken collectively, these disorders of the bodily self, involving either body parts or the entire body, have provided the most important insights for the scientific and conceptual understanding of the biological origins of the human sense of self-identity. Indeed, they directly point at the very anatomy of the self, which involves structures and networks devoted to multisensory integration, spatial cognition, vestibular processes, and action planning, diversely comprising parietotemporal, subcortical, and frontal structures of both hemispheres [15, 69, 70].

## Literary Case Studies

Equipped with this theoretical, experimental and clinical toolbox, we can now turn to an overview of selected cases from the literary double canon (see table 2 for an overview of works cited). Traditionally, when these works have been approached through the lenses of neurological science, it has been mainly under the suggestion that their authors might themselves have experienced phenomena similar to those depicted in their fiction (e.g. [7, 9]). While this might well be sometimes the case, this approach is not the one primarily taken in this chapter. Instead we suggest that the double is not necessarily a pathological and thoroughly abnormal experience, but a quite natural emanation of our normal cognitive architecture and sense of bodily self.

*Minor Doubles: Fragmentation and Splitting*

We start our review with cases of minor or incomplete duplications, involving shadows, reflections, body parts, and objects. Adalbert von Chamisso's *Peter Schlemihl* (1814) and Hans Christian Andersen's *The Shadow* (ca. 1840) are stories about individuals whose shadow have taken on an autonomous life and progressively usurp the place of the original self. They use a pattern familiar in later stories of full-blown doppelgängers: first there is a state of deprivation, either induced by or leading to a phenomenon of duplication or splitting; next the detached element grows independently until it becomes fully autonomous; the plot then follows the incremental process of substitution and usurpation on the part of the new entity towards the original self; and finally the story usually ends with a full-blown exchange, or switching of personalities, or altogether annihilation of the original self. In E.T.A. Hoffmann's *Die Abenteuer der Sylversternacht* (1815), a similar scenario is developed with a fugitive mirror reflection, the other age-old physical manifestation of the double [92].

In a parodic take of these tales, which were themselves derived from earlier widespread cultural folktales [93], Russian writer Nikolaï Gogol wrote *The Nose* (1835–1836), a story in which the nose of a mediocre and vain protagonist decides one morning to leave and lead a life of its own. The nose-deprived character later meets his rebellious olfactory organ parading in high-rank uniform as a pompous and self-conceited bigwig, and feels utterly humiliated as he tries to explain his predicament to the authorities [94]. Another of Gogol's short stories, *The Overcoat* (1842), takes a similar path, but using a piece of garment as the repository and embodiment of the protagonist's conceited self. The most famous of such stories, of course, is Oscar Wilde's *The Picture of Dorian Gray* (1890), in which a narcissistic and immoral man becomes obsessed by his portrait. He soon notices that his image in the picture seems to grow old and accumulate the physical marks of his infamy, while he remains remarkably youthful and handsome over the years [35]. Cases of artificial humans or machines that embody the fears, hubris and obsessions of their creators are also

**Table 2.** List of disorders and examples

| Disorder | Literary illustration (from text) |
|---|---|
| Minor doubles: fragmentation and splitting of the bodily self | *Peter Schlemihl* (1814): Adalbert von Chamisso<br>*The Shadow* (ca 1840): Hans Christian Andersen<br>*Die Abenteuer der Sylversternacht* (1815): E.T.A. Hoffmann<br>*The Nose* (1835–1836); *The Overcoat* (1842): Nikolaï Gogol<br>*The Picture of Dorian Gray* (1890): Oscar Wilde<br>*The Golem* (1915): Gustav Meyrink<br>*Frankenstein* (1818/1823): Mary Shelley<br>*The Strange Case of Dr. Jekyll and Mr. Hyde* (1886): R.L. Stevenson<br>*The Black Cat* (1843); *The Tell-Tale Heart* (1843): E.A. Poe<br>*The Cloven Viscount* (1952): Italo Calvino |
| Autoscopic hallucination | *Dichtung und Wahrheit* (1811–1833): Johann Wolfgang von Goethe<br>*Le docteur Héraclius Gloss* (1875?); *Lui?* (1883): Guy de Maupassant<br>*At the End of the Passage* (1890): Rudyard Kipling<br>*The Grayling Fisher* (1921): Jean Sarment |
| Heautoscopy and the doppelgänger | *The Devil's Elixir* (1814); *The Sandman* (1816): E.T.A. Hoffmann<br>*The Double* (1846/1866); *The Brothers Karamazov* (1880): Fyodor Dostoevsky<br>*William Wilson* (1839): E.A. Poe<br>*The Death of Baron Jesus Maria von Friedel* (1908): Hanns Heinz Ewers<br>*The Private Memoirs and Confession of a Justified Sinner* (1824): James Hogg<br>*The Secret Sharer* (1919): Joseph Conrad<br>*Despair* (1936): Vladimir Nabokov<br>*O homem duplicado* (2003): José Saramago<br>*Le chevalier double* (1840): Théophile Gautier<br>*Borges and I* (1960): Jorge Luis Borges |
| Feeling of a presence | *Inferno* (1896–1897): August Strindberg<br>*Ferdydurke* (1937): Witold Gombrowicz<br>*The Horla* (1896–1897): Guy de Maupassant<br>*The Jolly Corner* (1908): Henry James |
| Out-of-body experience | *Connaissances par les gouffres* (1961): Henri Michaux<br>*The Hound of the Baskervilles* (1901–1902): Arthur Conan Doyle<br>*The Star Rover* (1915): Jack London<br>*La lampe* (1892): Gaston Danville<br>*The Stolen Body* (1898); *The Remarkable Case of Davidson's Eyes* (1895): H.G. Wells<br>*Seeing* (1995): Greg Egan |
| Near-death experience | *A Tale of the Ragged Mountains* (1844): E.A. Poe<br>*The Bridge-Builders* (1893): Rudyard Kipling<br>*The Dream of a Ridiculous Man* (1876): Fyodor Dostoevsky |

often mentioned in studies of the double. Among these, Gustav Meyrink's *The Golem* (1915) and Mary Shelley's *Frankenstein* (1818/1823) are the foremost illustrations.

Although *The Strange Case of Dr. Jekyll and Mr. Hyde* (1886) involves the full transformation of one character into another, in the novel there is an episode reminiscent of body part disownership, illustrating the increasing unpredictability and ambiguity of the switching process between the scientist and the monster, spreading from body part to full body awareness [30]:

. . .my eyes fell upon my hand. Now the hand of Henry Jekyll was professional in shape and size: it was large, firm, white and comely. But the hand which I now saw, clearly enough [. . .] lying half shut on the bedclothes, was lean, corded, knuckly, of a dusky pallor and thickly shaded with a swart growth of hair. It was the hand of Edward Hyde [. . .] [B]ounding from my bed, I rushed to the mirror. At the sight that met my eyes, my blood was changed into something exquisitely thin and icy. Yes, I had gone to bed Henry Jekyll, I had awakened Edward Hyde.

In Edgar Allan Poe's *The Black Cat* (1843), the inner conscience of the protagonist is projected in the huge cat Pluto while he is slowly driven into madness. Interestingly, the cat itself would later produce its own double. In another of Poe's short stories *The Tell-Tale Heart* (1843), the guilty conscience of the protagonist is quite literally represented as his beating heart, which he starts hearing as if projected in external space and ultimately compels him to confess a murder.

Another remarkable story of the double, yet difficult to categorize, is Italo Calvino's *Il visconte dismezzatto* (The Cloven Viscount; 1952). The author took the notion of splitting of the self at face value and had his character literally cut in half by a bombshell. The left-half and the right-half then each lead a separate life. The right-half is the evil one: he frantically cuts in half everything that stands in his way. The left-half is the good one and strives to repair his counterpart's misdeeds. Unsurprisingly, each side falls in love with the same girl, and in the process of fighting for her they can eventually be reunited.

All these stories of fragmentary splitting, projection, and duplication are of course works of complete fantasy. Yet they are strikingly reminiscent of several unilateral or nonlateralized disorders of the bodily self, such as somatoparaphrenia, dysmorphophobia, depersonalization, personification of a body part, and internal heautoscopy (see reviews in [66, 67]), even including cases similar to Calvino's extreme splitting of the body image [78]. Moreover, they provide, so to speak, the creative background to ongoing scientific investigations of the mechanisms of the bodily self, including principles of shadow integration [95], mirrored self-perception [96, 97], body part localization and recognition [57, 58], perception of internal and autonomous bodily functions [98], and even extension, incorporation, and psychological embodiment of clothes [56, 99, 100]. We think that such common interests between clinical and scientific research on the one hand and literary creations on the other hand are strongly suggestive of deeper cognitive mechanisms underlying both domains.

### *Autoscopic Hallucination*

The first nonclinical description of an autoscopic hallucination is probably that of Aristotle, who reported the case of a man (later identified as Antipheron) in, of all places, his treatise on *Meteorology* (Book III, part 4). Indeed, an explanation for the phenomenon is provided in terms of atmospheric factors combined with eyesight deficiency:

Air must be condensed if it is to act as a mirror, though it often gives a reflection even uncondensed when the sight is weak. Such was the case of a man whose sight was faint and indistinct. He always saw an image in front of him and facing him as he walked. This was because his sight was reflected back to him. Its morbid condition made it so weak and delicate that the air close by acted as a mirror, just as distant and condensed air normally does, and his sight could not push it back.

Another frequently cited example is Johann Wolfgang von Goethe's personal account, reported in *Dichtung und Wahrheit* (1811–1833): 'I saw, not with the eyes of the body but with those of the spirit, my own self returning again on horseback along the same path, and indeed in clothes such as I had never worn [. . .] As soon as I had aroused myself from this dream, the shape had entirely disappeared.' Alfred de Musset, Percy Bysshe Shelley, Gabriele D'Annunzio, and Nathaniel Hawthorne, among others have likewise reported such experiences, sometimes allegorically, sometimes quite explicitly.

An undated story of the Turkish trickster Nasreddin Hodja illustrates the absurdity of autoscopic experiences: 'Nasreddin went to the market to sell two beautiful watermelons from his garden. As he walked, one fruit under each arm, he saw at a corner of the path, walking before him, a man wearing the exact same clothes as his and likewise carrying two watermelons. "By Allah!" he shouted, "if that is not me, I wonder who else it could be!" For a moment he sped up his walk, but a few steps later completely gave up catching himself. "Actually", he wondered, "what use could it be to catch myself up?" (quoted in [101]).

Apparitional experiences of the self can also be found, not surprisingly, in the occult literature; however, they tend to belong to categories such as 'phantoms of the living' or 'bilocation', and are usually reported by external witnesses rather than by the victim of the phenomenon. An oft-cited example took place in 1845 in what is now Latvia, where Ms. Emilie Sagée (or Octavie Saget, according to Camille Flammarion), a 32-year-old teacher, taught French at a girls' boarding school. The girls were astonished to see on multiple occasions Ms. Sagée present in several places at the same time, including one episode where the teacher was seen in the garden through the class window, and suddenly appeared duplicated as a flimsy image in the classroom armchair. There was no mention of Ms. Sagée ever meeting her own double, although she seemed quite familiar with the phenomenon as she could only sigh when she was fired from the establishment – the 19th time since she became a teacher at 16 [102].

The fearful potential of autoscopy was fully developed with the advent of fantastic literature and horror stories near the turn of the 19th century. Famous examples include two of Maupassant's short stories. The alleged autoscopic episodes are very similar, but worth comparing. In *Le docteur Héraclius Gloss* (1875?) the main character thinks his double is waiting for him in his office:

[. . .] in front of the fire, with his back turned towards the door through which he entered, he saw. . . Doctor Héraclius Gloss, attentively reading his manuscript. There was no possible doubt. . . . It was indeed himself. . . . His long dressing gown of antique silk with large red flowers was over his shoulders and on his head was his black velvet Greek cap embroidered with gold. The doctor understood that if his other self turned towards him, that if the two Héraclius were to come face to face, the one who trembled in his skin at that moment would be struck dead before its replication.

Likewise, in *Lui?* (1883):

> I noticed somebody sitting in my armchair by the fire, warming his feet, with his back to me [. . .] I saw him quite distinctly; his right arm was hanging down and his legs were crossed; the position of his head, which was somewhat inclined to the left of the armchair, seemed to indicate that he was asleep. 'Who can it be?' I asked myself. I could not see clearly, as the room was rather dark, so I put out my hand to touch him on the shoulder, and it came in contact with the back of the chair. There was nobody there; the seat was empty. I startled, good gracious!

Sollier listed Guy de Maupassant as his case No. 8 of 'external autoscopy' on the grounds that the writer is said to have reported autoscopic experiences to his friends (see [103] and below). Both literary cases, however, despite their being frequently quoted as such, depart somehow from the classical autoscopy, which involves a clear visual recognition of oneself. Yet these examples highlight the apprehension of seeing one's visual double and the inner conviction that a sensed presence might just be oneself. In the first case, the protagonist does not dare to uncover the identity of his 'double' (which turns out to be merely his monkey). In the second case, the 'double' vanishes as soon as the protagonist tries to touch him, and he concludes that he had a hallucination; yet he becomes obsessed by this event, and in the end realizes that the 'person' in the chair really was a manifestation of his own loneliness.

A more straightforward autoscopic double can be found in Rudyard Kipling's *At the End of the Passage* (1890), where a character is found dead with 'terror beyond the expression of any pen' in his eyes. Earlier he was left alone in a hostile and monotonous environment:

> Hummil turned on his heel to face the echoing desolation of his bungalow, and the first thing he saw standing in the verandah was the figure of himself. He had met a similar apparition once before, when he was suffering from overwork and the strain of the hot weather. 'This is bad, – already,' he said, rubbing his eyes. 'If the thing slides away from me all in one piece, like a ghost, I shall know it is only my eyes and stomach that are out of order. If it walks – my head is going.' He approached the figure, which naturally kept at an unvarying distance from him, as is the use of all specters that are born of overwork. [. . .] When he came in to dinner he found himself sitting at the table. The vision rose and walked out hastily. Except that it cast no shadow it was in all respects real.

The ending suggests that Hummil was scared to death by his visual double.

An autoscopic hallucination portrayed in a theatrical play can be found in Jean Sarment's *Le pêcheur d'ombres* (The Grayling Fisher; 1921). An amnesiac and broken-hearted character suddenly sees himself in external space:

> Ah! There I am. [. . .] There, in the mirror [there is of course no mirror] . . . Oh! Do I look stupid! [. . .] And sad! [. . .] I did not know I was so sad. [Speaking to the imaginary mirror:] Come on, smile! Don't you want to smile? [. . .] No; the more I try, the more stupid I look! [. . .] Ah! This

is too much! [. . .] Go away! Go away, will you! [. . .] [He shoots his pistol in front of him] I have made a little hole in the mirror, but I look just as stupid as before! [. . .] One should come up with a mirror system that could send back the bullet. . .

The play ends with the character actually committing suicide.

Literary depictions of autoscopy are abundant and varied, sometimes difficult to distinguish from the related categories heautoscopy and the feeling of a presence. The cases reported here illustrate the notion of recognizing oneself in an external – sometimes real or supernatural, but most frequently hallucinated – person. Psychological affinity between the first and second self is rather weaker than in full-blown stories of the doppelgänger, and like its neurological counterpart, autoscopic hallucination in literature is usually short lived. The first clinical case of autoscopy was reported by Arthur Wigan [104] describing in 1844 a 'gentleman who saw his own self'. Wigan's report was quite colorful and is worth quoting as it predates many literary renditions of the phenomenon. It is also quite unusual in that the patient was able to voluntarily make his double appear:

> I knew a very intelligent and amiable man, who had the power of thus placing before his eyes *himself*, and often laughed heartily at *his double*, who always seemed to laugh in turn. This was long a subject of amusement and joke, but the ultimate result was lamentable. He became gradually convinced that he was haunted by himself, or (to violate grammar for the sake of clearly expressing his idea) by his *self*. This other self would argue with him pertinaciously, and to his great mortification sometimes refute him, which, as he was very proud of his logical powers, humiliated him exceedingly. He was eccentric, but was never placed in confinement or subjected to the slightest restraint. At length, worn out by the annoyance, he deliberately resolved not to enter on another year of existence [. . .] – waited, pistol in hand, the night of the 31st of December, and as the clock struck twelve fired it into his mouth.

It is quite remarkable that the notion of the double as a harbinger of death can be found both in literary portrayals and in clinical cases of autoscopic hallucinations (and heautoscopy as well, see below). Probably the idea can be traced back to Ovid's myth of Narcissus in his *Metamorphoses* (ca. 8 AD), in which a young man died for the love of his own image (for the relationship between autoscopy and narcissism, see [10, 34]). Autoscopy can either lead to death – by suicide, fear, or otherwise – or be triggered by proximity with death or by states of deep depersonalization, depression, exhaustion, isolation, or loss of bodily feelings which are akin to mental, physical, or social annihilation [83]. This association is further suggested by conceiving suicide as an 'escape from the self' [105] and by not infrequent cases of suicides perpetrated in front of mirrors (as was the case of French psychiatrist Gaëtan de Clérambault, see also [106, 107]).

*Heautoscopy: The Doppelgänger*

If one considers heautoscopy the clinical analogue of the doppelgänger motif, then it certainly represents one of the most prevalent neurological disorders portrayed in literature. E.T.A. Hoffmann is often credited as having almost single-handedly perfected the doppelgänger theme and pinned down its main characteristic features. His first novel, *The Devil's Elixir* (1814), has an incredibly complicated and intricate plot condensing all the key elements of the double motif, including the notions of guilt, self-knowledge, sin, temptation, the demonic, and the limits of free will. *The Sandman* (1816) is perhaps more straightforward. The main character Nathaniel is obsessed by Coppelius and Coppola, two unrelated characters who haunt his thoughts. The novel remarkably enunciates the central elements of the double, as Nathaniel is warned of his self-destructive tendencies by his closest friends, who perspicaciously point out that these figures he is obsessed with really represent 'phantoms of [his] own ego' and that their 'power must have assumed within [him] the form of [himself]; indeed have become [himself], for otherwise [he] would not listen to it'. The power Coppelius holds on Nathaniel exists only because of his belief in him. Unable to resist his self-projected anxieties and fears, he ends up in the madhouse and finally puts himself to death by leaping off a tower after having seen, for the last time, his doppelgänger.

Perhaps the best-known story of the doppelgänger is *The Double*, Fyodor Dostoevsky's second novel (1846, revised in 1866). The tale has been said to reflect the author's personal experience of autoscopic phenomena on the grounds that he suffered from epilepsy. However, whereas several of his symptoms have been thoroughly documented, there is no evidence that he underwent an experience even remotely like that of his protagonist Golyadkin. The hero is a self-conscious, suspicious, vain, ambitious, and envious man, who starts his day by looking satisfactorily at his reflection and then acting as if he is 'somebody else' in order to escape people's scrutiny. As it turns out, Golyadkin is torn between his superficially glowing image of himself and inner feelings of despair, paranoia, doubt, and self-contempt. After having been thrown out of a prestigious ball, deeply humiliated, he contemplates suicide nearby a river, when he suddenly feels a presence. At first he sees no one, but then crosses twice the path of an individual whom he recognizes as himself. This 'Golyadkin Jr.' is 'another Mr. Golyadkin, but exactly the same as himself.' They soon share the same house and work at the same office, indeed they even share the same name. Although they get along pretty well at first, the double soon starts usurping the first Golyadkin's personality and humiliating him. Evidently, the double represents Golyadkin's glowing self-image; he is proud, arrogant and contemptuous, only this attitude is now turned against himself instead of others. Of course, in typical doppelgänger lore, all the mischievous and immoral activities of the second self will be ascribed to the original, while the second self is allowed to become widely popular. Golyadkin realizes that the situation is getting out of hand, and he writes to his double: 'Either you or I, but both of us together is impossible!' The double is ever more intrusive, threatening and offensive, and Golyadkin's identity and sanity start to crumble. During a second scene of humiliation at a party, he even hallucinates 'that an endless string of Golyadkins all exactly alike were bursting in through the doors of the room.' He must then be taken to a mental asylum.

Dostoevsky was probably the first to introduce the element of humor in the double motif. Although a quite tragic and verging on the pathological case report, the story can at times read like an absurdist farce much in the vein of Gogol's earlier work.

Paranoia and the sin of pride are at the forefront of this novel mixing of psychological and supernatural elements. The writer will revisit the theme on many occasions [108], perhaps most notably in *The Brothers Karamazov*, where Ivan receives regular visits from the Devil, whom he soon identifies as a projection of his own self: 'You're the embodiment of myself, but only of one side of me – of my thoughts and feelings, but only the most vile and stupid [. . .] All that is base, rotten and contemptible in me!'

Another famous story of rigorously identical doubles is Poe's *William Wilson* (1839). In this case, however, the double represents the good side of conscience instead of the bad one. Indeed, William Wilson is a depraved individual, 'prey to the most ungovernable passions'. He first meets his double at school, and realizes that not only do they look alike, but they also have similar temperaments and were born on the same date (January 19, like Poe himself). Wilson becomes increasingly uneasy with this constant presence of his inner conscience, and tries to escape by travelling abroad were he can live a life of infamy as he pleases. However, again and again he will inexplicably stumble across Wilson II, usually at the very moment he is about to perform some evil deed. In the end he sees no other choice than to kill this intrusive figure:

> I would submit no longer to be enslaved [. . .] I felt a light hand placed upon my shoulder, and that ever-remembered, low, damnable whisper within my ear [. . .] In a few seconds I forced him by sheer strength against the wainscoting, and thus, getting him at mercy, plunged my sword, with brute ferocity, repeatedly through and through his bosom [. . .] What human language can adequately portray that astonishment, that horror which possessed me at the spectacle then presented to view? [. . .] A large mirror, – so at first it seemed to me in my confusion – now stood where none had been perceptible before; and as I stepped up to it in extremity of terror, mine own image, but with features all pale and dabbled in blood, advanced to meet me with a feeble and tottering gait [. . .] It was Wilson; but he spoke no longer in a whisper, and I could have fancied that I myself was speaking while he said: 'You have conquered, and I yield. Yet henceforward art thou also dead [. . .] In me didst thou exist – and, in my death, see by this image, which is thine own, how utterly thou hast murdered thyself

A similar case of death by doppelgänger proxy can be found in *The Death of Baron Jesus Maria von Friedel* (1908), a short story by Hanns Heinz Ewers, which includes the interesting and rare twist that the double is of the opposite gender. Likewise, Wilde's Dorian Gray perishes as he attempts to shred his portrait.

An earlier story from Scottish[4] writer James Hogg is worth mentioning. *The Private Memoirs and Confessions of a Justified Sinner* (1824) is indeed one the most sophisticated treatments of the doppelgänger theme ever concocted. The story involves multiple perspectives, severable instances of doubling, physical mimicry and transformations, heautoscopy coupled with autoscopic hallucinations and the feeling of a presence, physical misidentifications of the intermetamorphosis type, psychological

[4] Mikorey [17] mentions that Griesinger (sadly, he does not provide a reference) held that the 'endemic' prominence of the 'hallucination of the double' in Scotland could be due to the (alleged) widespread presence of epilepsy in that country.

dissociation and depersonalization, alternate personalities, possession by the Devil, incorporation and fusion of the double within the self, and splitting of the self into twofold doubles. The following quote conveys the psychological complexity and precision of the novel:

> I generally conceived myself to be two people. When I lay in bed, I deemed there were two of us in it; when I sat up, I always beheld another person, and always in the same position from the place where I sat or stood, which was about three paces off me towards my left side [. . .] The most perverse part of it was, that I rarely conceived *myself* to be any of the two persons. I thought for the most part that my companion was one of them, and my brother the other; and I found, that to be obliged to speak and answer in the character of another man, was a most awkward business in the long run.

Not all doppelgänger stories are tales of terror, murder, persecution, and insanity. *The Secret Sharer* (1919) by Joseph Conrad, for instance, uses the motif rather positively. A young ship commander, somewhat insecure and feeling like 'a stranger to himself', rescues a man lost at sea, who turns out to be a criminal fugitive. The man is kept secretly in the captain's cabin and immediately a strong and mysterious psychological affinity develops between both men. Increasingly, there is confusion between both characters, they see themselves in each other and grow unsure as to which one is the captain and who is the criminal. In the end, the fugitive is put back to sea, and each character has grown stronger and more secure by having met their second self. Vladimir Nabokov's *Despair* (1936) turns the motif fully into a parody. The narrator Hermann becomes convinced that a tramp named Felix is his identical double. As it turns out, Felix is just another person, not even remotely resembling Hermann and having nothing to do with a doppelgänger. More recently, José Saramago exploited the theme with due respect to the classics, but adapting it to modern technology. In *O homem duplicado* (2003; translated somewhat thoughtlessly as *The Double*), a disgruntled teacher meets his second self in a home-video movie and becomes obsessed with tracking down the second-rate actor that looks like him.

Clinical manifestations of heautoscopy can be as dramatic and unsettling as their literary counterparts. 'Real life' cases suggestive of the doppelgänger have been carefully documented along the years and indicate the importance of multisensory integration, as well as somesthetic and vestibular mechanisms [13, 79]. The heautoscopic double, indeed, is foremost based on bodily and emotional functions, rather than visual processing per se. In one case reminiscent of the above extract from Hogg's *Confession of a Justified Sinner*, a patient with tuberculosis and meningitis, while lying on his side, saw 'two other himself' lying beside him in his bed, one above and one below the plane of the bed, in the same position and turning their back to him. He felt a strong belonging and corporeal affinity towards these doubles, 'as if there were some weight leaving his body to induce the phenomenon' [109]. In clinical cases, it is also frequent that the patient will project some of his ailment into the illusory double, one of the central features of the literary doppelgänger. Thus, very anxious patients can perceive a double who is about to die, and others will feel a strong urge to kill the double to get rid of their problems [109]. In *Le chevalier double* (1840) by Théophile Gautier, this empathetic resonance between self and double is emphasized as the main character and his second self fight to death, and each inflicted wound is felt by both at the same time. This phenomenon is reminiscent of recent observations on 'empathy for pain' and 'mirror allodynia' [110, 111], which could be facilitated by feelings of psychological and affective affinity [112].

As in literature, clinical cases of 'heterosexual heautoscopy', namely the experience of a double of the opposite gender, is rather rare. In one of few cases, a schizophrenic male patient felt 'the left side of his body exteriorize and take the shape of a woman's head, whom he considers his double'. The patient hated this 'apparition' and frequently harmed himself while trying to kill her [11]. In fact, as we have seen for autoscopic hallucinations, the notion of the double as a harbinger of death and promoter of suicide seems equally frequent, if not much more frequent, for tales of the doppelgänger and clinical cases of heautoscopy. A young patient with a history of epilepsy and a lesion in the left mesiobasal temporal lobe, for instance, jumped out of the window 'in order to escape the intolerable feeling of being divided in two.' Shortly before, he 'saw himself' lying in bed as he woke up, started a fight with his double, became suddenly confused as to which of both 'me' he was, and decided that the best way to put an end to the situation was to get rid of one of 'him' ([113]; see also [114, 115]).

Another case was explicitly compared to that of Golyadkin by the author reporting it. A man in his 50s once had an autoscopic hallucination at night, in which he saw an older double of himself. Years later, he entertained the delusion that a newly met person was that very double that appeared to him that night. At first, he had intense feelings of affinity for this 'second me', but soon became ambivalent and started to feel persecuted by this man. Hatred and suspicion then led to a strong feeling of looming disaster and impending death [11]. Visual doubles and doppelgängers looking younger or older than the original self are not infrequent in literature and clinical cases. The short story *Borges and I* (1960) by Jorge Luis Borges and *The Picture of Dorian Gray* (1890) by Oscar Wilde are prime examples. Just as the double typically involves a strong corporeal duplication which is spatially situated, there are many cases where the duplication additionally involves a temporal component [116]. In fact, there seems to be no obvious reason why the spatial duplication itself should stop at one item. Just like Golyadkin, at the bottom of despair, hallucinated 'an endless string of Golyadkins', there are clinical cases of so-called 'polyopic heautoscopy' where a multiplicity of 'doubles' is perceived, most frequently more than 3 and sometimes filling an entire room (review in [117]). A striking cinematographic example was portrayed in *Being John Malkovich* (Charlie Kaufman, 1999), where the actor-protagonist is projected into his own mind and discovers it is filled with replicas of himself, communicating through the restricted use of his own name. Perhaps one could conceive of the double as the 'rudimentary expression of an infinite swarm', waiting to proliferate [27].

*Feeling of a Presence*

The disturbing sensation of being alone and nevertheless feeling that there is someone nearby is perhaps the most familiar among autoscopy-related phenomena [91, 118]. In literary and clinical terms, however, it is much more that the fleeting impression everyone has felt at some time or another, and can indeed verge on absolute conviction [119]. The personal account of August Strindberg, given at length in his psychopathological memoir *Inferno* (1896–1897) is particularly striking in this regard, and in some respect reminiscent of Maupassant's fictional *The Horla* (see below).

The feeling of a presence is interesting in that the illusion is not primarily based upon the visual recognition of the double as oneself. Indeed, the 'presence' is most frequently not seen, and almost always explicitly identified as someone else or a 'shadow person', although it can well be sensed as a kind of 'alter ego' or 'guardian angel'. Yet the strong psychological affinity, the spatial proximity to one's body, its somesthetic qualities, and its frequent imitating behaviors all point to the notion that the double is really one's own projected and slightly mislocalized bodily self, although lacking a strong feeling of ownership. Moreover, the feeling of a presence (or 'false proximate awareness') is frequently associated with other autoscopic phenomena and disorders of the bodily self, either concomitantly or in direct succession.

Polish writer Witold Gombrowicz provides a literary example in *Ferdydurke* (1937), in which a feeling of a presence subsequently leads to a full-blown autoscopic hallucination:

> . . .suddenly the taste in my mouth turned bitter, my throat went dry – I realized that I was not alone. There was someone else in the room, in the corner by the stove where it was still dark – another person was there. But the door was locked. Not a person then, but an apparition. An apparition? The devil? A ghost? A dead person? I suddenly sensed that it was not someone dead but someone alive, and all at once my hair stood on end – I sensed another human, like a dog smells another dog. My mouth dry, my heart pounding, I was hardly able to catch my breath – when I realized that it was I standing by the stove [. . .] I peeked from under my covers at a face that was mine and yet it wasn't mine [. . .] Here were my lips. . . my ears. . . my nose, they were my home [. . .]. . . And how familiar! [. . .] I suddenly thought that it was not I. I felt like someone who unexpectedly looks into a mirror and for a split second does not recognize himself, so did the startling concreteness of the form surprise me and cut me to the quick.

The most popular story involving the feeling of a presence is certainly *The Horla* (1896–1897) by Guy de Maupassant. The narrator (or main character, according to an earlier version[5]) is haunted by an unseen presence. The tale is rich in psychiatric disturbances, including depersonalization, disownership, excessive agency detection,

[5] It is interesting that Maupassant should have written a previous version (1896) in the form of a clinical case report, where the main protagonist tells his strange story to an audience of medical students. Merely switching to the diary format (in 1897), while keeping essentially the same story save the ending, powerfully changed the significance and psychological impact of the tale, suggesting important mechanisms at work in the narrative format of stories of the double (see also James Hogg's *Confession of a Justified Sinner* for a change between third-person and first-person perspective).

and probably sleep paralysis. The realization that the 'double' really is a projection of the main protagonist is left ambiguous, but in the end, having been unable to get rid of the presence, he resolves to take his own life as the only solution left. The most famous episode in the story is the moment where the protagonist fails to see his own reflection in the mirror [a ploy Maupassant previously used in *Letter of a Madman* (1885)]:

> It was just like broad daylight, and I could not see myself in my mirror!. . . It was empty, profoundly clear, full of light! My image was not in it. . . and yet I, I was facing it! I saw the large limpid glass from top to bottom [. . .] I dared not make a movement, yet felt his presence nevertheless [. . .] he whom the imperceptible body had devoured my reflection.

Although often cited as the paradigmatic case of negative autoscopy, it is interesting that the phenomenon, at least as the protagonist interprets it, is due to the invisible sensed presence standing between the character and the mirror. It has often been reported that in writing *The Horla*, Maupassant was directly inspired by his own experience of insanity.[6] This idea, however, stands on the rather flimsy evidence that Maupassant ended up severely delusional (he did, but 6 years after publishing *The Horla*) and reported in a letter to his friend Paul Bourget that 'One out of two times, when I arrive home, I see my own double. I open my door and see myself sitting in my armchair. I know it's a hallucination at the very moment I experience it. Strange, isn't it? Without a bit of common sense, it would be quite frightening.' In an account reported 9 years after his death, Maupassant is also reported to have mentioned the following:

> Do you know that by staring for a long time at my own image reflected in a mirror, I sometimes feel that I am losing the notion of who I am? In those moments everything gets confused in my mind and I find it bizarre to see a head that I no longer recognize. So it seems strange to be who I am, that is to say: someone. And I feel that if that state were to last for more than a minute, I would go completely mad. My brain would gradually empty itself of all thoughts.

Yet his valet François Tassard reported in his memoirs the following claim about *The Horla*'s publication: 'I sent the manuscript of *The Horla* to Paris today; before the week is over you can be assured that all the papers will say that I am mad. They can write whatever they like, but I am perfectly sane and I knew very well what I was doing when I wrote that story. It is a work of the imagination that will engross readers and give them more than a shiver or two, for it is strange.' Indeed, *The Horla* was written at the height of Maupassant's creative powers and other works published around the same time are not suggestive in the least of a disturbed mind. Moreover, it should be recalled that Maupassant used a lot of treatments and drugs for his physical

[6] Indeed, the fictional character in *The Horla* is listed as case No. 12 in Sollier's treatise on autoscopic phenomena as if he were Maupassant himself [83]. The author highlights the importance of Maupassant's 'case' as it combines autoscopic hallucination, feeling of a presence ('simple cenesthetic hallucination') and negative heautoscopy, thereby illustrating the phenomenological continuity between these symptoms and suggesting a common (bodily based) mechanism underlying them.

ailments, including ether, mercury, chloral, antipyrine, leeches, cannabis, opium, arsenic, potassium iodide, tincture of colchicum, alcohol, cold showers, and sulfate water cures. Added to his well-known interest in the emerging neurological and psychiatric sciences and his passion for the occult and the unusual, it seems clear that reducing *The Horla* to a mere autobiography is a gross underestimation of Maupassant's extraordinary powers of imagination and creativity [103].

Henry James exploited a similar type of haunting phenomenon in *The Jolly Corner* (1908). In this novel, the psychological origin of the double is more explicit. An American expatriate returns to his family home after a 33-year leave in England. He first imagines what kind of a person he would now be had he never left, but soon this imaginary second self becomes an obsession, until he starts actually feeling its presence. From hunter of the double, he then becomes hunted by the ghostly figure, and to his terror ends up meeting his double. James thus raises the interesting questions of the influence of time, wasted opportunities, imagination, and counterfactual thinking on the emergence of the second self.

As a purely somesthetic (i.e. nonvisual) doppelgänger, the feeling of a presence has been conceptualized as 'heautoscopy without optical image' [119]. As such, it provides valuable insights as to the underlying mechanisms and differentiating factors of the broader set of autoscopic phenomena. Its phenomenological profile also suggests some combination of bodily based (somesthetic, vestibular, and motor) mechanisms and the spontaneous activation of social cognitive processes [120, 121]. Indeed, seizures and electrical stimulation at the left temporoparietal junction, an area of converging sensory integration, has recently been shown in a single case report to induce an irresistible urge to look to the right, accompanied with actual head and eye deviation towards that direction. It turned out, as the patient reported afterwards, that the reason she turned her head was that 'she thought a person was standing next to her' and 'she felt this presence as a threat' [122; see also 123].

It thus appears that bodily sensations and social imperatives interact tightly in the emergence of the feeling of a presence. After all, this illusion raises a question traditionally addressed by social psychologists: What does it feel like, and what does it imply, to have an *actual* human presence nearby? [124]. Because this experience is so frequent and seldom questioned, we tend to forget that the 'sensed presence', whether real or imaginary, is probably one of the most crucial experiences of our social species. It is thus not surprising that it can on occasions be excessively, or fail to be, activated, and that it should rely on a complex set of spatial, bodily, and social mechanisms. The continuity with other bodily disorders, such as peculiar cases of phantom limbs [75] and somatoparaphrenia [16, 67], sleep disorders [125] and disturbances of spatial and social cognition [126], its frequent occurrence in healthy individuals, in loners and in adventurers [91], as well as its abundant appearances in psychiatric cases and the occult literature, highlight the pervasiveness of this illusion as an anthropological phenomenon. As a consequence, the fact that many writers have ventured to exploit the motif in their fiction says more about the human mind in general than about their alleged mental disturbances.

*Out-of-Body Experiences*

At the end of the autoscopic phenomena continuum, the most dramatic and extreme manifestation of the second self happens during out-of-body experiences. Here, as it were, the projection and mislocalization of the bodily self is brought to full fruition. The individual does not merely perceive her second self; she *embodies* the second self. The world is then seen from the perspective of the exteriorized, elevated, self, and thus the physical body – the original self – becomes visible as an external element of the scene [89, 127, 128]. The phenomenon is widespread in the general population and across cultures, and has attracted considerable interest from parapsychologists, occultists, and religious writers; most available case reports derive from personal accounts or collected testimonies (e.g. [129]) and alleged 'methods' to induce and observe such states (e.g. [130, 131]). The phenomenon indeed seems to uniquely combine long-held beliefs and legends about the disembodied soul, powers of levitation, clairvoyance, the existence of hidden worlds, and of course the afterlife. The proximity of out-of-body experiences to shamanic voyages and drug-induced 'astral journeys' has long been recognized, and French poet Henri Michaux described in minute details his own disembodied experiences in *Connaissances par les gouffres* (Light through Darkness; 1961).

Literature has also contributed to the popularization of the out-of-body experience, although perhaps to a lesser degree than for the doppelgänger motif. Sir Arthur Conan Doyle, perhaps because of his interest in spiritualism, had his famous detective briefly touch the subject in *The Hound of the Baskervilles* (1901–1902) as an illustration of his fantastic powers of visualization. In the novel, Sherlock Holmes claims to have been to Devonshire at a time when it was obvious to Watson that he had not left his office. He explains: 'My body has remained in this arm-chair and has, I regret to observe, consumed in my absence two large pots of coffee and an incredible amount of tobacco. After you left I sent down to Stamford's for the ordnance map of this portion of the moor, and my spirit has hovered over it all day. I flatter myself that I could find my way about.'

Jack London provided a full-length novel account of out-of-body experiences in *The Star Rover* (1915), a story mostly referring to the reincarnation motif but providing interesting insights about the triggering of out-of-body experiences. A prisoner attempts to leave his body, as instructed by a fellow inmate:

> The trick is to [. . .] will yourself to die [. . .] The thing you must think and believe is that your body is one thing and your spirit is another thing. You are you, and your body is something else that don't amount to shucks. Your body don't count. You're the boss [. . .] You begin with the toes, one toe at a time. You make your toes die. You will them to die. And if you've got the belief and the will your toes will die. That is the big job – to start the dying. Once you've got the first toe dead, the rest is easy [. . .] When your body is all dead, and you are all there yet, you just skin out and leave your body. And when you leave your body you leave the cell. Stone walls and iron doors are to hold

bodies in. They can't hold the spirit in. [. . .] You are spirit outside of your body. You can look at your body from outside of it.

Literary out-of-body experiences are most prominent in fantastic and horror tales from the turn of the 19th century. Gaston Danville, a French writer with a strong interest in paranormal phenomena and psychopathology, described the phenomenon rather conventionally in *La lampe* (The Lamp, 1892): 'Suddenly, it seemed to me that a part of my being, mostly composed of my intimate personality, what seemed to constitute the very essence of me [. . .], let's call it my soul, became, detached from my body, which remained seated [. . .] Hovering above it, I thus looked at myself, from a bit above and to the right.' The character further describes feelings of lightness and joy, and the sensation of being a pure self. In characteristic fashion, the experience foreshadows his imminent death.

H.G. Wells also liked the motif and used it very creatively in several short stories. In *The Stolen Body* (1898), a character seeks to voluntarily leave his body in order to appear as a ghostly spirit to a friend. The experiment had been prearranged, much in the fashion of similar attempts by occult enthusiasts.[7] While the experiment is a success, something unexpected happens to the protagonist: as he is wandering out of his body, a lurking criminal spirit takes the vacant place, leaving the protagonist bodyless for the time being.

In another story, *The Remarkable Case of Davidson's Eyes* (1895), Wells imagined the consequences of dissociating bodily awareness from visuospatial perspective. As a result of an experiment gone wrong, a scientist suddenly finds himself contemplating a wonderful beach while his body stays at the laboratory. His eyes see a completely different world, and indeed from that perspective his own body is invisible to him. Yet he can freely move and can even communicate with his colleagues, as his sense of hearing also 'stayed' at the laboratory. This dissociated state lasts for several weeks, during which the scientist learns to progressively adapt to his condition. As he begins recovering, some objects from the 'real world' start appearing in the 'beach world', until his senses end up completely reunited. One could venture that this story provided the inspiration for Wells' *The Invisible Man* (1896) written shortly thereafter. Together with Maupassant's *Le Horla*, it also provides one of the few cases of negative heautoscopy.

More recently, science-fiction writer Greg Egan offered an entertaining mixture of *The Stolen Body* and *The Remarkable Case of Davidson's Eyes* in his short story *Seeing* (1995). The tale is also quite remarkable for the depth of its phenomenological detail and its scientific accuracy. A man who had an out-of-body experience in a hospital setting remains 'stuck' above his body, unable to regain his physical envelope. He can still move his physical body, yet the visual perspective remains that of a disembodied and hovering self. The character is acutely aware of the hallucinatory and

7 For instance, the poet W.B. Yeats and Maude Gonne; see also [132].

confabulatory nature of his visual experiences and is even able to conduct some experiments with medical staff. Visual targets shown to the 'me-above' are misreported, while those that are shown to the 'me-below' are accurately perceived, although in a 'blindsight' manner (i.e. he believes he is merely 'guessing'). The story strikes an ironic chord in light of the tired claims of 'veridical' perceptions in out-of-body states, and is probably the only one to join the skeptical perspective on the issue by pointing out the hallucinatory nature of these vivid percepts (e.g. [133, 134]).

The out-of-body experience in literature stands apart from most stories of the second self. Indeed, it deals less with notions of conflict, conscience, punishment, and persecution than with personal experimentation with the self and more generally the widespread cultural belief in a disembodied (and immortal) soul. As such, it is most likely derived from religious, mythological, and occult accounts rather than from clinical ones. Indeed, the scientific study of out-of-body experiences has had a revival only very lately, perhaps because of an academic taboo for questions related to paranormal lore. In this regard, it is quite remarkable to note some similarities with modern findings, such as the importance of mechanisms related to visual imagery, perspective taking and own body and motor imagery, as well as tendencies for dissociative experiences (e.g. [10, 135–140]). Likewise, Wells' and Egan's insights about the importance of visuospatial perspective and bodily self-identity as segregated functions predate current investigations of the out-of-body experience and related phenomena using techniques from virtual reality, allowing illusory self-projections, feelings of presence in artificial worlds, and even illusory swapping bodies with other persons [141–143; for an early account see 144].

*Near-Death Experiences*

Expanding from the out-of-body experience theme, many stories pushed the logic a step further, where not only the self leaves the body, but ostensibly visits the real or some spiritual world as the physical self dwells in a state of apparent unconsciousness or coma, or undergoes a highly stressful and threatening situation. This is the case, for instance, in Wells' short story *Under the Knife* (1896) and more recently in Alex Garland's *The Coma* (2004).

Edgar Allan Poe's *A Tale of the Ragged Mountains* (1844) provides details strikingly reminiscent of modern accounts of near-death experiences [80]. After having been lost for a day in the mountains, a man of 'singularly vigorous and creative' imagination, who also happens to be a morphine addict, tells a strange story. In the mountains, he entered a strange world filled with ancient characters and battles, and reports having been hit by an arrow at the right temple:

> An instantaneous and dreadful sickness seized me. I struggled – I gasped – I died [. . .] For many minutes [. . .] my sole sentiment – my sole feeling – was that of darkness and nonentity, with the consciousness of death. At length there seemed to pass a violent and sudden shock through my soul, as if of electricity. With it came the sense of elasticity and of light. This latter I felt – not saw. In an instant I seemed to rise from the ground. But I had no bodily, no visible, audible, or palpable

presence [. . .] Beneath me lay my corpse, with the arrow in my temple, the whole head greatly swollen and disfigured. But all these things I felt – not saw. I took interest in nothing. Even the corpse seemed a matter in which I had no concern. Volition I had none, but appeared to be impelled into motion, and flitted buoyantly out of the city, retracing the circuitous path by which I had entered it [. . .] I again experienced a shock as of a galvanic battery; the sense of weight, of volition, of substance, returned. I became my original self, and bent my step eagerly homeward – but the past had not lost the vividness of the real – and not now, even for an instant, can I compel my understanding to regard it as a dream.

Despite its stereotypical allure and, already by that time, overtired structure, the motif was introduced in almost identical terms in numerous literary works. Rudyard Kipling, for instance, casually inserted it in *The Bridge-Builders* (1893) in the context of a shipwreck:

In his mind Findlayson had already escaped from the boat, and was circling high in the air to find a rest for the sole of his foot. His body – he was really sorry for its gross helplessness – lay in the stern, the water rushing about its knees. 'How very ridiculous!' he said to himself, from his eyrie; 'that – is Findlayson – chief of the Kashi Bridge. The poor beast is going to be drowned, too. Drowned when it's close to shore. I'm – I'm on the shore already. Why doesn't it come along?' To his intense disgust, he found his soul back in his body again, and that body spluttering and choking in deep water. The pain of the reunion was atrocious, but it was necessary, also, to fight for the body.

Ernest Hemingway also experienced and used similar events in his writing, for instance in *A Farewell to Arms* (1929) and *The Snows of Kilimanjaro* (1936) (see [145]).

Even Dostoevsky had a go at it, in a lesser-known short story entitled *The Dream of a Ridiculous Man* (1876). A suicidal man falls asleep and has a vivid dream of shooting himself in the heart. He then is taken to his grave, ostensibly dead, painless, yet is aware of being dead. An out-of-body experience and astral journey in 'space' together with an unknown companion follows, in which he is entirely fearless and unaware of the passage of time, enjoying a deep feeling of peacefulness, and entering a different world depicted as a beautiful and welcoming replica of Earth, yet devoid of sin and sadness and imbued with a higher state of goodness, knowledge, and understanding. The character then experiences an intense feeling of oneness with all of humanity and nature. He also hears beautiful music and entertains the idea of a universal religion. The dream leaves a vivid and unforgettable impression on the protagonist.

Such accounts are strikingly reminiscent of the prototypical near-death experience as usually portrayed in New Age and religious literature [146, 147], and suggests indeed that the phenomenon as it is currently known is not merely influenced by the rather recent cultural enthusiasm for the topic [148]. Of course, this could either mean that the current prototypical motif is itself derived from these older literary accounts, or more likely that both types of accounts, modern and older ones, are derived from age-old religious and mythological accounts of the afterlife, themselves plausibly associated to constant forms of neuropsychological phenomena and cognitive constraints across ages and cultures [15, 90, 149, 150], including the other types of autoscopic phenomena described above. Scientific research on this complex topic is still in its infancy [80], having been considerably hindered by the parapsychological, religious, and popular highjacking of the issue [90]. Yet literary accounts have already pointed to the importance of dissociative states and bodily disturbances, and more importantly have recognized the powerful narrative appeal of these age-old experiences, helping to put them into words and consolidate in unmistakable shape this particular subset from the wide range of possible hallucinatory experiences [151].

## Framing the Literary Double in the Vocabulary of Cognitive Neuroscience

This extended review of literary contributions to the bodily self illustrates the richness of both the topic of the double in literature, and of the clinical and scientific research on the issue. At a deeper level are core neuropsychological mechanisms that for millennia have spawned strange experiences, philosophical puzzles, cultural representations, and beliefs, as well as immortal works of art. Only recently have science and medicine begun to catch up with the secrets of the second self. Yet despite exciting advances in recent years, coupled with increasingly sophisticated technology and methods, it is not too late to look back at the creative insights that writers have had over the years.

We have rather superficially pointed at analogies between literature, clinical disorders, and experimental approaches. The goal of the chapter was to provide a wide overview of the relevant issues, not a sharp and operant cognitive model of the double as portrayed in literature. This indeed would be unrealistic in light of the complexity and richness of the topic. Nevertheless, what the doppelgänger and related themes can tell today's scientists is still illuminating. The double, as we have seen, is frequently a projected or an intrusive figure, and is generally bodily based and spatially situated, oftentimes rather close to first self's body. It can be 'real' or 'illusory', 'internal' or 'external', 'subjective' or 'objective'. The double can physically or psychologically resemble the original self. It is often also a dynamic figure, changing as events go by, or becomes modulated according to specific needs and contexts. Between the double and original, there are relationships of complementarities and antagonisms, involving altruism, empathy, conflict, and rejection.

Quite independently of the supernatural nature of the double, these characteristics point to specific psychological and neurological mechanisms, which can be summarily and provisionally represented as the following principles:

- Privation: extending the body and embodying external artifacts decreases awareness of the physical counterpart; reciprocally, loss of awareness or function induces positive manifestations;
- Fusion: blurring the operations of normal mechanisms for self-other discrimination;

- Duplication: the bodily self and its components are fed several sets of conflicting information at the same time, eventually coalescing into separate and autonomous entities;
- Division, fragmentation, splitting: several bodily self-subcomponents are expressed in isolation from each other in a robust and continuous fashion;
- Substitution: a process of projection towards an external element (embodiment), or alternatively of complete incorporation of an external element (incorporation), has been successfully and durably achieved;
- Personification: the misguided and exaggerated activation of an agency/awareness attribution device directed at an external target or at own body parts;
- Switching: a symmetrical – simultaneous or progressive – process of self-other and other-self embodiment;
- Alternation: the dynamic activation of specific patterns of bodily and psychological states, which recurrently reach stable plateaus allowing transitorily identifiable functioning modes.

Philosophers, computational scientists, and experimental psychologists are already making ample use of similar principles [152]. For instance, the notion of 'body mereology' has proven fruitful to think about the ways in which the human body as a whole is processed and represented in relationship to isolated body parts and the presence or absence of action patterns [153]. Likewise, computational modeling of the out-of-body experience allows to factor in the relative importance of vestibular, somesthetic, and visual factors, and how they relate to the current position of the body [154]. In association with neuroimaging studies and methods from the behavioral sciences, the future looks promising for the scientific study of the core features of the literary double (e.g. [155, 156]).

## Conclusion: On the Origin of Doubles

Although Herdman [4] argued that the literary doppelgänger should comprise a strong supernatural element and not be a mere clinical delusion or hallucination, for lack of which the device would sink 'in decline' and 'in a state of decadence', it is clear that most novels, including the earlier ones, exploit this fundamental ambiguity between the subjective or objective nature of the double. Moreover, that illusory doubles have identifiable psychological, neurological, and psychiatric underpinnings does not detract from the fact that patients suffering from autoscopic phenomena will frequently consider their experiences as 'real'. Otherwise, autoscopic phenomena, including bilocation and disembodiment, would probably never have been so abundant in the occult literature. Therefore, given the scientific and historical evidence, the 'decline' of the double should probably be identified as the still widespread refusal to take seriously the neuropsychological significance of the double in the first place.

This persistence of supernatural beliefs is unfortunate. First, as we have mentioned above, beliefs in the paranormal have very likely hindered the scientific understanding of autoscopic phenomena. However and perhaps more importantly, scientific understanding may have been hampered because the supernatural view of autoscopic phenomena has failed to perceive the anthropological continuity between literature, mythology, medicine, and science in regard to the bodily self and its dysfunctions. Indeed, positing at the outset the existence of a disembodied soul and an afterworld immediately clouds interest in uncovering fine-grained mechanisms that could explain the emergence of such beliefs in the first place. Likewise, theorists of the literary double have argued that these fictional stories have inspired medical research, not the other way round [2, 4, 26], failing to see that clinical manifestations could have originally fueled the beliefs and folktales that in turn have inspired tales of the second self.

From where then does the idea of the double come from? On one account, the very motivation behind the creation of literary doubles derives from genuine pathological experiences, such as autoscopic phenomena or manifestations suggestive of 'split personality'. These pathological states, irrespective of their etiology, could have been experienced first-hand by authors, or alternatively could have reached cultural and mythological prominence by the time they inspired a writer. In another approach, the existence of pathologies involving doublings of the bodily self and splitting of identity on one hand, and cultural, mythological, and literary uses of stories, beliefs, and legends of the double on the other might both be horns of a common universal neurocognitive principle constrained by the very nature and architecture of the human mind (for discussions of cultural and medical influences on the emergence of specific symptoms and beliefs at the societal level, see [15, 157, 158]).

So the question of the nature and origins of the literary double could bear directly on the very cognitive dysfunctions producing pathological doubles. We speculate that common mechanisms might indeed underlie the creative production of doubles in the artistic domain, the belief in doubles in religious and occult traditions, and the symptoms involving doubles in neurology, psychiatry, and altered states of consciousness more generally. Taking this proposal full circle, it would then appear that these neuroanthropological constants are the multiple and dynamic neural and cognitive systems underlying our sense of the bodily self, in other words precisely those that induce the appearance of phantom limbs, unilateral disorders of perception, localization and ownership of limbs, autoscopic and heautoscopic doubles, sensed presences, and out-of-body experiences [17]. In healthy individuals, these same bodily systems can then be recruited to conceive of the second self, and use it as a convenient dummy device for daily functioning, the repository of beliefs and myths about the human condition, or the fascinating and entertaining doppelgänger of fiction.

## References


1 Keppler CF: The Literature of the Second Self. Tucson, University of Arizona Press, 1972.
2 Tymms R: Doubles in Literary Psychology. Cambridge, Bowes & Bowes, 1949.
3 Miller K: Doubles: Studies in Literary History. Oxford, Oxford University Press, 1985.
4 Herdman J: The Double in Nineteenth-Century Fiction. London, MacMillan Press, 1990.
5 Bargalló J: Hacia una tipología del doble: el doble por fusión, por fisión y por metamorfosis; in Bargalló J (ed): Identidad y alteridad: aproximación al tema del doble. Sevilla, Alfar, 1994, pp 11–26.
6 Troubetzkoy W (ed): La figure du double. Paris, Didier Erudition, 1995.
7 Pauly R: Le double en littérature et en médicine. J Med Bord 1949;126:309–323.
8 McCulloch WH: A certain archway: autoscopy and its companions seen in Western writing. Hist Psychiatry 1992;3:59–78.
9 Coleman SM: The phantom double: its psychological significance. Brit J M Psychol 1934;14:254–273.
10 Todd J, Dewhurst K: The double: its psychopathology and psychophysiology. J Nerv Ment Dis 1955;122:47–55.
11 Carp E: Troubles de l'image du corps. Acta Neurol Psychiatr Belg 1952;52:461–475.
12 Brugger P: Hostile interactions between body and self. Dialogues Clin Neurosci 2007;9:210–213.
13 Brugger P, Regard M, Landis T: Illusory reduplication of one's own body: phenomenology and classification of autoscopic phenomena. Cogn Neuropsychiatry 1997;2:19–38.
14 Rosset C: Le réel et son double. Paris, Gallimard, 1976.
15 Metzinger T: Out-of-body experiences as the origin of the concept of a 'soul'. Mind Matter 2005;3:57–84.
16 Brugger P: From phantom limb to phantom body. Varieties of extracorporeal awareness; in Knoblich G, Thornton I, Grosjean M, Shiffrar M (eds): Human Body Perception from the Inside Out. Oxford, Oxford University Press, 2006, pp 171–209.
17 Mikorey M: Fantômes et doubles. Paris, G. Doin, 1959/1952.
18 Blanke O: I and me: self-portraiture in brain damage; in Bogousslavsky J, Hennerici MG (eds): Neurological Disorders in Famous Artists – Part 2. Front Neurol Neurosci. Basel, Karger, 2007, vol 22, pp 14–29.
19 Boyer P: Intuitive expectations and the detection of mental disorder: a cognitive background to folk-psychiatries. Philos Psychol 2011;24:95–118.
20 Sperber D, Hirschfeld LA: The cognitive foundations of cultural stability and diversity. Trends Cogn Sci 2004;8:40–46.
21 Dehaene S, Cohen L: Cultural recycling of cortical maps. Neuron 2007;56:384–398.
22 Joshi ST (ed): Icons of Horror and the Supernatural: An Encyclopedia of Our Worst Nightmares. Westport, Greenwood Publishing Group, 2007.
23 Sangsue D: Fantômes, esprits et autres morts-vivants: essai de pneumatologie littéraire. Paris, José Corti, 2011.
24 Rogers R: A Psychoanalytical Study of the Double in Literature. Detroit, Wayne State University Press, 1970.
25 Guerard AJ: Concepts of the double; in Guerard AJ (ed): Stories of the Double. New York, JB Lippincott Company, 1967, pp 1–14.
26 Fonseca T: The doppelgänger; in Joshi ST (ed): Icons of Horror and the Supernatural: An Encyclopedia of Our Worst Nightmares. Westport, Greenwood Publishing Group, 2006, pp 187–213.
27 Jourde P, Tortonese P: Visages du double: un thème littéraire. Paris, Armand Colin, 2005.
28 Nabokov V: Strong Opinions. New York, McGraw-Hill, 1973.
29 Martín López R: Las manifestaciones del doble en la narrativa breve española contemporánea; thesis, Universidad Autónoma de Barcelona, Barcelona, 2006.
30 Dieguez S: Dr Jekyll et Mr Hyde: l'insupportable altérité. Cerveau Psycho 2010;42:76–81.
31 Christodoulou GN: The origins of the concept of 'doubles'. Bibliotheca Psychiatrica 1986;164:1–8.
32 Miyoshi M: The Divided Self: A Perspective on the Literature of the Victorians. New York, New York University Press, 1969.
33 Webber A: The Doppelgänger: Double Visions in German Literature. Oxford, Clarendon Press, 1996.
34 Rank O: Le Double. Paris, Petite Bibliothèque Payot, 1973/1919.
35 Dieguez S: Dorian Gray: la chute de narcisse. Cerveau Psycho 2011;44:80–86.
36 Rosset C: Fantasmagories. Paris, Minuit, 2006.
37 Dieguez S, Blanke O: Altered states of bodily consciousness; in Cardeña E, Winkelman M (eds): Altering Consciousness: A Multidisciplinary Perspective. Westport, Praeger, 2011, vol 2, pp 237–262.
38 Lopez C, Halje P, Blanke O: Body ownership and embodiment: vestibular and multisensory mechanisms. Neurophysiol Clin 2008;38:149–161.
39 de Vignemont F: Embodiment, ownership and disownership. Conscious Cogn 2011;20:82–93.
40 Wegner D: The Illusion of Conscious Will. Cambridge, MIT Press, 2002.

41 Marcel AJ: The Sense of Agency: Awareness and Ownership of Action; in Roessler J, Eilan N (eds): Agency and Self-Awareness: Issues in Philosophy and Psychology. Oxford, Clarendon Press, 2003, pp 48–93.
42 Gallagher S: Philosophical conceptions of the self: implications for cognitive science. Trends Cogn Sci 2000;4:14–21.
43 Neisser U: Five kinds of self-knowledge. Philos Psychol 1988;1:35–59.
44 Jeannerod M: The mechanism of self-recognition in humans. Behav Brain Res 2003;142:1–15.
45 Blanke O, Metzinger T: Full-body illusions and minimal phenomenal selfhood. Trends Cogn Sci 2009;13:7–13.
46 Markman K, Klein W, Suhr E (eds): Handbook of Mental Simulation and Human Imagination. Hove, Psychology Press, 2009.
47 Legrand D, Ruby P: What is self-specific? Theoretical investigation and critical review of neuroimaging results. Psychol Rev 2009;116:252–282.
48 Gibbs RW: Embodiment and Cognitive Science. Cambridge, Cambridge University Press, 2006.
49 Melzack R: Phantom limbs and the concept of a neuromatrix. Trends Neurosci 1990;13:88–92.
50 Berlucchi G, Aglioti SM: The body in the brain revisited. Exp Brain Res 2010;200:25–35.
51 Tsakiris M: My body in the brain: a neurocognitive model of body-ownership. Neuropsychologia 2010;48:703–712.
52 Maravita A, Iriki A: Tools for the body (schema). Trends Cogn Sci 2004;8:79–86.
53 Schilder P: L'image de notre corps. Paris, Gallimard, 1935.
54 Makin TR, Holmes NP, Ehrsson HH: On the other hand: dummy hands and peripersonal space. Behav Brain Res 2008;191:1–10.
55 De Preester H, Tsakiris M: Body-extension versus body-incorporation: is there a need for a body-model? Phenomenol Cogn Sci 2009;8:307–319.
56 Holmes NP, Spence C: Beyond the body schema: visual, prosthetic, and technological contributions to bodily perception and awareness; in Knoblich G, Thornton I, Grosjean M, Shiffrar M (eds): Human Body Perception from the Inside Out. Oxford, Oxford University Press, 2006, pp 15–64.
57 Botvinick M, Cohen J: Rubber hands 'feel' touch that eyes see. Nature 1998;391:756.
58 Tsakiris M, Haggard P: The rubber hand illusion revisited: visuotactile integration and self-attribution. J Exp Psychol Hum Percept Perform 2005;31:80–91.
59 Moseley GL, Olthof N, Venema A, Don S, Wijers M, Gallace A, Spence C: Psychologically induced cooling of a specific body part caused by the illusory ownership of an artificial counterpart. Proc Natl Acad Sci USA 2008;105:13169–13173.
60 Dieguez S, Mercier MR, Newby N, Blanke O: Feeling numbness for someone else's finger. Curr Biol 2009;19:R1108–R1109.
61 Aspell JE, Blanke O: Understanding the out-of-body experience from a neuroscientific perspective; in Murray CD (ed): Psychological Scientific Perspectives on Out of Body and Near Death Experiences. New York, Nova Science Publishers, 2009, pp 73–88.
62 Blanke O: Multisensory brain mechanisms of bodily self-consciousness. Nat Rev Neurosci 2012; 13:556–571.
63 Sforza A, Blanke O: Autoscopic phenomena: clinical and experimental perspectives; in Blom JD, Sommer IEC (eds): Hallucinations: Research and Practice. Berlin, Springer, 2012, pp 187–201.
64 Serino A, Haggard P: Touch and the Body. Neurosci Biobehav Rev 2010;34:224–236.
65 Menninger-Lerchenthal E: Der Eigene Doppelgänger. Bern, Huber, 1946.
66 Dieguez S, Staub F, Bogousslavsky J: Asomatognosia; in Godefroy O, Bogousslavsky J (eds): The Behavioral and Cognitive Neurology of Stroke. Cambridge, Cambridge University Press, 2007, pp 215–253.
67 Dieguez S, Annoni J-M: Asomatognosia: disorders of the bodily self; in Godefroy O (ed): Vascular Cognitive Impairment and Dementia: The Behavioral and Cognitive Neurology of Stroke, ed 2. Cambridge, Cambridge University Press, in press, chapter 13.
68 Blanke O, Arzy S, Landis T: Illusory reduplications of the human body and self. Handb Clin Neurol 2008;88:429–458.
69 Hécaen H, de Ajuriaguerra J: Méconnaissances et hallucinations corporelles. Paris, Masson, 1952.
70 Critchley M: The Parietal Lobes. New York, Hafner Press, 1953.
71 Lhermitte J: L'image de notre corps. Paris, L'Harmattan, 1939.
72 Bozzano E: Les phénomènes de bilocation. Paris, Jean Meyer, 1937.
73 Hilti LM, Brugger P: Incarnation and animation: physical versus representational deficits of body integrity. Exp Brain Res 2010;204:315–326.
74 Giummarra MJ, Gibson SJ, Georgiou-Karistianis N, Bradshaw JL: Central mechanisms in phantom limb perception: the past, present and future. Brain Res Rev 2007;54:219–232.

75 Khateb A, Simon SR, Dieguez S, Lazeyras F, Momjian-Mayor I, Blanke O, Landis T, Pegna AJ, Annoni JM: Seeing the phantom: a functional magnetic resonance imaging study of a supernumerary phantom limb. Ann Neurol 2009;65:698–705.
76 Shapiro MF, Fink M, Bender MB: Exosomesthesia or displacement of cutaneous sensation into extrapersonal space. AMA Arch Neurol Psy 1952;68:481–490.
77 Vallar G, Ronchi R: Somatoparaphrenia: a body delusion. A review of the neuropsychological literature. Exp Brain Res 2009;192:533–551.
78 Heydrich L, Dieguez S, Grunwald T, Seeck M, Blanke O: Illusory own body perceptions: case reports and relevance for bodily self-consciousness. Conscious Cogn 2010;19:702–710.
79 Blanke O, Mohr C: Out-of-body experience, heautoscopy, and autoscopic hallucinations of neurological origin: implications for neurocognitive mechanisms of corporeal awareness and self-consciousness. Brain Res Rev 2005;50:184–199.
80 Blanke O, Dieguez S: Leaving body and life behind: out-of-body and near-death experience; in Laureys S, Tononi G (eds): The Neurology of Consciousness: Cognitive Neuroscience and Neuropathology. Amsterdam, Elsevier, 2009, pp 303–325.
81 Brugger P, Mohr C: Out of the body, but not out of mind. Cortex 2009;45:137–140.
82 Brugger P: From haunted brain to haunted science. A cognitive neuroscience view of paranormal and pseudoscientific thought; in Houran J, Lange R (eds): Hauntings and Poltergeists: Multidisciplinary Perspectives. Jefferson, McFarland, 2001, pp 195–213.
83 Sollier P: Les Phénomènes d'Autoscopie. Paris, Alcan, 1903.
84 Devinsky O, Feldmann E, Burrowes K, Bromfield E: Autoscopic phenomena with seizures. Arch Neurol 1989;46:1080–1088.
85 Lunn V: Autoscopic phenomena. Acta Psychiat Scand 1970;46 (suppl 219):118–125.
86 Lukianowicz N: Autoscopic phenomena. Arch Neuro Psychiatr 1958;80:199–220.
87 Brugger P: Reflective mirrors: perspective-taking in autoscopic phenomena. Cogn Neuropsychiatry 2002;7:179–194.
88 Blanke O, Landis T, Spinelli L, Seeck M: Out-of-body experience and autoscopy of neurological origin. Brain 2004;127:243–258.
89 Blackmore SJ: Beyond the Body. An Investigation of Out-of-the-Body Experiences. Chicago, Academy Chicago Publishers, 1992/1982.
90 Dieguez S: NDE redux: skeptics need to reclaim, redefine and embrace near-death experiences. Skeptic 2008;14:42–43.
91 Geiger J: The Third Man Factor: Surviving the Impossible. New York, Weinstein, 2009.
92 Rosset C: Impressions fugitives: l'ombre, le reflet, l'écho. Minuit, Paris, 2004.
93 Thompson S: The Folktale. Berkeley, University of California Press, 1977.
94 Dieguez S: Le nez, une histoire complexe. . . Cerveau Psycho 2012;50:80–85.
95 Pavani F, Castiello U: Binding personal and extrapersonal space through body shadows. Nat Neurosci 2004;7:14–16.
96 Sforza A, Bufalari I, Haggard P, Aglioti SM: My face in yours: visuo-tactile facial stimulation influences sense of identity. Soc Neurosci 2010;5:148–162.
97 Dieguez S, Scherer J, Blanke O: My face through the looking-glass: the effect of mirror reversal on reflection-size estimation. Conscious Cogn 2011; 20:1452–1459.
98 Tsakiris M, Tajadura-Jiménez A, Costantini M: Just a heartbeat away from one's body: interoceptive sensitivity predicts malleability of body-representations. Proc Biol Sci 2011;278:2470–2476.
99 Faure H: Les appartenances du délirant: les investissements d'objets dans le vécu psychotique. Paris, R. Foulon, 1965.
100 Nemeroff C, Rozin P: The contagion concept in adult thinking in the United States: transmission of germs and interpersonal influence. Ethos 1994;22: 158–186.
101 Rosset C: Loin de moi: étude sur l'identité. Paris, Minuit, 1999.
102 Flammarion C: *La mort et son mystère: autour de la mort.* Paris, Ernest Flammarion, vol 2, 1921.
103 Dieguez S: Maupassant et la dissolution du soi; in Dieguez S (ed): Maux d'artistes: ce que cachent les oeuvres. Paris/Berlin, Pour la Science, 2010, pp 112–119.
104 Wigan AL: A new view of insanity: the duality of the mind proved by the structure, functions, and diseases of the brain, and by the phenomena of mental derangement, and shewn to be essential to moral responsibility. London, Longman, Brown, Green & Longmans, 1844.
105 Baumeister RF: Suicide as escape from self. Psychol Rev 1990;97:90–113.
106 Valli P: Suicide with fire-arms in front of the mirror: iconographic study. Minerva Medicoleg 1960; 80:165–167.
107 Riddick L, Mussell PG, Cumberland GD: The mirror's use in suicide. Am J Forensic Med Pathol 1989;10:14–16.
108 Kohlberg L: Psychological analysis and literary form: a study of the doubles in Dostoevsky. Daedalus 1963;92:345–362.

109 Hécaen H, Green A: Sur l'héautoscopie (à propos de quelques cas récents). Encéphale 1957;46:581–594.
110 Costantini M, Galati G, Romani GL, Aglioti SM: Empathic neural reactivity to noxious stimuli delivered to body parts and non-corporeal objects. Eur J Neurosci 2008;28:1222–1230.
111 Bradshaw JL, Mattingley JB: Allodynia: a sensory analogue of motor mirror neurons in a hyperaesthetic patient reporting instantaneous discomfort to another's perceived sudden minor injury? J Neurol Neurosurg Psychiatry 2001;70:135–136.
112 Montalan B, Lelard T, Godefroy O, Mouras H: Behavioral investigation of the influence of social categorization on empathy for pain: a minimal group paradigm study. Front Psychol 2012;3:389.
113 Brugger P, Agosti R, Regard M, Wieser WG, Landis T: Heautoscopy, epilepsy, and suicide. J Neurol Neurosurg Psychiatry 1994;57:838–839.
114 Siegel RK: Fire in the Brain. New York, Plume, 1992.
115 Anzellotti F, Onofrj V, Maruotti V, Ricciardi L, Franciotti R, Bonanni L, Thomas A, Onofrj M: Autoscopic phenomena: case report and review of literature. Behav Brain Funct 2011;7:2.
116 Arzy S, Blanke O: Out-of-body, out-of-time. Abnormal unity of body and self in space and time; in Buccheri R, Elitzur AC, Saniga M (eds): Endophysics, Time, Quantum and the Subjective. Hackensack, World Scientific Publishing Co, 2005, pp 507–530.
117 Brugger P, Blanke O, Regard M, Bradford DT, Landis T: Polyopic heautoscopy: case report and review of the literature. Cortex 2006;42:666–674.
118 Suedfeld P, Mocellin JS: The 'sensed presence' in unusual environments. Environ Behav 1987;19:33–52.
119 Brugger P, Regard M, Landis T: Unilaterally felt 'presences': the neuropsychiatry of one's invisible doppelgänger. Neuropsychiatry Neuropsychol Behav Neurol 1996;9:114–122.
120 Cheyne JA, Girard TA: The nature and varieties of felt presence experiences. Conscious Cogn 2007;16:984–991.
121 Nielsen T: Felt presence: paranoid delusion or hallucinatory social imagery? Conscious Cogn 2007;16:975–983.
122 Zijlmans M, van Eljsden P, Ferrier CH, Kho KH, van Rjen PC, Lejten FS: Illusory shadow person causing paradoxical gaze deviations during temporal lobe seizures. J Neurol Neurosurg Psychiatry 2009;80:686–688.
123 Arzy S, Seeck M, Ortigue S, Spinelli L, Blanke O: Induction of an illusory shadow person. Nature 2006;443:287.
124 Guérin B: Social Facilitation. Cambridge, Cambridge University Press, 1993.
125 Cheyne JA, Rueffer SD, Newby-Clark IR: Hypnagogic and hypnopompic hallucinations during sleep paralysis: neurological and cultural construction of the night-mare. Conscious Cogn 1999;8:319–337.
126 Kennedy DP, Gläscher J, Tyszka JM, Adolphs R: Personal space regulation by the human amygdala. Nat Neurosci 2009;12:1226–1227.
127 Gabbard GO, Twemlow AW: With the eyes of the mind: an empirical analysis of out-of-body states. New York, Praeger Scientific, 1984.
128 Irwin HJ: Flight of mind: a psychological study of the out-of-body experience. Metuchen, Scarecrow Press, 1985.
129 Rogo S (ed): Mind beyond the body: the mystery of ESP projection. New York, Penguin, 1978.
130 De Rochas A: L'extériorisation de la sensibilité: étude expérimentale et historique. Paris, Chamuel, 1895.
131 Lancelin C: Méthode de dédoublement personnel (extériorisation de la neuricité, sorties en astral). Paris, F. Sornot & F. Lanore, 1986/1913.
132 Broad CD: Lectures on psychical research. London, Routledge and Kegan Paul, 1967.
133 Dieguez S: NDE experiment: ethical concerns. Skeptical Inquirer 2009;33:44–48.
134 Augustine K: Does paranormal perception occur in near-death experiences? J Near-Death Stud 2007;25:203–236.
135 Blackmore SJ: Where am I? Perspectives in imagery and the out-of-body experience. J Mental Imagery 1987;11:53–66.
136 Terhune DB: The incidence and determinants of visual phenomenology during out-of-body experiences. Cortex 2009;45:236–242.
137 Braithwaite JJ, Samson D, Apperly I, Broglia E, Hulleman J: Cognitive correlates of the spontaneous out-of-body experience (OBE) in the psychologically normal population: evidence for an increased role of temporal-lobe instability, body-distortion processing, and impairments in own-body transformation. Cortex 2011;47:839–853.
138 Blanke O, Mohr C, Michel CM, Pascual-Leone A, Brugger P, Seeck M, Landis T, Thut G: Linking out-of-body experience and self processing to mental own-body imagery at the temporoparietal junction. J Neurosci 2005;25:550–557.
139 Irwin HJ: The disembodied self: an empirical study of dissociation and the out-of-body experience. J Parapsychol 2000;64:261–276.
140 Murray CD, Fox J: Dissociational body experiences: differences between respondents with and without prior out-of-body experiences. Brit J Psychol 2005;96:441–456.
141 Petkova VI, Ehrsson HH: If I were you: perceptual illusion of body swapping. PLoS One 2008;3:e3832.

142 Lenggenhager B, Tadi T, Metzinger T, Blanke O: Video ergo sum: manipulating bodily self-consciousness. Science 2007;317:1096–1099.
143 Slater M, Perez-Marcos D, Ehrsson HH, Sanchez-Vives MV: Towards a digital body: the virtual arm illusion. Front Hum Neurosci 2008;2:6.
144 Stratton GM: The spatial harmony of touch and sight. Mind 1899;8:492–505.
145 Dieguez S: 'A man can be destroyed but not defeated': Ernest Hemingway's near-death experience and declining health. Front Neurol Neurosci 2010;27:174–206.
146 Moody RA: Life after Life. Covington, Mockingbird Books, 1975.
147 Ring K: Life at Death: A Scientific Investigation of the Near-Death Experience. New York, Conward, McCann & Geoghegan, 1980.
148 Athappilly GK, Greyson B, Stevenson I: Do prevailing societal models influence reports of near-death experiences? A comparison of accounts reported before and after 1975. J Nerv Ment Dis 2006;194: 218–222.
149 Närhi J: Beautiful reflections: the cognitive and evolutionary foundations of paradise representations. Method Theory Study Religion 2008;20:339–365.
150 Siegel R: The psychology of life after death. Am Psychol 1980;35:911–931.
151 Marsh MN: Out-of-body and near-death experiences. Oxford, Oxford University Press, 2010.
152 Metzinger T: The Ego Tunnel. New York, Basic Books, 2009.
153 De Vignemont F, Tsakiris M, Haggard P: Body mereology; in Knoblich G, Thornton I, Grosjean M, Shiffrar M (eds): Human Body Perception from the Inside Out. New York, Oxford University Press, 2004, pp 147–170.
154 Schwabe L, Blanke O: The vestibular component in out-of-body experiences: a computational approach. Front Hum Neurosci 2008;2:17.
155 Ionta S, Heydrich L, Lenggenhager B, Mouthon M, Fornari E, Chapuis D, Gassert R, Blanke O: Multisensory mechanisms in temporo-parietal cortex support self-location and first-person perspective. Neuron 2011;70:363–374.
156 Bolognini N, Làdavas E, Farnè A: Spatial perspective and coordinate systems in autoscopy: a case report of a 'fantome de profil' in occipital brain damage. J Cogn Neurosci 2011;23:1741–1751.
157 Hufford DJ: The Terror That Comes in the Night. Philadelphia, University of Pennsylvania Press, 1982.
158 Hacking I: Mad Travelers: Reflections on the Reality of Transient Mental Illnesses. Charlottesville, University of Virginia Press, 1998.
159 Nabokov V: Lectures on Literature. New York, Harcourt, 1980/1948.

Sebastian Dieguez, PhD
Laboratory for Cognitive and Neurological Sciences, Unité de Neurologie
Département de Médecine, Université de Fribourg
PER 09 (salle 2.106), 5 chemin du Musée, CH–1700 Fribourg (Switzerland)
E-Mail sebastian.dieguez@unifr.ch

Bogousslavsky J, Dieguez S (eds): Literary Medicine: Brain Disease and Doctors in Novels, Theater, and Film.
Front Neurol Neurosci. Basel, Karger, 2013, vol 31, pp 116–125 (DOI: 10.1159/000343265)

# Van Gogh's Disease in the Light of His Correspondence

Piet H.A. Voskuil

Hans Berger Clinic for Epilepsy, Oosterhout, The Netherlands

**Abstract**

The literary quality of Vincent van Gogh's correspondence is widely recognized. He wrote expressively and evocatively, and had great literary knowledge. In this essay we follow his medical history in many quotes from in his letters to see how Vincent expressed his complaints, knowledge, and emotions connected with his disease. The symptoms became most clear after December 1888. In the beginning, Van Gogh hesitated to tell much about his ailment, but gradually painted in the letters his experiences, making use of the intermittent course of his cycloid psychoses. We will see an indication that, in the network that mediated Van Gogh's brain (dys)function, elements of synesthesia, prosopagnosia, and spatial agnosia might have been activated. Van Gogh's affinity for poetry, already in his early twenty's, makes the hypothesis of a, by epileptic discharges, kindled temporal lobe at most only part of the complex interpretation of this creative and suffering mind.



## The Correspondence

The correspondence of Vincent van Gogh (1853–1890) can be split into two parts: the letters he wrote himself (819 in all, 651 of them to his brother Theo and 7 to Theo and his wife Jo) and those he received (83, including 39 from Theo and 2 from Theo and Jo). His letters became widely known and ultimately received the interest and admiration they deserve. They are a rich source of information about Van Gogh's life story and work, and there was soon broad recognition of the literary qualities of his writing even by his contemporaries.

Gauguin described him once as 'a man obsessed by literature' and Van der Veen [1] found that Van Gogh mentioned more than 150 authors of some ten countries and had read at least 200 works in four different languages.

Van Gogh's colleague and friend Emile Bernard was so impressed by Vincent's literary style that he published extracts from his letters in the *Mercure de France* as early as 1893 and a collection of them in 1911. On that occasion he said: '. . .what does it matter if his style is not correct, it is alive and our indulgence will sense how to pay delicate attention to it.'

The poet W.H. Auden [2], who published an anthology with a brief foreword, wrote (1961): 'there is scarcely one letter by Van Gogh which I, who am certainly no expert, do not find fascinating.'

Jan Hulsker [3], for decades an authority on Van Gogh's correspondence, unreservedly placed the letters on the level of world literature: 'Vincent was able to express himself splendidly, and it is this remarkable writing talent that has secured his letters their lasting place in world literature, quite apart from their importance for the study of his life and work. . . . In many letters his emotions and beliefs are expressed so strongly and convincingly that a "real" writer could hardly have improved upon them.' This view is shared by Ronald de Leeuw [4] who speaks of 'the evocative power and unique integrity' of the letters.

Jansen et al. [5] in their splendid new complete and annotated edition of the letters (2009) say: 'If, under the essence of literature, one understands that it expresses the generally valid through the specific, the 'condition humaine', then it cannot be denied that Van Gogh's letters are indeed highly literary.'[1]

## The Disease

There is an on-going debate about the best diagnosis of Van Gogh's disease. The doctors who treated him diagnosed it as epilepsy. This was of course based on the concepts of this ailment in the 19th century. Felix Rey who treated him in the hospital in Arles (from Dec. 1888 to May 1889) was a fellow student of Aussoleil who wrote a thesis in 1890 on 'epilepsie larvée' (masked epilepsy). This terminology was given in a concept of Morel [6]. The observations of Rey are documented in letters to Theo. On December 29, 1888 he wrote:

> The day before yesterday he went to lie down in another patient's bed and would not leave it, despite my comments. In his night-shirt he chased the Sister on duty and absolutely forbids anyone at all to go near his bed. Yesterday he got up and went to wash in the coal-box.

On December 30, 1888 he wrote:

> When I tried to get him to talk about the motive that drove him to cut off his ear, he replied that it was a purely personal matter.

[1] In this chapter the quotes from the letters will be numbered as in the edition of Jansen et al. [5]. The English translation and annotation of this book can be found in the related website: www.vangoghletters.org.

On February 12, 1889 he wrote:

> He is less delirious, and he recognises me. He talks to me about painting, but sometimes he loses his train of thought and speaks nothing but disjointed words and jumbled phrases.

Acting on orders from the Chief of Police, Dr. Albert Delon examined Van Gogh on February 7, 1889. Delon was a member of the hospital board and employed as a doctor by the Bureau de Bienfaisance (L'Indicateur Marseillais 1889). He wrote the following in his report:

> I found this man in a state of extreme excitement, suffering from a true delirium, pronouncing incoherent words, only momentarily recognising the people around him. He is subject in particular to auditory hallucinations (he hears voices uttering reproaches against him) and to an 'idée fixe', according to which is supposed to have been the victim of an attempted poisoning.

In the medical files from the asylum Saint-Paul-de-Mausole in St. Remy where Vincent was admitted on May 6, 1889, we find detailed facts in the protocols concerning his admission to and dismissal from the asylum.

The asylum's physician, Dr. Theophile Peyron, examined Van Gogh and recorded his findings on the 9th and 25th of May 1889. On May 9, 1889 he wrote in the admissions register: 'I consider that Mr van Gogh is subject to attacks of epilepsy, separated by long intervals, and that it is advisable to place him under long-term observation in the institution.'

If one analyses the sources for description of the symptoms carefully in the light of modern insights into epilepsy, one must doubt the accuracy of Peyron's diagnosis. It is clear that beginning in December 1888, Van Gogh had eight episodic psychoses or according to others [7] better called cycloid psychoses. However, only in a few cases is there enough evidence of any relationship with epileptic seizures.

One seizure, which occurred early in 1890, was described by Poulet, one of Van Gogh's guards in St. Remy to the Van Gogh biographer Marc Edo Tralbaut [8]: 'Another day, when he went to fetch Vincent for dinner, Poulet found him with staring eyes and foaming lips; he had been trying to eat his paints. Three tubes of them.'

Another guard, Trabuc, might have witnessed a seizure on July 16, 1889. While studying that case we see that the sources of the medical history cannot always be taken for granted. We will discuss this in more detail later.

The aim of this chapter is not primarily to discuss Van Gogh's diagnosis (for this I refer the reader to earlier publications [9, 10]). To summarize some conclusions from studies of this author: In Van Gogh's case his personality disorder and later on the recurrent psychoses can be based on functional disturbances in networks of the prefrontal and limbic circuits of the brain. His personality showed elements of the Gastaut-Geschwind syndrome. The occurrence of symptoms was probably triggered

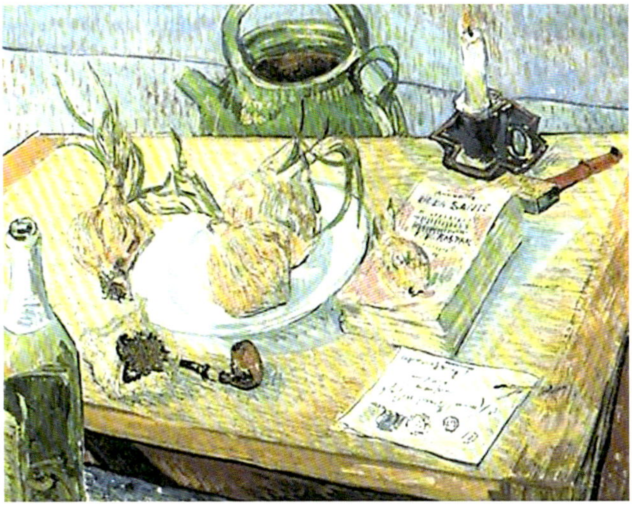

**Fig. 1.** Vincent van Gogh, *Still Life with a Plate of Onions* (begin January 1889, oil on canvas), Collection Kröller-Müller Museum, Otterlo, the Netherlands. Reprinted with kind permission. The book in the painting is *Annuaire de la Santé* (written by Dr. François Vincent Raspail and promoting camphor against hallucinations and nightmares). Van Gogh painted it (F 604/JH1656) shortly after his first admission. The envelope is probably Theo's letter which arrived on December 23, 1888, when Van Gogh cut off his left ear.

by interaction of genetic disposition and environmental factors such as emotional stress, alcohol, thujone (absinth), and physical exhaustion. According to developing knowledge, by consequences of periodic epileptiform discharges in the aforementioned networks, there might have been an interaction between these epileptic phenomena and paroxysmal disturbances of consciousness, behavioral changes, and episodic psychosis. Only on a few occasions in Van Gogh's medical history is the evidence for such an interaction convincing.

## The Disease in His Correspondence (Vincent's Anamnesis)

The earliest known letter is on September 29, 1872, and the last a few days before he died on July 29, 1890. He wrote much on health-related problems, but I must limit myself to a period starting with a letter on January 7, 1889.

On December 23, 1888 Van Gogh cut off part of his left earlobe. On that day he possibly received the letter from his brother Theo as depicted in 'Still life with onions and Annuaire de la Santé' (fig. 1), probably painted a few weeks later. In *The Art Newspaper* (2009), journalist Martin Baily speculated that the letter might have influenced the start of the psychotic state that developed on that day. He was admitted to the hospital Hôtel Dieu in Arles. On that occasion he did not want to speak much on his ailment and did not want to alarm his family too much.

> I've written a line to Mother and to Wil *which I addressed to our sister* with the sole aim of reassuring them, should you have happened to mention to them that I had been ill. For your part, simply tell them that I've been a bit ill like the time when I had the clap in The Hague, and that I got myself treated at the hospital. But that it's not worth the trouble of mentioning, since

I got off with a fright and that I was only in the aforesaid or mentioned hospital for a few days (732).

A few weeks later, he wrote:

Just a few words to tell you that I'm getting along so-so as regards my health and work.

Which I already find astonishing when I compare my state today with that of a month ago. I well knew that one could break one's arms and legs before, and that then afterwards that could get better but I didn't know that one could break one's brain and that afterwards that got better too.

. . .the unbearable hallucinations have stopped for now, reducing themselves to a simple nightmare on account of taking potassium bromide (743).

At the end of April 1889, shortly before he was admitted in St. Remy (on his own wish), Vincent wrote to his sister Wilhelmina (Wil):

In all I've had 4 big crises in which I hadn't the slightest idea of what I said, wanted, did.

Not counting that I fainted 3 times previously without plausible reason, and not retaining the least memory of what I felt then (764).

I can't precisely describe what the thing I have is like, there are terrible fits of anxiety sometimes – without any apparent cause – or then again a feeling of emptiness and fatigue in the mind (764).

Every day I take the remedy that the incomparable Dickens prescribes against suicide. It consists of a glass of wine, a piece of bread and cheese and a pipe of tobacco. It isn't complicated, you'll tell me, and you don't think that my melancholy comes close to that place, however at moments. . . (764).

On May 9, 1889 Van Gogh was admitted to the asylum Saint-Paul-de-Mausole in St. Remy. On the day of admission he wrote to his brother:

I wanted to tell you that I think I've done well to come here, first, in seeing the *reality* of the life of the diverse mad or cracked people in this menagerie, I'm losing the vague dread, the fear of the thing. And little by little I can come to consider madness as being an illness like any other. Then the change of surroundings is doing me good, I imagine.

As far as I know the doctor here is inclined to consider what I've had as an attack of an epileptic nature. But I haven't made any enquiries (772).

On July 16 while painting a quarry outside the asylum (fig. 2, 3) he had an attack witnessed by his guard Trabuc (fig. 4). Gastaut [11] described the seizure: 'it started with a contraction of one hand and a blank stare ['crispation de la main et un air haggard'] before he fell down.' Of course, this is very suspect for an epileptic seizure. Asked for his source, Gastaut told that after leaving his clinic in 1984 he had destroyed nearly all his archives (personal communication, 1988).

What do we know from Vincent's letters about this event? After a prolonged and intermittent recovery, on August 22 he wrote to Theo:

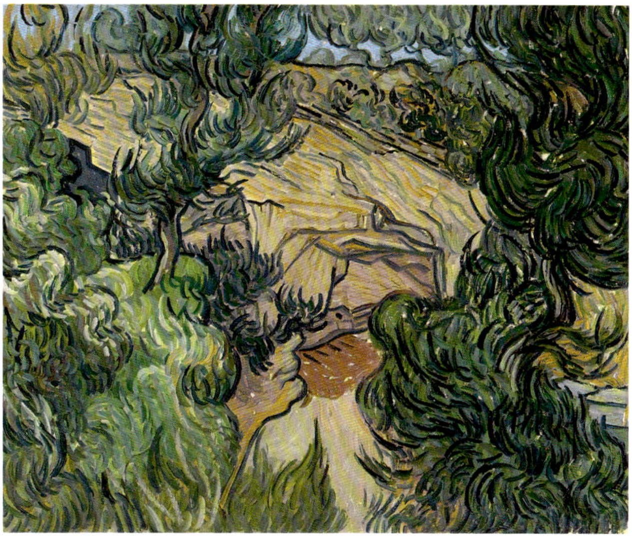

**Fig. 2.** Vincent van Gogh, *The Entrance to a Quarry*, 1889 (F744, JH1802). Reprinted with kind permission from the Van Gogh Museum Amsterdam, the Netherlands.

3

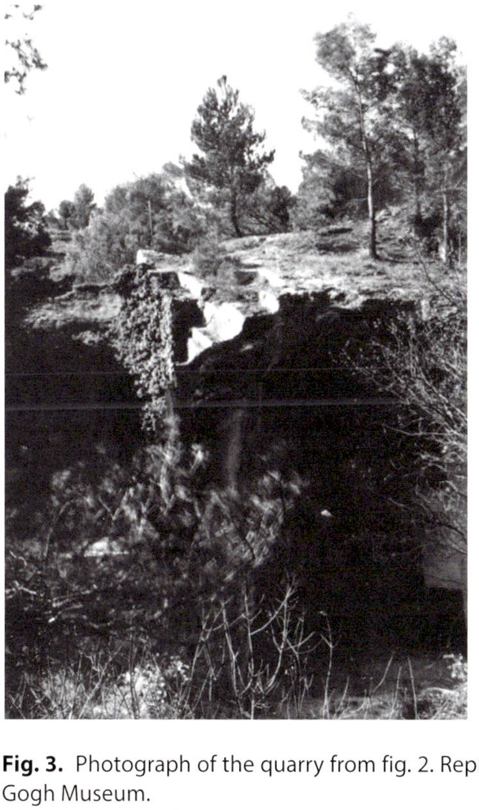

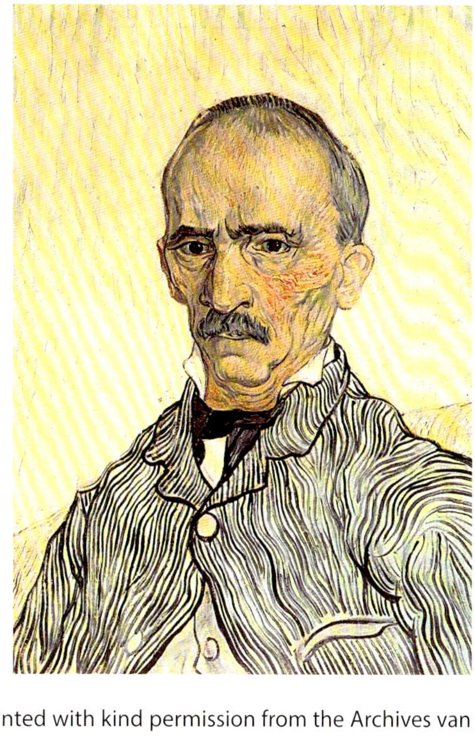

4

**Fig. 3.** Photograph of the quarry from fig. 2. Reprinted with kind permission from the Archives van Gogh Museum.
**Fig. 4.** Painting by Van Gogh of Charles-Elzéard Trabuc, 1889 (F629, JH1774). Kunstmuseum Solothurn, Solothurn, Switzerland. Reprinted with kind permission.

This new crisis, my dear brother, came upon me in the fields, and when I was in the middle of painting on a windy day. I'll send you the canvas, which I nevertheless finished. And it was precisely a more sober attempt, matt in colour without looking impressive, broken greens, reds and rusty ochre yellows, as I told you that from time to time I felt a desire to begin again with a palette like the one in the north (797) (fig. 5a).

. . .knowing that you wish me to write you a line I'm letting you know that it's very difficult for me to write, so disturbed is my mind. So I'm taking advantage of an interval (797) (fig. 5a).

For many days I've been absolutely distraught, as in Arles, just as much if not worse, and it's to be presumed that these crises will recur in the future, it is ABOMINABLE. I haven't been able to eat for 4 days, as my throat is swollen (797) (fig. 5b).

It appears that I pick up filthy things and eat them, although my memories of these bad moments are vague, and it appears to me that there's something shady about it, still for the same reason that they have I don't know what prejudice against painters here. I no longer see any possibility for courage or good hope, but anyway it wasn't yesterday that we found out that this profession isn't a happy one (797) (fig. 5b).

This medical history as told by Vincent is far from complete, but to finish it is good to show once more an example of his own extensive reading. In a long letter to his sister Wil, to whom he seems to have a special affection, he wrote on October 21, 1889:

'I had read an article on Dostoevsy, who had written a book, *Souvenirs de la maison des morts,* and that spurred me on to begin work again on a large study that I'd begun in the fever ward in Arles. But it's annoying to paint figures without models.'

In the same letter we find interesting indications for experiences in the field of prosopagnosia and spatial agnosia.

I've read another of Carmen Sylva's ideas [*Les pensées d'une reine*], which is very true: when you suffer a lot – you see everybody at a great distance, and as if at the far end of an immense arena – the very voices seem to come from a long way off. I've experienced this in these crises to such a point that all the people I see then seem to me, *even if I recognize them* – which isn't always the case – to come from very far away and to be *entirely different* from what they are in reality, so much do I then seem to see in them pleasant or unpleasant resemblances to people I've known in other times and places (812).

### A Complicated Mind

In 1884, Van Gogh gave painting lessons to Anton C. Kerssemakers (1846–1926) who was a tanner and amateur artist. In his *Reminiscences of Vincent van Gogh* Kerssemakers [12] wrote:

He [Vincent] was always comparing painting to music, and in order to gain an even better understanding of the value and nuances of the tones, he began to take piano lessons with an old music teacher who was also the organist in E[indhoven]. This did not last long, however because during the lessons Van Gogh incessantly compared the tones of the piano with Prussian blue and

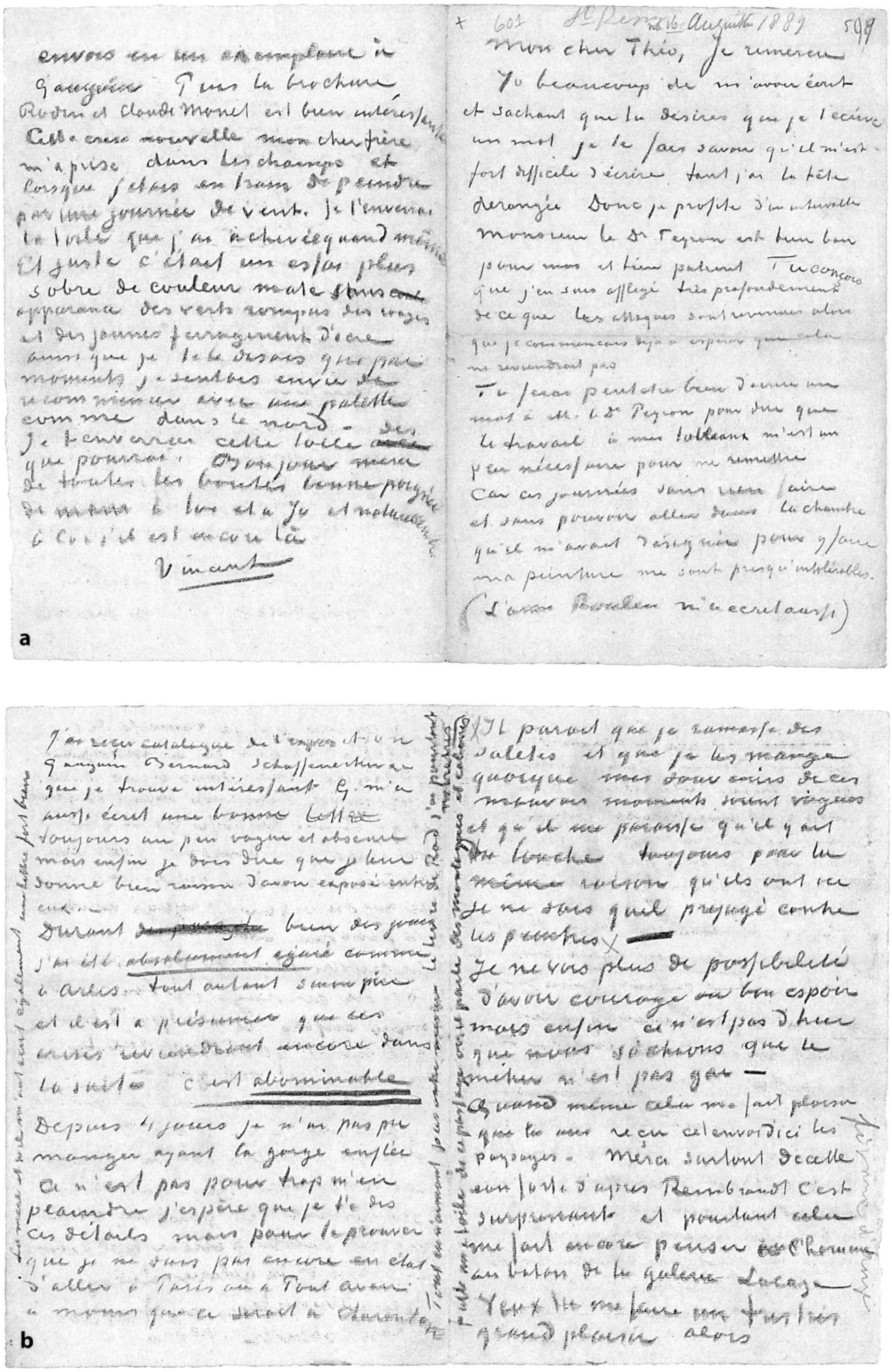

**Fig. 5. a,b** Letter 797 describes a crisis that occurred while painting a quarry on July 16, 1889. Reprinted with kind permission from the Van Gogh Museum Amsterdam, the Netherlands.

dark green, or dark ochre with bright cadmium, so that the good man thought he was dealing with a madman and became so afraid of him that he discontinued the lessons.

Is this a case of synesthesia? Maybe, but in Van Gogh's case we must never forget to look with the eye of an art historian, too. On October 10, 1930 another amateur art apprentice of Van Gogh, Dimmen Gestel [13] wrote:

> Toon Kers[semakers] and Van de Wakker [another apprentice] told me lately, how conscientiously Vincent studied chromatics from books by Delacroix and others, who related colours and music. I am told, that Vincent attached much importance to this and actually wished to convince himself, how far colours and tones were interrelated, and that's why he took piano-lessons from Van der Sande [= Hein van der Zande, 1820–1903].

Some authors (Gastaut [11], Trimble [14]) suppose that Van Gogh had personality traits of hypergraphia and hyperreligiosity, in keeping with the features of the Gastaut-Geschwind (Gastaut called it 'Waxman-Geschwind') syndrome, being part of a functional brain disorder by kindling of the temporal lobe in patients with epilepsy. Trimble even suggested that 'the prodigious output of his paintings (that averaged an oil painting approximately every other day in six years after 1884) was a variant of the hypergraphia.'

One can question whether this hypothesis of a kindled temporal lobe is not going too far afield in medical terms since already in 1875 Van Gogh was copying verses of poets he had read and compiling them in poetry albums for his brother Theo and the artist Matthijs Maris [15].

It is intriguing to see that in some way he already seems to predict his own fate in a copy taken from *L'oiseau*. This is a translation by Michelet of a poem by Friedrich Rückert (who was the maternal grandfather of Hans Berger, founder of the electroencephalography!). The lark is compared by Rückert to an artist:

> ... all its merits, all its defects in him are superabundant. He is mild and timid, mistrustful but not at all cunning. He takes no heed to his safety and travels alone. He is burningly jealous ...
>
> 'He will break his heart to sing' says one of his historians. He listens; he takes up his abode, especially where an echo exists, to listen and reply. Nervous to an excess, one sees him in captivity sometimes sleeping long through the day with perturbing dreams; sometimes struggling, starting up, and wildly battling. He is subject to nervous attacks and epilepsy. [...] Thus love and light are undoubtedly his point of departure; but art itself, the love of the beautiful, confusedly seen in glimpses, and very keenly felt, are a second aliment, which sustains his soul, and supplies it with a new inspiration. And this is boundless – a day opened onto the infinite.
>
> The true greatness of the artist consists in overshooting his mark, in doing more than he willed; and moreover in passing far beyond the goal, in crossing the limits of the possible, and looking beyond-beyond.
>
> Hence arise great sorrows, in inexhaustible source of melancholy; hence the sublime folly of weeping for misfortunes which he has never experienced (Translation into English by Wouter van der Veen [1]).

In conclusion, creativity and deep emotions live side by side in the same brain that mediated Van Gogh's disease. In this neurobiological framework, many facilitating and disturbing factors interacted in a complex causal relationship. Van Gogh's beautiful art in the form of letters, paintings, and drawings remain for us to enjoy.

## References


1 Van der Veen W: Van Gogh: A Literary Mind. Van Gogh Studies 2. Amsterdam, Waanders Publishers, Zwolle/van Gogh Museum, 2009.
2 Auden WH (ed): Van Gogh: A Selfportrait. Letters Revealing His Life as a Painter. New York, Marlowe & Company, 1961, p 5.
3 Hulsker J: The letters; in Van Uitert E, Hoyle M (eds): The Rijksmuseum Vincent van Gogh. Cat. Amsterdam. Amsterdam, Meulenhof/Landshoff, 1987, pp 51–58.
4 De Leeuw R: De brieven van Vincent van Gogh. Amsterdam, Bert Bakker, 2003, p 14.
5 Jansen L, Luijten H, Bakker N (eds): Vincent van Gogh – De brieven. Van Gogh Museum, Huygens Instituut. Amsterdam, Amsterdam University Press, 2009. www.vangoghletters.org.
6 Morel BA: D'une forme de délire,suite d'une surexicitation nerveuse se ratachant à une variété non encore décrite d'épilepsie (épilepsie larvée). Gazette hebdomadaire de medicine et chirurgie 1860;7:773–775, 819–821, 836–841.
7 Leonhard K, Beckmann (ed): Classification of Endogenous Psychoses and Their Differentiated Etiology, second revised and enlarged edition. Vienna, Springer, 1999.
8 Tralbaut ME: Vincent van Gogh. Lausanne, Edita, 1974, pp 288–290.
9 Voskuil P: Vincent van Gogh's malady: a test case for the relationship between temporal lobe dysfunction and epilepsy? J Hist Neurosci 1992;1:155–162.
10 Voskuil P: The illness of Vincent van Gogh (letter to the editor and author's response). J Hist Neurosci 2005;14:169–176.
11 Gastaut H: La maladie de Vincent van Gogh, envisagée à la lumière des conceptions nouvelles sur l'épilepsie psychomotrice. Annales Méd Psychol (Paris) 1956;2:1–43.
12 Kerssemakers A: Reminiscences of Vincent van Gogh; in: De Amsterdammer, weekblad voor Nederland (de Groene), April 14 and 21, 1912; in: Verzamelde brieven van Vincent van Gogh. Wereldbibliotheek 1974;3:92–97.
13 Gestel D: Vincent van Gogh en eenige persoonlijke herinneringen aan hem; in: Het Eindhovensch dagblad October 10th,1930; in: Verzamelde brieven van Vincent van Gogh. Wereldbibliotheek 1974;3:90–91.
14 Trimble M: The Soul in the Brain. The Cerebral Basis of Language, Art and Belief. Baltimore, John Hopkins University Press, 2007, p 153.
15 Pabst F (ed): Vincent van Gogh's Poetry Albums. Amsterdam, Waanders, Zwolle, Rijksmuseum Vincent van Gogh, 1988, p 16.



Piet H.A. Voskuil, MD
Neurologist
Torendreef 14
NL–4851 BH Ulvenhout (The Netherlands)
E-Mail p.voskuil@wxs.nl

Bogousslavsky J, Dieguez S (eds): Literary Medicine: Brain Disease and Doctors in Novels, Theater, and Film.
Front Neurol Neurosci. Basel, Karger, 2013, vol 31, pp 126–136 (DOI: 10.1159/000343255)

# Migraine and Metaphor

Joost Haan

Department of Neurology, Rijnland Hospital and Leiden University Medical Centre, Leiderdorp/Leiden, The Netherlands

**Abstract**

The metaphors of migraine make it a challenging source of inspiration for writers of fiction. The visual aura is a hallucination, the outside world – the so-called 'reality' – is distorted. The excruciating pain can stand for horror, punishment, and fate. Photophobia, phonophobia, and osmophobia underline visual, acoustic, and olfactoric stimuli. The protagonist sees, hears, and smells more, but not always better. Paradoxically, this increased awareness of 'reality' results in a need to seek isolation. Often, the end of a migraine attack is like a rescue. Immediately after an attack the fear of the next one begins. As migraine is hereditary, there are also aspects of solidarity, but shame and blame are nearby.



Many novels contain characters with migraine, in some of them migraine is a major theme. Descriptions of auras can be found in James Lasdun's *The Horned Man* and Siri Hustvedt's *The Blindfold. Alice in Wonderland* is associated with childhood auras. Metaphors of pain can be found in Thomas Mann's *Doctor Faustus* and Irvin Yalom's *When Nietzsche Wept*. Ian McEwan's *Atonement* contains a remarkable role for phonophobia. In Mark Salzman's *Lying Awake* migraine is the wrong diagnosis.

For many, migraine is a mysterious disease. Migraine sufferers look and behave normal and even during an attack hardly anything abnormal can be seen 'from the outside'. The most typical part of migraine – the aura – cannot be perceived by others [1]. As a consequence, a diagnosis of migraine is solely and completely based on the narrative of the patient. Migraine depends on language, but linguistic signs are arbitrary. The relation of words with reality is problematic [2].

Pain is strongly associated with metaphors [3, 4]. The same is true for the aura and the 'phobias' [5]. The various metaphoric aspects of migraine make it a challenging source of inspiration for fiction. What else do writers want than symbols of horror, punishment, rescue, distorted reality, unpredictability? Of the many novels that contain descriptions of characters with migraine, here some remarkable examples will be given.

## Misleading Phonophobia in Ian McEwan's *Atonement*

In Ian McEwan's novel *Atonement* [6], nothing is as it seems. During a family party the 13-year-old Briony Tallis witnesses the romance between her sister Cecilia and Robbie, the son of the cleaning lady. Briony secretly watches the two lovers, but does not understand exactly what is going on. She fills in the events with her fantasy. As later that evening a girl is raped, Briony sees a glimpse of the attacker running away. In her perception it must have been Robbie. This accusation causes a row of occurrences with serious life-long implications for many of the characters. Only in the end does Briony realize that she might have been wrong, and that it might all have been a part of her fantasy, but her atonement comes too late.

In chapter six of the novel, Emily Tallis, the mother of Briony and Cecilia, retreats to her room during the party. She feels a migraine attack coming.

> Not long after lunch, once she was assured that her sister's children and Briony had eaten sensibly and would keep their promise to stay away from the pool for at least two hours, Emily Tallis had withdrawn from the white glare of the afternoon's heat to a cool and dark bedroom. She was not in pain, not yet, but she was retreating before its threat. There were illuminated points in her vision, little pinpricks, as though the worn fabric of the visible world was being held up against a far brighter light. She felt in the top right corner of her brain a heaviness, the inert body weight of some curled and sleeping animal; but when she touched her head and pressed, the presence disappeared from the coordinates of actual space. Now it was in the top right corner of her mind, and in her imagination she could stand on tiptoe and raise her right hand to it. It was important, however, not to provoke it; once this lazy creature moved from the periphery to the center, then the knifing pains would obliterate all thought, and there would be no chance of dining with Leon and the family tonight. It bore her no malice, this animal, it was indifferent to her misery. It would move as a caged panther might: because it was awake, out of boredom, for the sake of movement itself, or for no reason at all, and with no awareness. She lay supine on her bed without a pillow, a glass of water within reach and, at her side, a book she knew she could not read. A long, blurred strip of daylight reflected on the ceiling above the pelmet was all that broke the darkness. She lay rigidly apprehensive, held at knifepoint, knowing that fear would not let her sleep and that her only hope was in keeping still.

Lying in her bed, she hears all kind of noises from the house and tries to interpret them. The house is creaking, Emily 'rested her palm against her forehead, and heard another tick as the building shrank tighter.' From below she hears a metallic clang, from upstairs the thud of feet. She hears energetic scuffling and something hard rattling across the floorboards.

Emily feels guilty, illness has stopped her giving her children all a mother should.

> Migraine, mother love and, over the years, many hours of lying still on her bed, had distilled from this sensitivity a sixth sense, a tentacular awareness that reached out from the dimness and moved through the house, unseen and all-knowing.

She hears the murmur of voices and a conversation that penetrates a wall, she hears doors opening and closing, a tread on the stairs, the sound of the trap on the gravel, someone struggling with luggage, a man's voice in the nursery, and she knows what all these sounds mean. 'She lay in the dark and knew everything.'

In the end, however, all her interpretations appear to be wrong. With her migrainous sensitivity to sound, she registers everything that is happening in her house, but it does not help her to interpret these perceptions correctly. On the contrary, she has no idea of the real drama that is taking place, and not only misses any true perception of the situation, but also appears (again) to be a bad (absent) mother for her daughters, even at this crucial moment in their lives.

McEwan's migraine metaphors are astonishing, from the pinpricks in Emily's visual field to the heaviness in her brain. Migraine is described as a sleeping animal, a lazy creature, a caged panther that – once awaked – causes 'knifing pains'. Briony incorrectly interprets the occurrences because of her youth and her excess of fantasy, Emily does the same because of her migraine. The following questions arise: 'What is reality and what fiction?', 'Whose atonement are we reading about?', and 'Must a migraine sufferer feel guilty?'

### An Aura as Hold: *The Horned Man* by James Lasdun

Lawrence Miller, the protagonist of the literary thriller *The Horned Man* by James Lasdun [7] is professor of Gender Studies at the Arthur Clay University, and also a member of the Sexual Harassment Committee of that university. Lately, he has got into trouble. His wife has left him, and now accuses him of stalking. Since the divorce, Lawrence lives alone and can hardly take care of himself. At work, he anxiously tries to avoid contact with female students, afraid that they will accuse him of sexual harassment. When he has to talk to one of them, he leaves the door of his room wide open, so that passers-by can look in, and witness that nothing irregular is taking place. Nevertheless, Lawrence blushes frequently during such conversations. A short affair with a female colleague ends in an accusation of rape. As a result of all these disturbances, Lawrence has to visit his (female and attractive) psychiatrist very often.

Then, strange things start to happen. A bookmark has been moved, there are unknown numbers on Lawrence's telephone bill, a coin disappears from his room. Lawrence finds out that his predecessor at the University – a woman – has been murdered; he finds her clothes in his room.

Then he gets an attack:

> Abruptly, before I had finished the story, a small, pulsating silver spot appeared in the corner of my field of vision.
>
> I hadn't experienced this phenomenon since I was twelve or thirteen, but I recognised it immediately, and put the book down with a feeling of alarm.
>
> The spot began to grow, as I had feared it would, flickering and pulsating across my vision like a swarm of angry insects. . . After a while all I could see were a few peripheral slivers of the ceiling and walls surrounding me. And then for a minute or two I became completely blind.

Shortly hereafter, his head begins to throb with an intense ache. He has to lay down on his bed in darkness. Sounds of the upper floor irritate him. Lawrence has an attack of migraine with aura. He knows these from his youth, but has not had them for a long time.

Even more strange occurrences follow. Without purpose, Lawrence is a voyeur of a woman in his own room, he talks to a woman in Central Park who later is murdered, he tries to find out who murdered his predecessor at the university but is accused himself, and he searches for his ex-wife in a shelter for victims of domestic abuse wearing woman's clothes.

Later in the story Lawrence has a second attack of migraine with aura. A flickering silver light spreads across his field of vision like 'a great, sunlit shoal of mackerel', and is followed by a pounding ache, hammering in his skull. Not long after this attack, a thick, white, horn-like protrusion grows out of his forehead. Miller is the horned man.

It is clear that Lawrence Miller is confused, and because of the first person narrative, we, the readers, are confused too. What is real, what is hallucination? Who is guilty? Who is the victim? In fact, the only 'realistic' and therefore understandable parts of the novel are the two perfectly described migraine attacks. In this enigmatic novel, only migraine offers a 'hold' to reality.

### A Wrong Diagnosis: *Lying Awake* by Mark Salzman and *The Dark Half* by Stephen King

In Mark Salzman's novel *Lying Awake*, Sister John of the Cross has what many headache sufferers fear: a brain tumor [8]. In 1969 she entered the Order of Discalced Carmelites. In the following years, it became clear that she was a shy and unremarkable member of the order. After several years she has lost her motivation and inspiration, and she has doubts about her vocation: 'her heart felt squeezed dry' and 'God thirsted, but she had nothing to offer.'

Then, in 1994, her attacks began.

> The left side of her vision got blurry, and her fingers felt stiff. The doctor had assured her that these were common migraine symptoms, and that the best thing to do when the headaches struck

was not to struggle against them. 'Just try to relax,' he said, 'breathe deeply and let it happen. Surrender to it. You're a contemplative; think of it as spiritual exercise.'

*Remember what Christ endured.*

*Hang on.*

The headache attacks become more frequent, from twice a month to every other day, they seem to come in cycles. Then the attacks start to be accompanied by hallucinations and visions of God. Sister John has ecstatic mystical experiences. When she writes these down, her books become a great success. She becomes of great importance for the order, as the books sell well. A second doctor is consulted when the attacks also lead to loss of consciousness. It becomes clear that Sister John suffers from epilepsy and headache from a temporal meningioma. After difficult considerations, she decides for an operation. Her 'migraine' and her epilepsy, but also her divine inspiration, disappear. She points to the bandage around her head. 'When they took this out, my muse went with it.'

*Lying Awake* is said to be an illustration of how narrative fiction can engage readers in exploring social, psychological, and spiritual dimensions of a patient's subjective experience of illness and suffering [9]. Among other important themes, it illustrates the fear patients suffering from headaches have of a 'serious' disease.

Murder and violence seem to be the 'muse' of Stephen King. In the thriller *The Dark Half*, the protagonist Thad Beaumont has suffered severe headache attacks since his youth [10]. The pain is unbearable, makes him nauseous, and forces him to lay down in a dark room. Before the attacks Thad hears the singing of a thousand birds. The doctor thinks of migraine, but after an epileptic fit this diagnosis is changed: Thad has a brain tumor. At operation the tumor appears to be 'benign', consisting of the remnants of Thad's rudimentary twin brother.

The headaches disappear, but a bloodcurdling story starts.

### Migraine Headache as Purification: *When Nietzsche Wept* by Irvin Yalom

The German philosopher Friedrich Nietzsche (1844–1900) probably suffered from migraine. He had as many as 120 attacks per year [11], so that 'any given year contained two hundred days of pain' [12].

> 'Do I in any way profit from this misery?' Nietzsche finally responded. 'I have reflected on that very question for many years. Perhaps I *do* profit. . . You suggest that the attacks are caused by stress, but sometimes the opposite is true – that the attacks dissipate stress. My work is stressful. It requires me to face the dark side of existence, and the migraine attack, awful as it is, may be a cleansing convulsion that permits me to continue.'

These words are not from Nietzsche himself, but from a fictive Nietzsche in the novel *When Nietzsche Wept* written by the American psychiatrist Irvin D. Yalom [13].

In the novel, Nietzsche is treated for his severe headache attacks by Joseph Breuer, a Viennese 'Nervenarzt'. The treatment is partially successful, but after initial consent, Nietzsche decides to stop it, because he does not want to get rid of his 'great liberator'. He sees the migraine attack as some sort of purification. Besides, he has problems with the patient-doctor relationship, which he can only see in terms of being in power or not, or being independent or not. Nietzsche does not want a treatment that is based on compassion.

Some doubt arises because the headache attacks become very severe:

> Monstrous crippling headaches; seasickness on dry land – vertigo, disequilibrium, nausea, vomiting, anorexia, disgust for food; fevers, heavy night sweats which necessitated two or three nightly changes of linen; crushing bouts of fatigue which at times approximated generalised muscular paralysis; gastric pain; hematemesis; intestinal cramps; severe constipation; haemorrhoids; and disabling visual problems. . . Visual scintillations and scotoma, which often preceded a headache; intractable insomnia; severe nocturnal muscle cramps; generalised tension; and rapid, inexplicable mood shifts.

Up to now, Nietzsche's treatments consisted of diets, cold water baths, resting cures, chloral hydrate, morphine, and veronal. Breuer proposes a treatment with 'talking cures', supported by ergotamine and magnesium. However, the psychotherapeutic sessions turn the doctor-patient relationship upside down. The conversations with Nietzsche bring Breuer in a deep crisis. He fears getting old, is afraid of dying, becomes uncertain when making choices, and misses his mother. Nietzsche becomes Breuer's therapist. In the end, however, Breuer is 'cured' – not by Nietzsche, but by Breuer's young friend Sigmund Freud who cures him by means of hypnosis.

In the final scene of the book, Nietzsche has a migraine attack. Breuer's treatment, consisting of coffee, ergotamine, and magnesium stops the attack, but not the emotions. Nietzsche's tears after the attack symbolize his love for Lou Salomé, his loneliness, and his relief of earthly problems.

For the 'real' Nietzsche, his headaches were part of the 'terror and horror of existence' [12]. Human beings can live with suffering, but not when it is meaningless.

> Only great suffering is the ultimate emancipator of the spirit. . . Only great suffering; that great suffering, under which we seem to be over a fire of greenwood, the suffering that takes its time – forces us philosophers to descend into our nethermost depths (from *Nietzsche contra Wagner*, cited in [12]).

Kain [12] explains the relation between Nietzsche's topics 'suffering' and 'eternal recurrence'.

> Now imagine that at your worst moment, your loneliest loneliness, a demon appears to you or you imagine a demon appearing to you. And this demon tells you that you will have to live your life over again, innumerable times more, and that everything, every last bit of pain and suffering, every last migraine, every last bout of nausea and vomiting, will return, exactly the same, over and over and over again.

Nietzsche decided that he would not change one single detail of his life, not one moment of pain. He decided to love his fate. For the 'real' Nietzsche, as well as for Yalom's fictive one, migraine appears to be the great liberator.

## Migraine versus Syphilis in Thomas Mann's *Doctor Faustus*

Adrian Leverkühn is infected by *Treponema pallidum*, the microorganism that causes syphilis. He has let himself be infected on purpose. On one hand, syphilis causes a lot of horrible symptoms, but on the other also a sort of creative madness, original sources of inspiration, which was what Leverkühn was searching for. He also suffers from migraine, as his father [14].

> Afflicted creature that I am, had lain in the dark all the day with tedious headache, having often to retch and vomit, as comes with severe visitations, but toward evening came bettering, all unhoped and of a sudden. Could hold down the soup the mother brought me. . .

The story of Leverkühn is told by his friend Serenus Zeitblom, who starts to write in 1943, shortly after the first defeats of the German army in World War II. Zeitblom reflects on German history and culture, he thinks of Luther, von Goethe, and Beethoven, but in the first place he remembers his friend who died in 1940. Leverkühn died after a long disease, nursed by his mother for ten years, fully demented as a result of syphilis. Before that time, he created masterpieces such as *Apocalipsis cum Figuris* and *Dr. Faustus' Lamentation*. Zeitblom (and Mann) make the life of Leverkühn symbolic for the German people. The infection is 'nazism', the outcome is known.

Leverkühn has had migraine since he was 14. Because of his migraine he was declared unfit for military service (!). After the willful infection with syphilis in 1906, the frequency of the migraine attacks increases.

> Leverkühn, to whom I reported these same impressions, was extraordinarily ill at the time – suffering from something like the degrading tortures, the pinching agonies of red-hot tongs; yet there was no need to fear directly for his life, though it seemed to have reached a low point, so low that he merely eked out his existence, barely dragging himself from one day to the next. He had come down with an intestinal condition that even the strictest diet could not relieve; every few days it would return, beginning with a violent headache, followed by hours, sometimes days of vomiting, even on an empty stomach – the sheerest misery, undignified, devious, and degrading, each attack ending in complete exhaustion and persistent sensitivity to light.

In *Doctor Faustus* [14], syphilis and migraine become connected. Various explanations are possible for this association, from the example of Nietzsche (who was thought to suffer from both migraine and syphilis) to migraine caused by syphilis (which is unlikely, as Leverkühn had migraine before he acquired syphilis). Another explanation is that both diseases symbolize aspects of the history of the German people: syphilis stands for 'guilt' (nazism) and migraine for 'fate' (as it is hereditary). It seems that the inimitable Thomas Mann found a new, important migraine metaphor.

### Aspects of Pediatric Migraine: Alice in Wonderland

There is no mention of migraine in Lewis Carroll's *Alice's Adventures in Wonderland* and *Through the Looking Glass* [15, 16]. Headache only occurs in two scenes, but in both a diagnosis of tension-headache is more likely [5]. During an interrogation, the King gets a stabbing headache and asks his wife to take over. In another scene, Tweetledum refrains from fighting a duel with his twin brother Tweedledee, as 'today he has a headache (and toothache)'.

Nevertheless, Alice and her creator have been inextricably associated with migraine. There are some reasons for this. First, the books contain some original hallucinations that have not ceased to fascinate the readers and to remind them of some sort of migrainous experiences. Second, Lewis Carroll (real name Charles Lutwidge Dodgson) is by some experts thought to have suffered from migraine himself, a diagnosis that is still under discussion.

> 'Curiouser and curiouser!' cried Alice (she was so much surprised, that for the moment she quite forgot how to speak good English); 'now I'm opening out like the largest telescope that ever was! Good-bye, feet! (for when she looked down at her feet, they seemed to be almost out of sight, they were getting so far off).

Microsomatognosia, metamorphopsia, prosopagnosia, micropsia, and macropsia are fascinating neurological phenomena that are often associated with pediatric migraine. In 1952, the American headache specialist Lippman [17] described these hallucinations in children with migraine. He recognized a resemblance with some of the descriptions in the books of Lewis Carroll and introduced the eponym, 'Alice in Wonderland syndrome.'

As said, there is no mention of headache that fulfills the criteria of migraine in the two books. There is no mention of nausea, vomiting, photophobia, or phonophobia. For the various instances of distorted (visual) reality in the books, multiple alternative explanations are possible.

After the 'birth' of the Alice in Wonderland syndrome, however, the discussion mainly concentrated on the question whether the author did suffer from migraine himself (summarized in [18]). This question seems as difficult to answer as unimportant. Charles Lutwidge Dodgson was a complex and enigmatic person. He was very shy, and had a special relationship with young girls, his 'child-friends'. He never had a relationship with a woman, and lost his interest in girls when they reached the age of 13. He wrote 98,721 letters to – and was a fervent amateur photographer of – little girls. Dodgson once made a self-diagnosis of 'bilious migraine', but this cannot be checked with the present migraine criteria. In his diaries, he describes a total of six attacks with visual phenomena, among which are flashes and scotomata, but always without headache. Without exception, however, these attacks occurred after the publication of the Alice books, and cannot be seen as their inspiration.

Why – in my opinion – it is not of importance whether the writer suffered from migraine or not is because the 'the writer is dead' [19]. After a text is written, the intention of the author – and certainly also his biography – stops to be of importance. It is the reader who determines the meaning and the value of the text. In the case of Alice, one can interpret the text as containing elements of migraine, but – for example – a diagnosis of a feverish dream or delirium is also possible. Nevertheless, the 'migraine-interpretation' has led to an useful eponym, independent of the true meaning of the text or the biographic details of the author.

## The Feeling of Migraine: *The Blindfold* by Siri Hustvedt

The American writer Siri Hustvedt suffers from migraine herself, as can be read in her various entries on the internet, but also in her autobiographic essay *The Shaking Woman* [20]. She is married to the postmodern American writer Paul Auster, and is seen as a postmodern writer herself. This means – in her case – that her books contain a continuous play with 'reality'. The protagonists are confused, and so are the readers. Hustvedt's books remind us of the fact that words, language, and linguistic signs are by definition unreliable [2].

In *The Blindfold,* Hustvedt tells the story of Iris Vegan, a student of literature (!) in New York [21]. The story is presented in reversed chronological order. Iris makes a study of one of the protagonists of the novel *Middlemarch* by George Eliot (who also suffered from migraine). In the first chapter, she works for Mr. Morning and has to make a catalogue of objects that had belonged to a woman that has been murdered. In the second chapter, Iris has a difficult relation with Stephen, but secretly likes Stephen's friend George (!) more. At the end of a photo session with George, she runs away because she is afraid of the expression on his face, 'like a person who has just eaten well'.

Shortly thereafter, she gets a migraine attack.

> The image was changing. With more curiosity than alarm, I noticed a small black hole in the face. How can that be? I said to myself. It wasn't there before. But not for a moment did I doubt its reality. The hole grew, eating away the left eye and nose, and then the dread came, cold and absolute, a terror so profound it created a kind of paralysis. I was transfixed. The hole was devouring the entire image, the face and hair, the shoulders, breasts, and torso, and I saw only the arm stumps hanging there alone for an instant, and then they too were engulfed, but like a person in a dream I couldn't cry out. There was no sound in me, and I watched as the hole began to swallow the picture's frame. . . It was bonded to my hands, a part of my limbs, and then I was blind. . . It was over, and I could feel pain in my head. I suffer from migraine and am susceptible to nervous tricks and minor hallucinations, but I have never been able to write of these aberrations

that are purely neurological, because while they are happening, I am convinced that I am seeing the truth, that the terrible fragility and absence I feel is the world – stark and unclothed. That nakedness is irretrievable.

The number of attacks increases enormously and in chapter three Iris is admitted to a hospital. 'As migraineur, I had low status. Admittedly, I was a bad case: I had pain in my head for seven months almost without respite. Sometimes it was mild, sometimes brutal.' Nevertheless, she feels guilty because the other patients have more serious diseases. As she keeps on worrying, a psychiatrist is called. This doctor spoke kindly in a low voice. He has a white beard that Iris finds 'reassuring'. She worries about the costs, and sighs: 'He looked expensive to me, and I kept wondering if his sympathy was covered by my insurance.'

In the fourth and last chapter of the novel it becomes clear that the occurrences of the first three chapters have been told in a reversed order. First she was in the hospital, then she had the relation with Stephen and finally she worked for Mr. Morning. The reason for this reversal does not become clear. In the last chapter, Iris belongs to people who wear masks and blindfolds, probably as symbols of their self-protection. She tells her story to Paris, a superficial and decadent dandy. He ridicules her, and they have a fight. Iris escapes. After the last sentence of the book, the reader is left puzzled: 'Then I took off my shoes and ran to the IRT, ran, as they say, like a bat out of hell.'

The postmodernist Siri Hustvedt tells her story in a reversed chronological order. She calls her protagonist Iris (which is, of course, Siri spelled backwards) and gives descriptions of migraine attacks a very prominent place in the narrative. An interpretation is difficult, but could the backbone of the story be a migraine attack backwards? In part four, the blindfold could stand for the visual aura, in part three, the hospital symbolizes the headache phase, part two the social consequences of having migraine, and finally part one, the recovery phase.

Who has a better explanation?

## References


1. Schott GD: Exploring the visual hallucinations of migraine aura: the tacit contribution of illustration. Brain 2007;130:1690–1703.
2. de Saussure F: Course in General Linguistics. New York, Columbia University Press, 2011.
3. Loftus S: Pain and its metaphors: a dialogical approach. J Med Humanit 2011;32:213–230.
4. Frank AW: Metaphors of pain. Lit Med 2012;29: 182–196.
5. Haan J, Meulenberg F: Migraine als Muze (Migraine as a Muse). Amsterdam, Belvédère, 2009.
6. McEwan I: Atonement. London, Jonathan Cape, 2001.
7. Lasdun J: The Horned Man. London, Jonathan Cape,2002.
8. Salzman M: Lying Awake. New York, Alfred A. Knopf, 2000.
9. Glannon W: Medicine through the novel: Lying Awake. J Med Ethics Med Humanit 2005;31:31–34.
10. King S: The Dark Half. New York, Viking, 1989.
11. Jones JM: Great pains: famous people with headaches. Cephalalgia 1999;19:627–630.
12. Kain PJ: Nietzsche, eternal recurrence, and the horror of existence. J Nietzsche Stud 2007;33:49–63.

13 Yalom ID: When Nietzsche Wept. A Novel of Obsession. New York, HarperCollins Publishers, 1992.
14 Mann T: Doctor Faustus. 1947. English translation, Alfred A. Knopf/Vintage, 1999.
15 Carroll L: Alice's Adventures in Wonderland. London, Chadwick and Sons, 1865.
16 Carroll L: Through the Looking Glass, and What Alice Found There. London, MacMillan, 1871.
17 Lippman CW: Certain hallucinations peculiar to migraine. J Nerv Ment Dis 1952;116:346–351.
18 Restak RM: Alice in migraineland. Headache 2006;46:306–311.
19 Barthes R: S/Z. Paris, Seuil, 1970.
20 Hustvedt S: The Shaking Woman. New York, Henry Holt and Company, 2010.
21 Hustvedt S: The Blindfold. New York, Norton Paperback, 1993.

Joost Haan, MD, PhD
Department of Neurology
Rijnland Hospital
NL–2353 GA Leiderdorp (The Netherlands)
E-Mail jhaan@rijnland.nl

Bogousslavsky J, Dieguez S (eds): Literary Medicine: Brain Disease and Doctors in Novels, Theater, and Film.
Front Neurol Neurosci. Basel, Karger, 2013, vol 31, pp 137–168 (DOI: 10.1159/000345526)

# Stranger than Fiction: Literary and Clinical Amnesia

Sebastian Dieguez · Jean-Marie Annoni

Laboratory for Cognitive and Neurological Sciences, Département de Médecine, Hôpital de Fribourg, Université de Fribourg, Fribourg, Switzerland

**Abstract**

This chapter broadly covers literary uses of amnesia and memory disorders. Amnesia in fiction offers authors an efficient and dramatic device to tackle themes such as identity, personal liberty, or guilt. We argue against the common complaint that fictional amnesia is scientifically inaccurate, pointing out that the goals of literature are different from those of science, that amnesia is still poorly understood, and that real-life cases can sometimes be stranger than fiction. The chapter provides examples from the neuropsychological literature, media reports, mythology, historical cases, detective stories, war stories, theatrical plays, and other genres. Special attention is given to retrograde and dissociative amnesia, as these are the most frequent types of amnesia portrayed in fiction, while other types of memory disorders are more shortly treated. We argue that the predominance of disorders affecting autobiographical memory in fiction is in itself a revealing fact about the mechanisms of human memory, illustrating how fictional treatments of pathology can inform back neurological and psychological research. 

## Memory, Amnesia and the Novel

### *Memory and Literature*

The topic of memory is at the very heart of every literary endeavor. Authors write to tell stories: tales of ancient times, reports of recent events, and anticipations of what is to come. Imaginary events, places, and persons are conjured out of stored individual and collective knowledge, and then reworked through the powers of creativity. We uncover our past to put it under the glare of the present, to retrospectively interpret its course, and to explore the building up of our very sense of identity. Novels are all about memory, and it is from this human capability that all novels flow.

Perhaps most famously, Marcel Proust has embodied the pervasive presence of memory in literature by grounding his 'immense building' – *In Search of Lost Time* (1913–1927) – on the very notion of remembrance [1, 2]. From a humble little madeleine, the involuntary surge of long forgotten memories leads the narrator on a quest to become an accomplished writer. The philosopher John Locke, in his *Essay Concerning Human Understanding* (1689), famously reduced the notion of personal identity to that of self-consciousness, by which he meant what we would call today episodic or autobiographical memory: we feel that we are *someone* because of our memories, and because we know these memories refer back to *us*. We are, in this sense, quite literally our memory store. Although Locke's argument has led to much controversy and charges of circularity and confusion, the idea that remembering our past is a central constituent of our identity remains a key tenet of our daily practices and literary conventions. To understand *who* someone is, one needs to know at least something about her past.

This emphasis on individual memory – especially in its involuntary manifestations [3] – as the crux of the authentic self can be contrasted with frequent literary uses of memory as a collective phenomenon. History, culture, society, and family are cornerstones of our sense of identity, just as much as, and inseparably from, our personal remembrances. We are selves among other selves, we interact with our elders, we transmit to our youngest, we read books and sing songs, we tell each other stories, we pay tribute to long gone heroes, and we visit monuments and museums. Literature in itself is an important part of this collective memory. It builds on distributed knowledge, widespread obsessions and passions, as well as shared traumas; in turn, literature contributes by perpetuating and consolidating this common knowledge, becoming its universal repository.

### *Literature and Failings of Memory*

From these tight links between memory, literature, and the self, it should come as no surprise that failures of memory have been since time immemorial of great interest to writers, poets, and playwrights, as well as clinicians, psychologists, and philosophers. Failings of memory, indeed, reveal the very architecture and functions of this capacity [4–6].

Writers in antiquity have often exploited this revealing feature of memory impairments. For instance, Greek and Roman authors from around the 7th century BC (e.g. Hesiod) to the 1st century BC (e.g. Virgil, Ovid, Seneca) wrote about the myth of Lethe, the river of forgetfulness. Lethe was closely associated with sleep, night, and death, and as a feminine divinity stood opposed to Mnemosyne, the goddess of memory, mother of the muses. The river Lethe was one of several that flowed through the underworld. Whichever soul – mortal or immortal – drank from its water immediately experienced complete oblivion, and thus was freed from his or her earlier self and fit for reincarnation [7]. Life, existence, and identity were in those times conceptually close to the notion of remembering, and amnesia offered the possibility of rebirth as a different entity.

Homer's *Odyssey*, composed around the 8th century BC, is in a broad sense a story about memory and identity. The return to Ithaca means for Odysseus not only retrieving his home, his wife, and his close ones, but is foremost about reclaiming his own identity. The main danger along his journey is not that of dying, but that of forgetting his true self and the reason for his quest. When Odysseus sends three of his men to scout the land of the Lotus-eaters, these creatures 'did them no hurt, but gave them to eat of the lotus, which was so delicious that those who ate of it left off caring about home, and did not even want to go back and say what had happened to them, but were for staying and munching lotus with the Lotus-eater without thinking further of their return'. The lotus flower induces amnesia, and so does the song of the Sirens: 'If any one unwarily draws in too close and hears the singing of the Sirens, his wife and children will never welcome him home again, for they sit in a green field and warble him to death with the sweetness of their song'. Here forgetfulness is induced by the nostalgia of past deeds, as flattery and vanity freeze the victim in an inauthentic self and prevents one from attending to one's future [8, 9]. Impairment of memory, thus, was akin in antiquity to a failure to be true to oneself and therefore revealed the importance of memory for having a sense of self and responsibility. Further, the destructive power of the song of the Sirens reveals that memory is not merely tuned to the past, but serves to look forwards, to reach one's goals and to act on the material world.

In *The Recognition of Śakuntalā*, a classic Indian play from around the 4th century AD written by Kālidāsa, a young girl – Śakuntalā – recently married to King Dusyanta is cursed by having her husband forget her entirely: 'Who is she, this veiled creature [. . .] Could I have married her? I no longer know [. . .] however hard I try, I don't remember marrying this lady. So how can I accept her when she's obviously pregnant, and I have no reason to believe it's anything to do with me?' The only antidote would be for Śakuntalā to show him her wedding ring, which would have him instantly recover his memory. The ring is momentarily lost, but it will eventually show up by chance in the belly of a fish. The tale is interesting as it portrays the crucial importance of memory for social interactions and emotions such as love. Moreover, here the main character is not amnesiac, rather she is the one forgotten by an amnesiac. To have an identity, we need to be able to remember our past, but just as importantly we also need to be remembered by others. Finally, the story also highlights the arbitrariness of memory failure, which can strike at any moment like a curse, and likewise be restored seemingly miraculously.

## Stranger than Fiction? Neurological and Literary Amnesia

### *Literary Amnesia as Mythology*

As hinted in the previous sections, literary amnesia is a fruitful device and metaphor to explore topics as varied as the sense of identity, social relatedness, the possibility of rebirth, the need for an authentic self, or the capability to look forwards. These uses reveal intuitive conceptions of memory from times when the science of memory and research on amnesia were in their infancy and still the province of poets, philosophers, and theologians. From a medical standpoint, however, they seem entirely naïve as to the actual mechanisms and subtleties of memory loss. With the advent of neurological and psychiatric sciences in the second half of the 19th century, as well as the multiplication of published case reports of amnesiac patients, literary characters began displaying amnesia in a more clinical than mythological context. Still, were they any closer to our current knowledge of memory (dys)functions than the ancient depictions?

In this chapter, we will not address as such the matter of clinical accuracy of literary amnesia. Nevertheless, it is true that neurologists, psychologists, and psychiatrists can oftentimes be much chagrined by how their disciplines are depicted in fictional works. Sally Baxendale [10], for instance, deplored that the treatment of amnesia in movies is disconnected from clinical and scientific knowledge, or at best 'neurologically improbable'. Specifically, she notes that the overwhelming majority of cinematic amnesiacs display extremely severe impairment for recalling information preceding amnesia onset, contrasting with fully preserved capacities for encoding and learning new information. This pattern of profound retrograde amnesia coexisting with perfect or near-perfect anterograde memory, Baxendale notes, is the opposite of the most common pattern in organic amnestic syndromes (i.e. anterograde impairment with better recall of remote events). Moreover, the etiology of real-life cases with amnestic syndrome is overwhelmingly organic (e.g. encephalopathies, strokes, closed-head injuries, penetrating wounds, neurosurgery), whereas in movies psychological triggers of amnesia are dominant. Baxendale also criticizes the frequent, complete, and dramatic recovery of memories in film, oftentimes following a second traumatic event (or even a second head injury), a séance of hypnosis, or more simply an encounter with a familiar object, person, or place from the past. Baxendale finally argues that these cinematic 'myths' are misleading to the public: people have an idea of amnesia 'more in keeping with a psychiatric than an organic cause' and perhaps entertain exaggerated hopes as to the chances of recovery or improvement of amnestic syndromes.

Similar observations probably led Laird Cermak, a pioneer of modern memory research, to coin the term 'TV amnesia' for those fictional and dramatic depictions of retrograde amnesia, perhaps having in mind the most contrived portrayals in soap-operas and sit-coms (quoted in [11]).

*Looking for Oneself? Amnesia Stranger than Reality*

Now it is certainly the case that many literary uses of amnesia stretch the limits of clinical plausibility. One thinks of the frequent ploy in crime and mystery novels of having an amnesiac character investigate his own past. This approach is rather successfully exploited in Patrick Modiano's *Rue des boutiques obscures* (Missing Person;

1978), in which we follow an amnesiac turned detective in his quest to find his lost identity, and foremost to understand the reasons for his complete loss of autobiographical memories. The narration jumps from one cue to the other, with the lingering possibility that the character might actually be completely misled by every meager 'lead'. However, flashes of fragmented memories progressively start building a coherent picture. Ultimately, they fail to provide a sense of closure as the story ends ambiguously [12]. The potentially misleading nature of recollected 'memories' has been most explicitly used in Diego Marani's *New Finnish Grammar* (2000), the story of a soldier found unable to speak and severely amnesiac. An empathetic doctor believes him to be a Finnish compatriot, and sets out to teach him the Finnish language and send him back to Helsinki, his assumed homeland. As it turns out, this assumption has been completely wrong from the outset: the man never had the slightest relationship to Finland.

An extension of the amnesiac-looking-for-his-own-identity ploy is to have the protagonist discover that he is the author of the very crime he happens to be investigating. This is actually the plot of what is often considered the first crime novel, Wilkie Collins' *The Moonstone* (1868). A man investigating the theft of a diamond discovers that he is the culprit, having himself stolen the stone in a dissociative state induced by the involuntary intake of laudanum. As he does not remember any of the events during this trance-like episode, he must still figure out exactly what he did with the diamond. Canadian scientist and novelist Grant Allen was probably the first to extend the idea to its fullest form in *Recalled to Life* (1891). Following the murder of her father, a girl loses all prior autobiographical memories: 'I began life all over again, with that terrible scene of blood as my first birthday and practical starting point.' Turned detective, she sets out to investigate that fateful event and eventually discovers that she herself was the killer, and that the murder caused her dense psychogenic amnesia.

More recently, Anne Perry launched with *The Face of a Stranger* (1990) a whole series of novels featuring an amnesiac detective. Detective William Monk has lost all autobiographical memories following a hansom accident. As his investigations unfold, all the while attempting to hide his amnesia to everyone, Monk makes further discoveries about his past and has flashes of childhood memories. In the first installment, these fragmentary recollections happen to be relevant for the murder he is currently investigating, and soon begins to wonder whether he might be the very culprit he is looking for. David Goodis' *Nightfall* (1947), takes the opposite stance. A man unwittingly involved in a bank robbery must prove he is innocent by producing a case with the stolen money. Unfortunately, he suffers from 'regressive amnesia', precluding him from remembering just what happened to that case. The novel includes references to neurology and psychoanalysis.

Perhaps the most extraordinarily convoluted of such stories is *The Long Wait* (1951) by Mickey Spillane. In this action-thriller, amnesia is mixed with physical misidentification. The main (amnesiac) character thinks all along he is exacting revenge for a look-alike friend who died attempting to save his life in an accident. As it turns out, the protagonist actually *is* this friend, and is thus seeking revenge for himself.

As far-fetched as many of these fictional depictions of amnesia are, the possibility of relearning one's past, as it were from a third person perspective – a process different from spontaneous (i.e. from the first-person perspective) recovery – has been reported in several real-life cases. One patient, for instance, relearned his entire life up to the onset of retrograde amnesia at age 19, 'as if he had read a book about his life', by piecing together the information gathered from his parents. This knowledge about himself was never felt as genuine memories though, rather they seemed to him like abstract facts [13; see also 14].

*Literary Amnesia as Thought Experiments*

It is true that most cases of real-life amnesia would make for poor fiction, or at least rather poor entertainment as compared to the few examples listed above. From this point of view, the claim that fictional amnesia is unrealistic or even utterly outlandish is not entirely unwarranted. However, it should be clear that the purpose of fiction is not to provide accurate depictions of scientific and medical knowledge. What is more, comparing fictional cases to the average clinical case is an unfair and incorrect way to approach the question. The real issue is not whether cases of literary amnesia seem usual or not to the clinician, but whether they are at least plausible and work for a general audience. An assessment of plausibility thus must refer not to the average case, but should extend to unique and extraordinary cases. And an assessment of functionality would ask whether the depiction of fictional amnesia is acceptable and understandable to the audience, whether it performs its assigned job in the plot structure, and how it helps to put forward the broader message of the work at hand.

Asking these questions thus allow not only investigating folk-conceptions of memory, but also keeping in focus the scope and limits of real-life amnesia as well. For instance, the mere fact that literary amnesiacs overwhelmingly suffer from retrograde amnesia with no anterograde impairment, and that the loss of memory most often involves all information about self-identity rather than other domains, perhaps says something important about intuitive conceptions of memory. Likewise, that cases such as these should be very rare in real clinical settings also says something about the actual mechanisms of memory. In short, rather than conceiving of literary amnesia as inaccurate fantasies, it could be more productive to see it as a type of thought-experiment.

*Real-Life Amnesia Stranger than Fiction*

A more provocative argument against the complaint that fictional amnesia is unrealistic or inaccurate is that, in fact, it might well be the case that real-life amnesia is sometimes much more perplexing and surprising than its literary counterpart. Amnesia research has a longstanding tradition of controversy and puzzling observations [15–18], indeed, perhaps more than any other symptom, raising suspicions of counterfeiting [19]. Over the years, many types of amnesia and memory disorders have been described, countless case reports have been published, and many theories have emerged. Clinicians soon noticed that amnesia often presents itself as a strikingly fragmented phenomenon, and since the early days of modern research virtually all types of dissociation have been reported. Taking the onset of disorder as the defining flagpole for the phenomenology of amnesia, and contrasting this time-frame with the ever-moving present, clinicians have noticed that the memory impairment can affect both remote and recent events, or concern specifically only one of the two. The concepts of anterograde and retrograde amnesia have been influential ever since [15]. Amnesia can also involve a very narrow time-frame; these cases of focal, isolated, or lacunar amnesia most frequently concern events surrounding a triggering event or injury, but can also affect a specific period of the patient's life, while leaving all other memories intact. The question of etiology, understandably, has also been at the forefront of amnesia research. Yet, despite recent advances in the cognitive neurosciences, many puzzling questions remain on the anatomical basis of amnesia, the importance of psychological factors, and the interaction between these different levels. Indeed, despite much claims to the contrary [20], the distinction between organic and psychogenic amnesia is alive and well. Why do some psychological traumas and mild head injuries lead to dramatic impairments of memory in some patients, but not in the overwhelming majority of those who suffer such common ailments?

Because we still do not fully understand the mechanisms of these different phenomena, it seems premature at this stage to criticize or condemn literary works as inaccurate regarding their portrayal of memory disorders. This also holds from a more theoretical standpoint, as regards the domains of memory storage and retrieval. In most literary cases of amnesia, the impairment is one of access to past, and especially personal, information. Yet even in real-life organic amnestic syndrome, access to ostensibly lost information can sometimes be demonstrated using implicit methods [21, 22].

Consider now the classic distinctions between episodic, semantic, autobiographical, and procedural memory. As it happens, authors of fiction, whether they have been medically informed or not, often instinctively draw fine-grained distinctions between these different domains. One famous example is the character Jason Bourne from the Robert Ludlum novels. Despite having lost all personal information and his very sense of identity, Bourne maintains his skills as a highly trained CIA covert assassin, which indeed allows him to survive and to pursue his quest to recover his identity. In real-life cases, such dissociations can appear in all sorts of combinations, sometimes defying the most imaginative fictions. For instance, Sellal et al. [14] reported a patient with a retrograde amnesia covering 10 years and concerning autobiographical and semantic memory. Yet the patient never lost his sense of identity and could recognize all his relatives. He also had a striking ability to quickly relearn all the lost information. Intriguingly, he also suffered from a striking loss of procedural skills, such as using a computer and signing his name, and wrote with an altered and juvenile handwriting. In contrast, a patient reported by Hennig-Fast et al. [23] had a complete loss of identity following an episode of dissociative fugue, yet retained perfect knowledge for past public events and, despite having no knowledge whatsoever of having these skills, could use a computer, play the guitar, and even sign his own name, which he claimed not to know (for reviews of dissociations in retrograde forms of amnesia, see [24–26]).

Real-life amnesia is also often accompanied by other neurological and cognitive impairments, most frequently entirely neglected in fiction. Take for instance the feature of confabulation, a defining component of Korsakoff's syndrome and, indeed, sometimes the most prominent symptom in cases of confabulatory amnesia [27]. The complication here is that patients take these intrusive memories, or even flat-out fantasies, to be true. To them, their ongoing reality takes place in a parallel world or disjointed time-course, making them effectively time- or alternate reality-travelers. Such a feature is not so infrequent in the neurological ward, yet authors of fiction have seldom exploited its potential (*Korsakov* by E. Fottorino, 2004, is one exception).

Finally, although patterns of memory recovery in fictional amnesia often seem contrived and excessively convenient, we will see below that dramatic examples do exist in the clinical literature, again pushing the boundaries of our knowledge about how memory works.

*The Narrative Potential of Real-Life Amnesia*

There is an additional and most important aspect that makes the topic of amnesia especially fit for literature, and that is the very method of assessment for memory disorders. Facing complaints of memory, or a patient lacking knowledge of her memory impairment, there is only one way a clinician can go about documenting the nature and extent of the disorder: put simply, one has to *investigate*. This is of course true of all medical ailments, but certainly the assessment of amnesia – and especially the most puzzling cases – most often takes the form of a real detective work. To establish the presence and severity of amnesia, the clinician has, one way or the other, to know at some point the specific features of the patient's life events, her preferred domains of knowledge, her habits, and her previous skills. Not only must the patient be thoroughly interrogated and tested on a regular basis, but it soon becomes almost necessary to interrogate her close relatives, friends, and colleagues, perhaps also gather some personal belongings of the patient such as photographs, lists of names, addresses, schools, and events known to have been familiar to the patient. Now, if the clinician has to do this task, it is perhaps not so contrived that under some circumstances the patient herself might be led to perform such an investigation.

More generally, the very striking presentation of amnesia lends itself to deep metaphysical questions about identity and the self, as well as one's place in time and society. This is very often the broad message in stories of literary amnesia, but there is no reason it should not affect patients and their relatives in much the same way. Cases of very severe anterograde amnesia – patients forever stuck in the present, such as

H.M. – indeed raise some unsettling thoughts about what it must be like to be unable to remember that one is unable to remember [28].

For these reasons, it is not surprising that at least some neurological and psychiatric cases occasionally read like mysteries, thrillers, or dramas. Every now and then, an individual is found wandering some place and claiming not to know his or her own name, address, identity, or whereabouts. The media issues a photograph of that person and asks 'Do you know this (wo)man?', the police and medical experts are involved, witnesses begin to appear, further questions arise regarding motives, etiology, and identity, and a real-life mystery is born [29–31]. Other cases are less of a mystery as far as the issue of past identity is concerned than as regards dramatic changes in personality. Such a story has recently made the news. When 27-year-old Chris Birch recovered from a stroke, he found himself unable to recall most of his previous life. . . and gay. Previously a party boy, beer drinker, rubgy and motorbike fan, and bank employee, he swapped banking for hairdressing, discovered a new sexual orientation and is now barely able to identify with his earlier self [32]. The possibility to restart an entirely different life is a frequent topic of literary amnesia, but as can be seen, real-life cases are not entirely impossible.

Plenty of striking cases can also be found in the medical literature. One of us, for instance, has reported the case of a transsexual patient struck by severe retrograde amnesia following a thalamic stroke, several months after (male-to-female) surgical sexual reassignment had been performed. Now a woman, the patient had no recollection whatsoever of her new condition, and believed she was still a man (and behaved as such) [33].

Consider also the case of a man who became completely mute and presented with a 10-year span of retrograde amnesia in the aftermath of a high-voltage electric shock [34]. To cope with his speech impairment, the patient entered a school for the deaf and became a fluent user of sign-language. However, about 2 years later he suffered a minor head injury due to slipping on the ice and immediately recovered from mutism. Yet the retrograde amnesia persisted, and the patient became (and still is) a passionate advocate for the deaf community.

Another striking case in the neuropsychological literature was reported by Glisky et al. [35]. A 33-year-old male was found in the area of Tucson, Arizona (USA), speaking with a German accent and unable to recall his own name and identity, or anything about his whereabouts. After his photograph was displayed on television, it appeared that the man came from Germany a few months ago with a considerable amount of money and wearing expensive clothes. He was unable to speak in his mother tongue, and indeed denied having any knowledge of German. His only memory was the vague recollection that someone shot at him with a gun. On his return to Germany, the man was arrested upon disembarking for a business-related crime and had difficulties speaking German fluently for some weeks.

As can be seen from these few examples, specific cases of real-life amnesia would very easily lend themselves to fictional treatments. Indeed, some of them would probably seem even less likely than purely fictional cases. As we will see in the next section, some real-life cases were actually so striking that they achieved historical status, in turn inspiring a whole range of literary works. This is the now classic case of amnesiac soldiers suddenly emerging from oblivion, and of the incredible Bruneri-Canella affair in Italy.

## History Meets Neurology and Literature

### *The Living Unknown Soldier: Anouilh and Giraudoux*

Literary cases of amnesia often serve to emphasize the importance of memory as a collective duty [5, 36]. George Santayana famously wrote: 'Those who cannot remember the past are condemned to repeat it.' This trope was quite prominent in French literature in the between-wars years, and a peculiar anecdote has been most influential in helping to catalyze the idea. The aftermath of World War I was painful beyond imagination. In France alone, millions had died or disappeared, an entire generation was broken, and a country had to be rebuilt almost from scratch. Of those who survived and returned, many presented a wealth of puzzling mental and physical disorders [37]. Yet from this unbearable collective trauma, the most pressing questions concerned the role of memory in coping with such an event: forgetting seemed to be the only way forwards, yet remembering was the honorable thing to do for the sacrificed. In this conflicting context, something almost unimaginable happened: the dead suddenly came back from the battlefield.

About 300,000 persons were reported missing on the French side after the Great War, many were unidentifiable bodies and soldiers who, for whatever reason, simply vanished without a trace [38]. Their families and relatives very often entertained the hope to see them again someday. Now this hope was suddenly reawakened with the news that a handful of disappeared soldiers were in fact alive, yet not only impossible to identify, but unable to recall their own identity. There were ten such amnesiacs in 1919, or 'poor fools' or the 'living dead' as the press labeled them. A photograph of six of them was published in the local press in 1920 and later at the national level in 1922 (fig. 1). Among the six was a man called Anthelme Mangin – an unreliable name he himself provided – and it was his story that would entrance the public for many years to come (the Mangin feuilleton would only come to an end with his death in 1942). Mangin was first institutionalized in 1918 at the departmental asylum of Bron, in the Aveyron area. When his case became publicized, the entire country became curious about his real identity and more than 300 families officially required additional information about him, hoping to recognize a long forgotten son or husband. Most of them, of course, were quickly disillusioned, but at least 20 claimants became convinced that Mangin really was the man they longed for. Unfortunately, the process of identification was not easy. Mangin turned out to be wholly uncooperative with the claimants. His attitude was puzzling to the doctors who examined him as well. The diagnosis was that of 'negativistic dementia' in the context of a syndrome of 'dementia praecox', a conclusion, interestingly enough, independently reached by the French and German doctors who examined him. Mangin was apathetic and utterly indifferent to his situation; he did not seem in the least interested in finding his real identity and remained wholly unaffected by the manifestations of joy from the persons claiming to recognize him. Despite extensive testing and innumerable court-ordered expert appraisals, Mangin's real identity, very likely that of one Octave Monjoin, would never be officially recognized.

The particulars of this extraordinary case were not unnoticed by contemporary authors of fiction. Indeed, such a simple and dramatic premise lent itself to countless variations and developments. In the heyday of the Mangin case, as five families led a bitter fight in the courtrooms for his ownership (and that of his war pension), Jean Anouilh wrote *Le voyageur sans bagage (*The Traveller without Luggage; 1937), a quite successful play that would launch his career as a promising young playwright.

Gaston – labeled in the list of characters simply as 'amnesiac' – has forgotten everything about his past ever since he was found injured during the war, and from then on leads a peaceful existence at an asylum. However, he is reclaimed by several families as a possible relative, and thus is in the process of visiting their homes in the hope that some connection with his real identity could be made. This situation is not to his liking: 'You know, I've seen so many misguided old ladies, kissing me with their wet noses; and mistaken elderly men rubbing me to their beards. . . . Imagine a man with close to four hundred families [. . .] determined to cherish him. That's a lot.' Claimants for Mangin had to file an official request to Dr. Feynarou, his main caregiver. Then he would carefully examine the case at hand, and only if it seemed strong enough he would organize a direct confrontation at the asylum. In Anouilh's play, the process is advanced enough that Gaston himself can be brought to visit the homes of a handful of solid claimants, hoping the immersion process will trigger the surge of old memories. Chief among these families are the Renauds, who indeed will turn out to be his real relatives. Interestingly, in 1937, the same year that *Le voyageur sans bagage* was played, a similar approach was attempted on Mangin. He was brought to the village he was assumed to have grown up in. Despite some traces of recognition, the experiment was not conclusive (see below for successful cases of memory retrieval following recognition of familiar events, both in literary and real-life cases). Another 'therapy' to induce memory recovery common to Mangin and Gaston was the use of 'fixation abscesses', namely the injection of oil of turpentine. The method had no effect (or at least not the one intended) on either, and was soon altogether abandoned by the medical world [38].

Pharmacological methods for memory recovery, however, are still sometimes attempted in clinical settings. Sodium amytal, sodium pentothal, or lorazepam interviews have been conducted in amnesiac patients with the aim of unearthing otherwise inaccessible memories. Pujol and Kopelman [39], for instance, have reported the successful use of lorazepam in a patient with complete loss of identity,

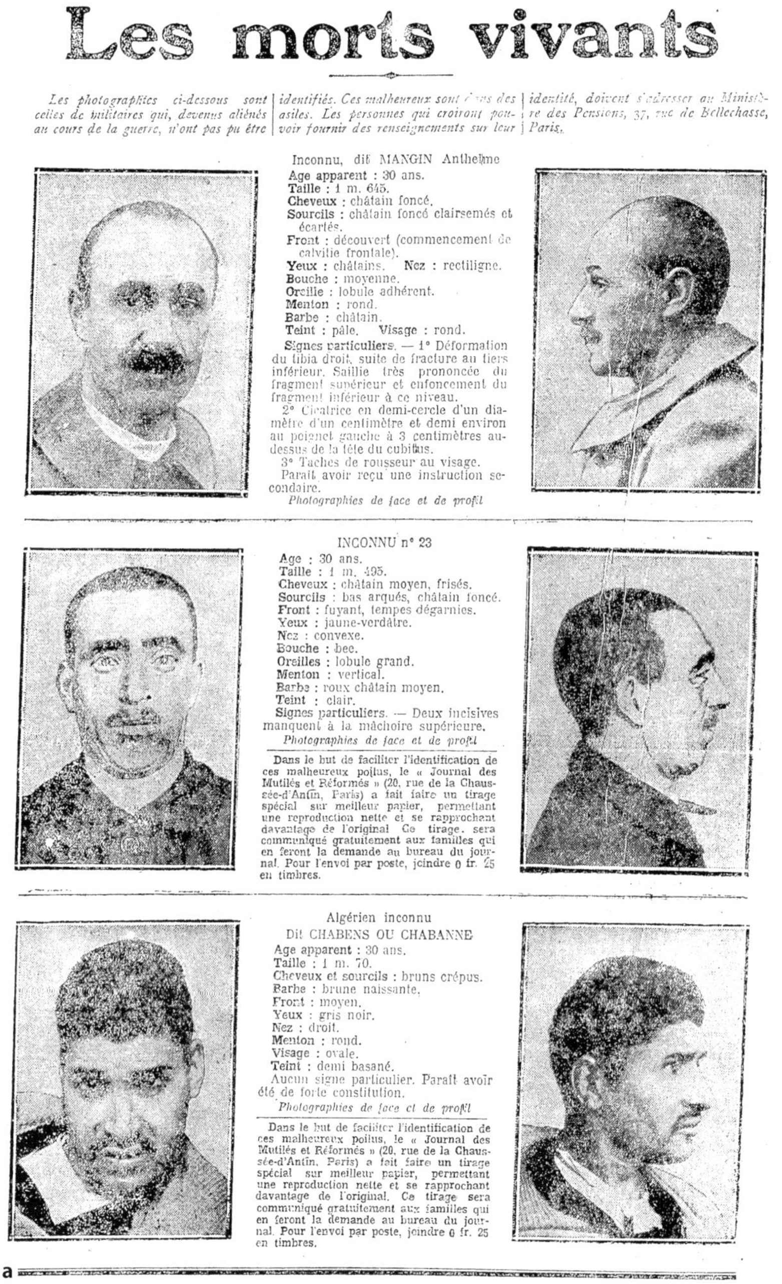

# Les morts vivants

*Les photographies ci-dessous sont celles de militaires qui, devenus aliénés au cours de la guerre, n'ont pas pu être identifiés. Ces malheureux sont dans des asiles. Les personnes qui croiront pouvoir fournir des renseignements sur leur identité, doivent s'adresser au Ministère des Pensions, 37, rue de Bellechasse, Paris.*

Inconnu, dit MANGIN Anthelme

**Age apparent** : 30 ans.
**Taille** : 1 m. 645.
**Cheveux** : châtain foncé.
**Sourcils** : châtain foncé clairsemés et écartés.
**Front** : découvert (commencement de calvitie frontale).
**Yeux** : châtains. **Nez** : rectiligne.
**Bouche** : moyenne.
**Oreille** : lobule adhérent.
**Menton** : rond.
**Barbe** : châtain.
**Teint** : pâle. **Visage** : rond.

**Signes particuliers.** — 1° Déformation du tibia droit, suite de fracture au tiers inférieur. Saillie très prononcée du fragment supérieur et enfoncement du fragment inférieur à ce niveau.

2° Cicatrice en demi-cercle d'un diamètre d'un centimètre et demi environ au poignet gauche à 3 centimètres au-dessus de la tête du cubitus.

3° Taches de rousseur au visage.

Paraît avoir reçu une instruction secondaire.

*Photographies de face et de profil*

INCONNU n° 23

**Age** : 30 ans.
**Taille** : 1 m. 495.
**Cheveux** : châtain moyen, frisés.
**Sourcils** : bas arqués, châtain foncé.
**Front** : fuyant, tempes dégarnies.
**Yeux** : jaune-verdâtre.
**Nez** : convexe.
**Bouche** : bec.
**Oreilles** : lobule grand.
**Menton** : vertical.
**Barbe** : roux châtain moyen.
**Teint** : clair.

**Signes particuliers.** — Deux incisives manquent à la mâchoire supérieure.

*Photographies de face et de profil*

**Dans le but de faciliter l'identification de ces malheureux poilus, le « Journal des Mutilés et Réformés » (20, rue de la Chaussée-d'Antin, Paris) a fait faire un tirage spécial sur meilleur papier, permettant une reproduction nette et se rapprochant davantage de l'original. Ce tirage sera communiqué gratuitement aux familles qui en feront la demande au bureau du journal. Pour l'envoi par poste, joindre 0 fr. 25 en timbres.**

Algérien inconnu
Dit CHABENS OU CHABANNE

**Age apparent** : 30 ans.
**Taille** : 1 m. 70.
**Cheveux et sourcils** : bruns crépus.
**Barbe** : brune naissante.
**Front** : moyen.
**Yeux** : gris noir.
**Nez** : droit.
**Menton** : rond.
**Visage** : ovale.
**Teint** : demi basané.

Aucun signe particulier. Paraît avoir été de forte constitution.

*Photographies de face et de profil*

**Dans le but de faciliter l'identification de ces malheureux poilus, le « Journal des Mutilés et Réformés » (20, rue de la Chaussée-d'Antin, Paris) a fait faire un tirage spécial sur meilleur papier, permettant une reproduction nette et se rapprochant davantage de l'original. Ce tirage sera communiqué gratuitement aux familles qui en feront la demande au bureau du journal. Pour l'envoi par poste, joindre 0 fr. 25 en timbres.**

a

**Fig. 1.** The unknown living soldier. **a** Amnesiac patients reported in the *Journal des Mutilés et Réformés*, February 25, 1922. The text is titled 'The living dead' and starts 'The photographs below are of soldiers who, having become insane during the war, could not be identified.' Mangin is depicted at the top together with a list of his physical details.

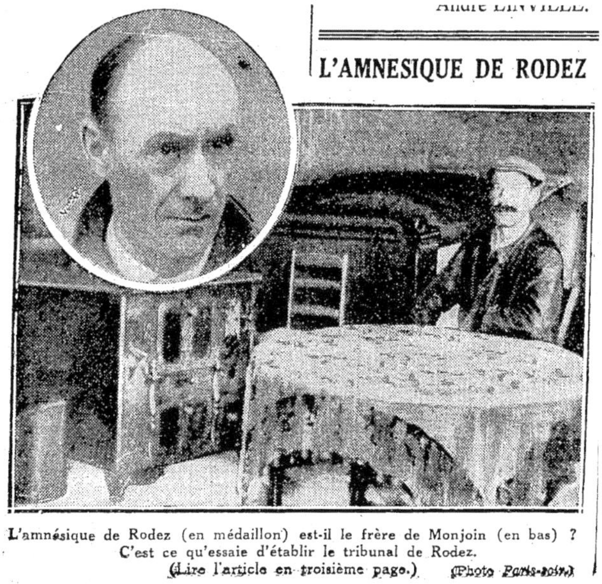

L'AMNESIQUE DE RODEZ

L'amnésique de Rodez (en médaillon) est-il le frère de Monjoin (en bas) ?
C'est ce qu'essaie d'établir le tribunal de Rodez.
(Lire l'article en troisième page.) (Photo Paris-soir.)

b

**Fig. 1. b** The Mangin case was followed up for many years. Here in the February 3, 1935 issue of *Journal des Mutilés et Combattants*, Mangin's probable brother has been identified and the case is still in the courts.

autobiographical, and semantic amnesia, as well as expressive dysphasia. The drug allowed him to retrieve the precipitating event of his psychogenic disorder (i.e. being kidnapped in the boot of a car), and subsequently recovered all of his memories, as well as speech capacities. Glitsky et al. [35], using sodium amytal in their patient (described above) only obtained unreliable information, while Levine et al. [40], using the same procedure with a patient with dense and isolated retrograde amnesia following a severe traumatic brain injury, obtained some information previously inaccessible to the patient, but of a rather fragmentary nature and with no long-term effects on the memory impairment. There has been a report of complete recovery of past memories during (but only during) the effect of sodium amytal, and Stuss and colleagues were able to induce a complete and permanent recovery with the same procedure (i.e. outlasting the effect of the drug; both cases cited in [41]). A literary example is found in *Mine Own Executioner* (1945) by Nigel Balchin, in which a psychoanalyst uncovers repressed war memories in a disturbed veteran using sodium pentothal.

Whereas Anthelme Mangin became the symbol of a wounded country and a living paradox embodying unfulfilled hope, Jean Anouilh's amnesiac exploits the story in a more personal way. In the play, amnesia becomes an allegory for individual freedom, the opportunity to become whoever one wants to be regardless of birth, class, family, society, and nation. Gaston hates Jacques Renaud, his older self, and forcefully rejects all the overwhelming evidence that he is indeed this person. Unlike Mangin, Gaston suffers a pure retrograde amnesia with otherwise very well preserved cognitive functions. This allows Anouilh's character to rebel against his well-meaning enemies and his earlier self, and to exploit his predicament to his own advantage (see [42] for a discussion on the Gaston-Mangin connections).

Anouilh, as it turns out, was also inspired by Jean Giraudoux's *Siegfried* (first published as a novel in 1922 and adapted as a theatrical play in 1928). This story of another war amnesiac was itself inspired by real-life cases such as Mangin, but possibly also by the author's own brother who suffered from spells of transient amnesia following a bombardment [5]. In the story, 'Siegfried' is found naked and unconscious on the battlefield, and is rescued by a German nurse. When he wakes up, his memory is entirely blank; the man is like a newborn that has to be taught virtually everything from scratch. He is thus 'brought up' as a German. This endeavor is so successful that he ends up as a prominent and charismatic politician in postwar Munich. Meanwhile, in France, a man reads an article written by Siegfried in a German newspaper and somehow immediately recognizes the writing style of Jacques Forestier, a writer friend of his that disappeared during the war. As it turns out, Siegfried's real identity is indeed that of Jacques Forestier, and the novel as well as the play portray the character as the embodiment of a possible reconciliation between France and Germany, a most ambitious and courageous artistic stance in those early years after the war.

Thus, in Giraudoux's *Siegfried*, contrary to Anouilh's plea for self-assertiveness and individual freedom, amnesia is used for a broader political goal. Himself a prominent Germanophile, diplomat, and war veteran, Giraudoux took his message of peace to heart, and the ploy of amnesia helped him encapsulate his ideas in a powerful and persuasive format. The amnesiac, in his purity and innocence, embodies a modern version of the noble savage, and allows addressing the absurdity of human conflicts, the malleability of national identity, the relatedness of all human beings, and the possibility of rebirth, and therefore of reconciliation. Although he realizes that he has become both German and French, Siegfried does not choose a camp: 'I refuse to carve trenches inside myself' [5, 7, 38].

*Other Literary Amnesiacs from World War I*

Although much less prominent than Giraudoux or Anouilh's, there have been a number of other literary amnesiacs in France very likely inspired by Mangin's case and other reports of war-related amnesia (fig. 2). Abel Moreau's *Le fou* (1926), for instance, takes place in 1924 and was obviously directly prompted by press releases of unknown amnesiacs. Indeed, it begins with a portrayal of ten war amnesiacs living together in the same asylum. None of them know who they are, not even their own names. One day, as 'Lucien' reads the newspaper to the other 'fools,' an item describing the discovery of eight dead soldiers down a deep trench in the woods suddenly strikes him. The cadavers are unidentifiable, but the names were recovered on surrounding equipment. Lucien becomes very troubled and agitated, as he begins to realize that the cadavers are those of his former unit; and printed on the list, he recognizes his real name: 'Létang Casimir. . . that's me!' From this moment he remembers everything and sets out to return to his village. However, times have changed, most

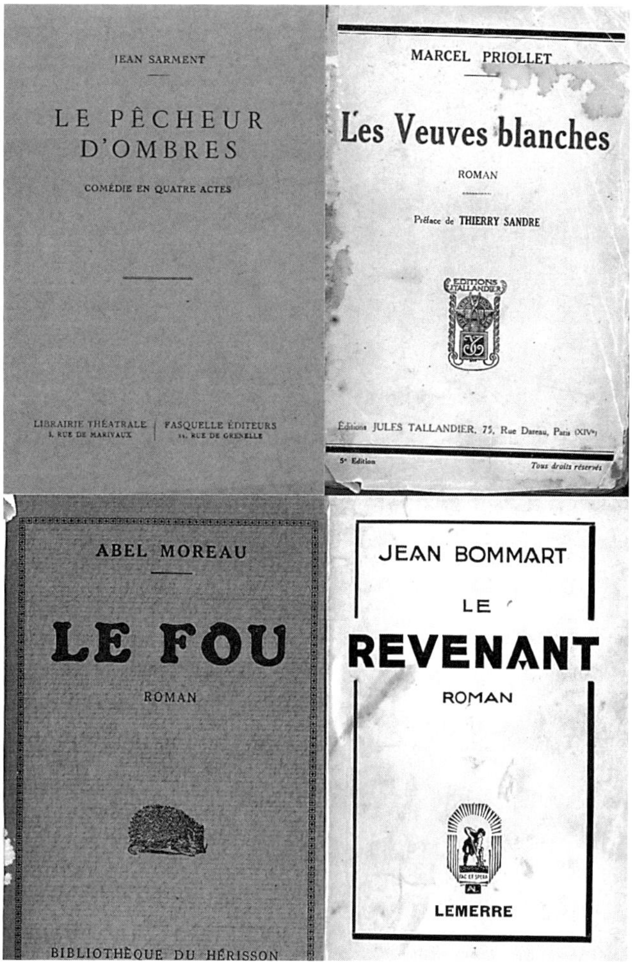


**Fig. 2.** Literary amnesiacs of World War I. The Great War was especially fertile in cases of literary amnesia. Between 1921 and 1937, a number of books explored the difficulties of amnesiac soldiers in dealing with their forgotten past and in coping with the present. Left to right and top to bottom: Jean Sarment's *Le pêcheur d'ombres*; Marcel Priollet's *Les veuves blanches*; Abel Moreau's *Le fou*; and Jean Bommart's *Le revenant* (Sebastian Dieguez, personal collection).

of those he knew are dead and no one is waiting for him. His wife has since then remarried. He has not only been amnesiac, he was thoroughly *forgotten* ever since his disappearance. In the end, he cannot cope with his new life, and returns to the asylum to live in oblivion and happiness with his fellow amnesiacs. No details are provided as to the causes of amnesia, and a doctor makes only a short appearance providing no help whatsoever. The pattern of memory recovery in Moreau's character is strikingly similar to that of an early case reported by Marie-Yves-Gérard Molin de Teyssieu [43]. The case is that of Louis D., a young man who lost all memories including his own name following a shell explosion. In the absence of recovery, the administration provided him with a new identity, and he was sent home to start a new life. However, some time later, in a strange course of events, he was charged for identity theft. Nearly 3 years after the onset of amnesia, with no discernible improvement but well-preserved cognitive abilities, he stumbled upon a familiar name while browsing a client listing at his new job. The name turned out to be that of a childhood friend, and from that moment he recovered the entire 'chain of memories' leading to full restoration of his past and identity.

In a book published the same year as *Le fou*, the consequences of amnesia in a missing soldier are told, so to speak, from the other side. Marcel Priollet's *Les veuves blanches* (The White Widows; 1926) tells the quest of a young girl for her disappeared fiancé. Lieutenant René Darty has been reported dead during a German attack in July 1918, yet Jeannine d'Ablainval, the girlfriend, fiercely believes him to be alive somewhere. René is indeed eventually located in a small town in Germany, near the French border. He does not recognize Jeannine or his mother, seems indifferent to his situation, and, much like Giraudoux's 'Siegfried', believes he is German. Professor Doctor Sigfried Zevort, 'one of Switzerland's medical glories', is able to examine him and concludes that the patient suffers from 'traumatic retrograde amnesia.' René is then kidnapped and brought back to France, and the book concludes with a chapter entitled 'Pauvres savants' (Poor scientists). In these final pages, two renowned doctors are negatively portrayed: Dr. T.L. Swift from the University of Pennsylvania (USA), and Professor Perugini, from corso Cavour, Milan. Both discuss René Darty's case, 'a traumatic retrograde amnesia, with total loss of memory and psychic asthenia [. . .] a ghost of a man, without memory or will.' We also learn that 'English, French and American doctors, neurologists and psychiatrists' have already examined the patient. All proposals for rehabilitation have failed: he 'must relearn everything' from scratch, including written language, using 'the system employed for inattentive or retarded children'. Jeannine is worried about the course of events; René's mental state indeed seems to deteriorate with this approach. She begins reading for herself about amnesia, and an interesting paragraph lists the following works, *Les maladies de la mémoire* by Ribot, *Sémiologie des affections du système nerveux* by Déjerine, *Blessures du crâne et du cerveau* by Chatelin and Martel, and *Psychologie de l'attention* by Nayrac, indicating that the author also did his homework. She integrates all of this knowledge about 'that mysterious and complicated machine that is the human brain', and concludes that the best hope for memory recovery is the 'method of evocation', namely, instead of having the patient relearn everything, he should be immersed 'in a grave situation, a considerable event that might have provoked a profound emotion' which would hopefully 'wake up, so to speak, a flow of memories.' Dr. Swift is dismissive about the idea: 'this method of evocation, which actually is mostly grounded on legends, has long been abandoned.' However, Jeannine carries out the project, and she arranges a meeting with her 'phantom fiancé' in the very place – same time, same season – where they shared their first kiss before René left for the war, carefully attending to all the details of the original event. The stratagem works, René has a 'shock' and his 'dementia receded to the depth of his rekindled pupils'. René fully retrieves his memory and personality, Jeannine becomes a doctor, and love has accomplished the miracle that science was unable, or unwilling, to achieve.

The novel thus has a happy ending, but it also vehemently decries the French attitude of forgetfulness and lack of due respect towards the veterans and the dead: 'People forgot. . . . Did this – this incredible thing – merely exist to eventually disappear from men's memory? The law of remembrance was being violated [. . .] But then. . .if *this* counted for so little, does it mean that there will always be wars?'

The ploy of sudden and complete memory recovery following an elaborate staging of an emotional and familiar event was most forcefully used by Balzac in *Adieu*, a short story from 1830. A lover sets out to restage in minute details the entire battle of Berezina to awaken the senses of an amnesiac and catatonic girl. The enterprise works too well, however, as the emotional surge ironically kills the woman.

The method of 'evocation', although dismissed as based on 'legends' in *Les veuves blanches* and catalogued as 'myths' of amnesia by Baxendale [10], was actually documented by Lucchelli et al. [41] in 2 patients. The first one had a surge of all his lost autobiographical life when, 1 year after amnesia onset due to a thalamic stroke, he found himself on an operating table for a pacemaker implantation and suddenly remembered having been in a similar situation some 25 years before, for a hernia operation. The second patient had a similar surge of lost memories 1 month after a car accident, as he was playing tennis and suddenly remembered having made a similar mistake in another match, years before. By analogy to the famous proustian episode, the authors dubbed such observations the 'petites madeleines phenomenon', and they suggest that sudden recovery of forgotten memories in cases of retrograde amnesia are most likely to happen in the context of an unplanned event that closely resembles a forgotten one, and in which the patient is currently playing an active role. Memory is then restored in an automatic chain of associations.

The pattern of amnesia in all the stories described up to now is rather stereotypically that of a pure and complete retrograde amnesia, mostly involving a loss of personal identity covering the entire life. *Le revenant* (The Ghost; 1932) by Jean Bommart, introduces an interesting twist to this pattern. The story takes place in 1931, 15 years after World War I veteran Jacques Brette, now 40-years-old, was sent home following a shell explosion that left a piece of shrapnel in his brain (at the right frontoparietal junction, we are told). Recovery was very good, however, and he became a bank accountant, got married, and had a child. War is but a distant and vague memory to him now; he leads a ranged, monotonous, and boring life, obedient to his domineering wife and lacking any desires or ambition. One day though, he comes across a former friend from the trenches and they start sharing war memories. Brette becomes overexcited and flooded by memories, and as he walks the streets, fully immersed in the vivid details of the events that led to his war wound, he is hit by a taxi. Unconscious, bleeding abundantly from the left temple, he is taken to the hospital. On first assessment, Professor Baudot detects no fracture but is worried about the effects of the trauma on the shrapnel located inside his head. Brette survives, but when he wakes up, it is soon apparent that he believes himself to be at the military hospital in 1916, when he first woke up from his war wound 15 years ago. As a result, he does not recognize or remember anything about his wife, kid, or job, and immediately retrieves his youthful personality and the manly manners and language of the trenches. Moreover, he is anosognosic. This specific pattern of amnesia, thus, allows (so to speak) the patient, author, and reader to travel back in time, and in the process denounce France's progressive forgetfulness and neglect of her war heroes. The patient is encouraged to write down his memories of the war, which constitute a fair part of the book and are strikingly precise and vivid. Dr. Baudot proposes a mechanism explaining how the 'partial amnesia' leads to reminiscences from the war, basically combining Ribot's law, frontal disinhibition, and a triggering psychological event. The brain, 'liberated' from 'weak memories' and 'the guide of reason', is flooded by the emotional and powerful memories of the battlefields, which were reactivated shortly before the onset of amnesia. Although memory of the last 15 years remains severely impaired for the rest of the novel, anosognosia resolves as the patient is progressively persuaded that the war is over. He is discharged and the doctor's recommendation is that he should act with his wife as if he is no longer amnesiac and resume his job at the bank; the rationale being that immersing the patient in his everyday life should help the reemergence of lost memories. Ultimately, he cannot endorse this role; the character he is required to be soon becomes 'the other', leading to marital problems and an inability to adapt to 'civilian life'. A living 'anachronism' with a double personality, Brette eventually chooses to restart his life from where he left it in 1916, entirely denying the past 15 years and leaving France behind for new adventures in Indochina.

The idea of a possible 'rebirth' is thus close to Jean Anouilh's concern, but the trick here is to bring into sharp focus, using a focal amnesic lacuna of 15 years, the real self that the protagonist had been and had subsequently forgotten due to the routine of quotidian life. Vivid reminiscences and incredibly detailed flashes (ecmnesia) from the past have been reported by Thomas-Antérion et al. [44] in a patient suffering from extended retrograde amnesia after having fallen from a chair. The patient had very strong recollections of how a neighborhood looked like 15 years earlier, but could not currently orient himself in that same place, due to the many changes that occurred in the meantime. Interestingly, his healthy relatives who knew the same place were unable to provide such precise details. He also was the only person who vividly remembered all the specifics of an unremarkable class meeting that took place 15 years earlier.

### *The Bruneri-Canella Affair and Pirandello*

The case of the missing French amnesiacs, as we have seen, inspired a wealth of literary works and led to creative uses of the topic of amnesia. In Italy, a similar story achieved a central status at the interface of literature and neuropsychiatry, yet was in many ways much stranger than most fictional and clinical cases. On the February 6, 1927, the picture of a bearded man appeared in the weekly *Domenica del Corriere* with the caption 'Who knows him?' (fig. 3). This man was arrested one year before as

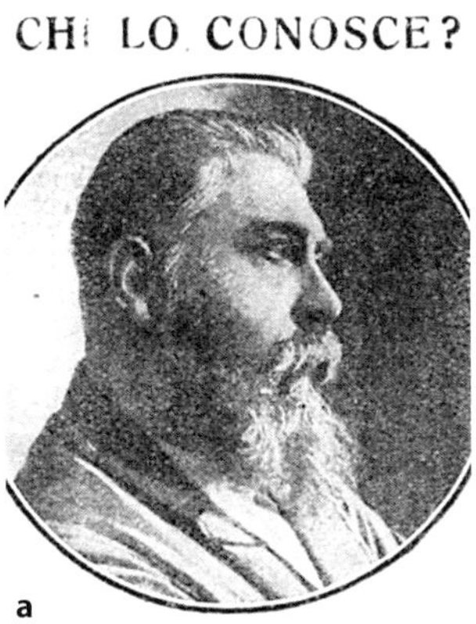


a

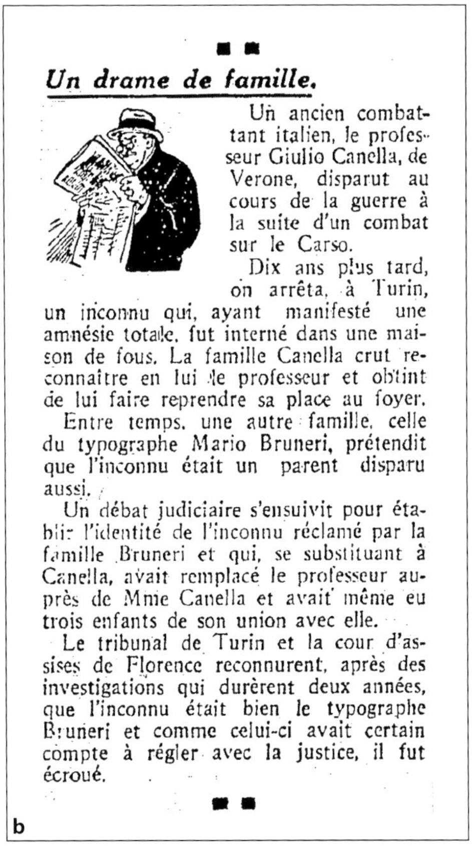

**Un drame de famille.**

Un ancien combattant italien, le professeur Giulio Canella, de Verone, disparut au cours de la guerre à la suite d'un combat sur le Carso.

Dix ans plus tard, on arrêta, à Turin, un inconnu qui, ayant manifesté une amnésie totale, fut interné dans une maison de fous. La famille Canella crut reconnaître en lui le professeur et obtint de lui faire reprendre sa place au foyer.

Entre temps, une autre famille, celle du typographe Mario Bruneri, prétendit que l'inconnu était un parent disparu aussi.

Un débat judiciaire s'ensuivit pour établir l'identité de l'inconnu réclamé par la famille Bruneri et qui, se substituant à Canella, avait remplacé le professeur auprès de Mme Canella et avait même eu trois enfants de son union avec elle.

Le tribunal de Turin et la cour d'assises de Florence reconnurent, après des investigations qui durèrent deux années, que l'inconnu était bien le typographe Bruneri et comme celui-ci avait certain compte à régler avec la justice, il fut écroué.

b

**Fig. 3.** The Bruneri-Canella affair. **a** Picture of the 'Collegno amnesiac' originally published in *Domenica del Corriere*, February 6, 1927. First recognized as professor Giulio Canella, the man turned out to be Mario Bruneri (from Archivi Storici della Psicologia Italiana). **b** Extract from *Journal des Mutilés et Combattants*, January 3, 1932. The Bruneri-Canella affair reached France only after Pirandello's play *Come tu mi vuoi* (1930) made it famous, and was merely allotted the space of a brief news item (compare to the 20-year-long treatment of the Mangin affair in the very same newspaper). Giulio Canella was a distinguished professor of philosophy (codirector in 1909 of the newly founded Rivista di Filosofia neo-scolastica, Florence), while Mario Bruneri was a modest typographer and a felon.

he was caught stealing a funeral urn from a Jewish cemetery in Turin. He was agitated and impulsive, and could not produce any information about himself. Considered unstable, the man was brought to the asylum in Collegno, and became known ever since as 'Lo smemorato di Collegno' (the Collegno amnesiac). As many soldiers were also reported missing in Italy during the years 1915–1918, the photograph was 'recognized' by many people. Among them, Renzo Canella had suspicions that the man could be his brother, Professor Giulio Canella – a learned and distinguished man reported missing in action in 1916. The brother had some doubts about the identity of the mysterious amnesiac, but Professor Canella's wife, Giulia Canella, subsequently claimed absolute certainty that the amnesiac was her husband. The mystery man was thus discharged, and resumed life with his loving (and wealthy) spouse. All was thus for the better, until it transpired that much evidence pointed against the Canella identity, and in favor of another lead, namely one Mario Bruneri, a modest typographer and incidentally a con-man under police investigation. Despite the quickly vanishing case for Giulia Canella, she strongly held to her belief and her fierce dispute with Bruneri's wife, who lately appeared on the scene, was brought to the courts. The Italian public got entranced by this battle and soon split camps between *Canelliani* and *Bruneriani*. In 1931, a final judgment ruled that the man's real identity was that of Mario Bruneri, and that the whole affair was basically an elaborated fraud. Incredibly, though, Giulia and Mario stayed together and fled to Brazil.

The case was hugely instrumental in the development of forensic techniques and psychological research in Italy. But its dramatic development was also ripe for fictional adaptations, and indeed, one year before its judicial closure, playwright and novelist Luigi Pirandello produced *Come tu mi vuoi* (As You Desire Me; 1930), a play ostensibly inspired by the Bruneri-Canella affair. The story is notable for introducing one of the very few female amnesiacs in literature, simply referred to as 'the unknown woman' throughout the play. She is strikingly beautiful and remembers nothing about her past. Not that she seems to care: she has decided to use her predicament to become not who *she* wants to be – like the protagonists in *Le voyageur sans bagage* and *Le revenant* – but rather who *others* want her to be. As she is literally no one, she is ready to play whichever role would please those that claim to recognize her. Pirandello exploits the topic of amnesia in an extraordinarily sophisticated way, juggling with the concepts of memory, identity, past, present, similarity, difference, love, desire, and rejection. The unknown woman becomes a metaphor of the blank page, on which an author can do as he pleases with his characters. Long before *Come tu mi vuoi*, the topics of identity and authorship were the well-established trademarks of Pirandello's work; it is thus not surprising that an author so fascinated by cases of mistaken identity and questions about the nature of the self (see the chapter by Paciaroni and Kilcline [this vol., pp. 69–76]) would be enthralled by the real-life story of the Collegno amnesiac, and that an entire school of 'the theater of memory' would emerge from such a striking congruence between fiction and reality [45].

## Literature Meets Theory: The Conundrum of Dissociative Amnesia

We now turn to a more theoretical question pertaining to the relationships between literary and clinical amnesia. Up to now, we have examined how literature has exploited the topic of amnesia and how real-life cases of amnesia are sometimes very close to, and indeed have served as sources for, artistic works. However, one might also ask whether the very existence of amnesia in literature can tell us something about the historical reality and the scientific understanding of memory disturbances.

In this regard, Pope et al. [46] famously (or notoriously) challenged readers to 'find a case of dissociative amnesia for a traumatic event in any fictional or nonfictional work before 1800'. The goal was to examine whether 'dissociative amnesia' was documented throughout history in the same way as other mental disturbances such as depression or hallucinations. If there is no trace to be found of such a striking disturbance in novels or plays predating its medical description, then this would count, the authors argued, as evidence that dissociative amnesia is not a 'natural neuropsychological phenomenon', but rather a culture-bound (i.e. 'pseudoneurological') syndrome. The broader question is one familiar to clinicians and memory researchers: can a psychological trauma, in the absence of detectable organic damage, really induce severe memory impairment, or are we dealing in such cases with instances better ascribed to the nebulous area ranging from malingering to hysteria?

We have described above a few literary cases, mostly from the 20th century, that would perhaps count as dissociative amnesia (e.g. Pirandello's 'unknown woman'; Moreau's 'le fou'). A more direct example can be found in Jean Sarment's *Le pêcheur d'ombres* (The Grayling Fisher; 1921), a poorly known play that could nevertheless, at least partly, have inspired Giraudoux and Anouilh's amnesiacs. Jean is a 25-year-old man who has been living with his brother and mother in a state of deep apathy since he was found wandering near a train station some four years earlier. His family hopes to make him recover his senses by inviting Nelly, a young girl whom he was in love with and seems to be the cause of his current state. Jean does not remember much of his past and has a very fragmentary sense of identity, but he appears to be happy and serene in his current state, whereas previous to his 'crisis' he was a brooding and impulsive man. The 'experiment' has a strange outcome: Jean immediately recognizes Nelly, but without the slightest emotional reaction. The two get along very well, Nelly liking his new personality. Progressively, with her help, his past begins to unfold, first in short flashes and later in floods of memories. Unfortunately, the memories also include the sorrow caused by her previous rejection; he starts brooding again and misses his previous state of oblivious indifference. Meanwhile, his brother becomes jealous of this newfound love; a bachelor older than Jean, he'd rather keep Nelly to himself. To this aim, he decides to confess the nature of the 'experiment', presenting it as a trick performed only to help him recover his memory, and adds that Nelly is actually a substitute, a completely different person he actually never met before. Although this is a lie, Jean believes it and rejects Nelly, who cannot convince him of her true identity and real love for him. The play ends with Jean's suicide.

This story highlights the benefits of amnesia and illustrates the malleability of memory and identity in defenseless amnesiac patients. Most importantly, it rather explicitly depicts a sentimental break-up as the triggering event for severe retrograde amnesia, involving not only the character's autobiographical memory, but also semantic knowledge and procedural skills (Jean cannot remember famous persons or events and is unable to play the piano or write poetry as he previously did). Whereas many other instances of literary amnesia are only vague about the issue of etiology, here a purely psychological cause is highlighted. As a matter of fact, broken hearts leading to psychogenic amnesia have been reported in the clinical literature (e.g. [47]). Most recently, Baird and McKay [48] described such a patient, whose story includes a mystery twist of sorts. A 25-year-old man woke up one day on his bathroom floor, unable to recall who and where he was. Two years earlier, the patient was deeply affected by a break-up with his then fiancée, and had trouble recovering from this devastating setback. As it turns out, upon his current admission to the hospital, his mother found a diamond ring in his belongings and it was subsequently found that the patient purchased it 3 weeks before the onset of his amnesia, as Valentine's Day was nearing. The patient claimed to have no recollection of this ring, and its intended recipient could not be identified. The authors hypothesize that their patient suffered from a second rejection and that this event precipitated the dissociative episode.

It seems almost self-evident why such cases, though medically puzzling, would make for good fiction. Amnesia introduces a de facto ellipse in the narrative flow; the author, the reader, and the protagonists must, as it were, work together to fill in the missing information in order to make sense of the ongoing events. From this perspective, the challenge from Pope et al. [46] is certainly warranted: if such cases have always existed, then they must have come to the attention of early authors of fiction.

From their review, Pope et al. [46] found that dissociative amnesia was very frequent in modern works, but could only trace a few from the 19th century, such as Dr. Manette in Dickens' *A Tale of Two Cities* (1859) and the preacher Penn in Kipling's *Captain Courageous* (1896) [they do not mention countess Stéphanie de Vandières from Balzac's *Adieu* (1830); see above]. The issued challenge brought back no convincing example (despite more than 100 responses) previous to the year 1800, and so the authors concluded that dissociative amnesia is 'a cultural product of its time, rather than an actual neurological disorder in the brain'. The condition, they suggest, is intrinsically linked to the advent of romanticism, the emergence of hypnosis, and the developing notion of the unconscious, all cultural phenomena positing that under some circumstances the human mind can split in order to protect itself against unwanted memories. Perhaps the disorder also prospered due to the popularity of authors such as Freud and Janet, and even, the authors point out, because of 'its convenience as a dramatic device'.

The challenge award (USD 1,000), however, was later conceded to retired English teacher, poet, and editor George Simmers for his submission *Nina, ou la folle par amour* (1786), an opera written by Benoît-Joseph Marsollier (music by Nicolas Dalayrac), the story of a woman who becomes amnesiac after seeing her lover killed by a rival [49]. They also acknowledged the case of the Présidente de Tourvel in Choderlos de Laclos' *Les liaisons dangereuses* (1782), who suffers from a brief (30 min) episode of amnesia and confusion upon awakening in a deep state of depression (letter CXLIX).

The challenge itself has not gone unchallenged, for instance on the grounds that the required criteria for cases of dissociative amnesia were unclear or too stringent, that classic cases such as Shakespeare's *King Lear* (~1603–1606) were dismissed too hastily from the contest, and that the year 1800 cutoff was arbitrary [50]. Moreover, the debate did not consider important advances in the cognitive neuroscience of dissociative (or psychogenic) amnesia, which highlights possible neural mechanisms responsible for the 'blocking' of certain memories (e.g. [51]). Despite these shortcomings, the challenge raised interesting questions at the interface of art and neuropsychiatry. Using historical literature as a database to investigate the nature of mental disorders is a commendable and promising project (one indeed pursued throughout the present volume). Not only can works of art be inspired by real-life medical cases, but literary products and traditions can in turn inform medical researchers, theorists, and historians, and perhaps even prompt the emergence and consolidation of previously inexistent conditions [52, 53].

## Other Literary Memory Disorders: Anterograde, Semantic and Collective Amnesia, Excesses of Memory

This chapter has mainly focused on literary depictions of retrograde amnesia, as this is by far the most prominent representation of memory disorders in fiction (the next section will provide an attempt to explain this feature). In this section we outline other types of literary memory disturbances.

*Dementia and Anterograde Amnesia*
Anterograde amnesia is very rarely portrayed in fiction; strikingly, it never accompanies retrograde amnesia in the stories presented herein. Interestingly, the works that do introduce anterograde amnesia are all rather recent and neurologically informed, as if the authors were willingly taking a stance against the all too popular form of isolated retrograde amnesia.

Martin Suter's *Small World* (1997) is an apt example. The book presents an accurate portrayal of dementia of the Alzheimer type, including a credible neuropsychological assessment and many anecdotal observations that are familiar to clinicians and caregivers of such patients. The main protagonist, Conrad Lang, 65 years of age, starts displaying early signs of disorientation, forgetfulness, and misidentification. A diagnosis of Alzheimer's disease is made, and as the disease progresses he is increasingly aware of long forgotten memories from his early years, allowing him to understand what happened when he was 5-years-old and uncover the secrets of the wealthy family in which he was raised. The reminiscence of very remote memories in Alzheimer's disease is informed here by Ribot's law and the phenomenology of ecmnesia, and allows for an original and poignant plot structure.

A more personal and harrowing account of the destructiveness of Alzheimer's disease was provided the same year by Annie Ernaux's strikingly crude, precise, and unapologetic depiction of her own mother's dementia, including the tragic experience of being forgotten by a loved one (*Je ne suis pas sortie de ma nuit*, 1997).

More recently, a fictive type of anterograde amnesia was depicted in Steven J. Watson's successful first novel, *Before I Go to Sleep* (2011). The main character of this story, a 47-year-old woman, can store new memories only up to 24 h, after which she forgets everything. Every morning, she thus wakes up as a blank slate and has to piece together, again and again, every fragment of her life. She keeps a diary to facilitate this painful process, and incidentally discovers that she might not be the person her relatives tell her she is, as well as the actual cause of her debilitating condition. Although largely a work of the imagination, the character was inspired by the amnesic patient H.M., the paradigmatic case of severe anterograde amnesia [28].

The most sophisticated use of anterograde amnesia in fiction comes from the movie *Memento* (USA, 2000, directed by Christopher Nolan), in which the main character cannot encode any new information and yet has to solve a convoluted mystery. The narrative structure uses a reversed chronological order, effectively allowing the audience to experience the same disorder as the protagonist.

More allegorical forms of ongoing forgetfulness and distortions of memory are scattered in Malcolm Lowry's *Under the Volcano* (1947), which depicts in painstaking detail the phenomenological effects of alcoholic intoxication [54]. Likewise, Eric Fottorino explores the intermingling of fantasy and reality through the confabulating mind of a narrator with Korsakoff's syndrome, perhaps the only novel portraying this disorder (*Korsakov*, 2004).

*Semantic and 'Collective' Amnesia*

Semantic amnesia is rarely depicted in literature. One notable exception is Gabriel Garcia Marquez's *One Hundred Years of Solitude* (1967), at least according to one recent interpretation. Rascovsky et al. [55] indeed made an analogy between one of the symptoms of the 'insomnia plague' that strikes the inhabitants of the city of Macondo and the clinical syndrome of semantic dementia, first recognized 8 years after the publication of the novel. Just like real-life patients suffering from semantic dementia, the characters of the novel are afflicted by the progressive loss of 'the name and notion of things'. An interesting consequence of this impairment is the strategies used to cope with it: 'With an inked brush he marked everything with its name: *table, chair, clock, door, wall, bed, pan*. He went to the corral and marked the animals and plants.' A cow would later be wearing a sign indicating 'This is the cow. She must be milked every morning so that she will produce milk, and the milk must be boiled in order to be mixed with coffee to make coffee and milk.' Eventually, an antidote allows the recovery of the meaning of things, and the characters can contemplate the full absurdity of being surrounded by labeled objects.

Whereas amnesia in *One Hundred Years of Solitude* allows its author to explore the anxieties of a postcolonial Latin America reclaiming a culture for itself, George Orwell's *Nineteen Eighty-Four* (1949) takes a political and epistemological stance against the voluntary manipulation of meaning and memory by the powers that be. The principles of doublethink, newspeak and memory hole, all coined by Orwell, illustrate the malleability and vulnerability of memory processes. Pathology at the individual level is here extended to the collective level, and offers a striking anticipation of the so-called 'memory wars' (e.g. [56]) and current concerns about widespread misinformation [57].

*Excesses of Memory*

Besides syndromes of amnesia, literature has also explored the other face of memory abnormality, namely its uncontrolled excesses. The classic illustration is Jorge Luis Borges's *Funes the Memorious* (1944), the story of a man plagued by his inability to forget even the minutest details of his existence. Borges takes the condition to its most absurd extremities, as Funes also remembers every episode of remembering, therefore infinitely and uselessly multiplying his memories. What is more, he is unable to conceive of abstract entities; to him, a dog really is a multiplicity of the same dog seen from different perspectives and in different circumstances. The story can be read as an allegory illustrating the importance of forgetting and the tyrannical aspects of memory in mental life, and ultimately the role of the artist as a skilled synthesizer of the only relevant aspects of reality [58]. Some real-life cases of extraordinary mnemonists have been described [59] and recently some persons with extensive and almost perfectly reliable autobiographical memories have been reported under the new clinical entity 'hyperthymestic syndrome' [60, 61].

On a related note, literature has much more frequently portrayed the effects of obsessive and intrusive memories [for instance in Stefan Zweig's *The Royal Game* (1942) and Primo Levi's *If This Is a Man* (1942)], illustrating the painful flashbacks in cases of posttraumatic stress disorder, and poetry and prose have made ample use of the déjà vu experience [62, 63]. Likewise, the sudden intrusion of involuntary or so-called 'panoramic' memories have often been exploited as a subjective flash-back device [e.g. Hemingway's *Snows of Kilimanjaro* (1936), see [64]].

## The Folk Neuropsychiatry of the Amnesiac Character

This chapter has examined a wide array of memory disorders in fiction (table 1) and offered comparisons with cases taken from history and clinical science. We have argued that the view that literary amnesia is clinically inaccurate or far-fetched is at best too simplistic, and at worst misguided. Instead of asking whether cases of literary amnesia are clinically accurate or realistic, we should instead ask what are the uses of amnesia in literature and how do authors and readers conceive of memory and its disorders. As such, cases of literary amnesia become valuable data, just like real-life cases but for different reasons. Literary amnesia covers a wider range of questions encompassing the topics of self-identity, social relationships, and culture at large.

**Table 1.** Fictional works portraying amnesiac characters cited in text (for depictions of amnesia in movies, see Baxendale [10])

| Works cited in text | Author | Year |
|---|---|---|
| *Odyssey* | Homer | ca. 700 BC |
| *The Recognition of Śakuntalā* | Kālidāsa | ca. 350 BC |
| *King Lear* | W. Shakespeare | ca 1603–1606 |
| *Les liaisons dangereuses* | Choderlos de Laclos | 1782 |
| *Nina, ou la folle par amour* | Benoît-Joseph Marsollier | 1786 |
| *Adieu* | Honoré de Balzac | 1830 |
| *A Tale of Two Cities* | Charles Dickens | 1859 |
| *The Moonstone* | Wilkie Collins | 1868 |
| *Recalled to Life* | Grant Allen | 1891 |
| *Captain Courageous* | Rudyard Kipling | 1896 |
| *Le pêcheur d'ombres* | Jean Sarment | 1921 |
| *Siegfried* | Jean Giraudoux | 1922/1928 |
| *Le fou* | Abel Moreau | 1926 |
| *Les veuves blanches* | Marcel Priollet | 1926 |
| *As You Desire Me* | Luigi Pirandello | 1930 |
| *Le revenant* | Jean Bommart | 1932 |
| *The Snows of Kilimanjaro* | Ernest Hemingway | 1936 |
| *Le voyageur sans bagage* | Jean Anouilh | 1937 |
| *The Royal Game* | Stefan Zweig | 1942 |
| *If This Is a Man* | Primo Levi | 1942 |
| *Funes the Memorious* | Jorge Luis Borges | 1944 |
| *Mine Own Executioner* | Nigel Balchin | 1945 |
| *Nightfall* | David Goodis | 1947 |
| *Under the Volcano* | Malcolm Lowry | 1947 |
| *Nineteen Eighty-Four* | George Orwell | 1949 |
| *The Long Wait* | Michael Spillane | 1951 |
| *One Hundred Years of Solitude* | Gabriel Garcia Marquez | 1967 |
| *Rue des boutiques obscures* | Patrick Modiano | 1978 |
| *The Bourne Trilogy* | Robert Ludlum | 1980, 1986, 1990 |
| *The Face of a Stranger* | Anne Perry | 1990 |
| *Small World* | Martin Suter | 1997 |
| *Je ne suis pas sortie de ma nuit* | Annie Ernaux | 1997 |
| *New Finnish Grammar* | Diego Marani | 2000 |
| *Korsakov* | Eric Fottorino | 2004 |
| *The Mysterious Flame of Queen Loana* | Umberto Eco | 2004 |
| *Before I Go to Sleep* | S.J. Watson | 2011 |

One way to look at fictional amnesiacs is to see them as thought experiments. An author can freely experiment with his characters, and ask what would be the consequences if such and such cognitive capacity suddenly were to disappear. Amnesiac characters thus allow pushing the limits of what can be done in a real laboratory, and by the same token reveal intuitive conceptions about the human mind. In this concluding section, we take these two approaches in turn.

*Amnesiac Characters as Fictional Experiments: Uses of Amnesia*

What is the amnesiac character used for in literature? Whether an author decides to simply tell the story of an amnesiac, to exploit the condition for secondary motives, or (probably most frequently) both, the choice of this very specific condition remains to be explained. After all, stories of protagonists with aphasia, Parkinson's disease, or anosognosia are few, despite these disorders being arguably much more frequent than pure retrograde amnesia. As we argued in the opening section, however, amnesia is tightly linked to literature because the very theme of memory is indissociable from fiction. The amnesiac character can thus serve as an exploratory device of this intrinsic link, plunging the depth, as it were, of narration by excising (or knocking out, a geneticist might say) its core element: remembrance. Amnesia therefore becomes in literature a discourse about fiction and reality, bringing to the fore what is left of humanity and the world when the very act of remembering is removed.

This revealing function of literary amnesia offers insights on a variety of topics, and provides in the process a tentative portrait of the amnesiac character in general[1].

One central theme, perhaps the most frequent and important, is that of identity and self-preservation. The primary effect of being unable to remember one's past is to become immensely vulnerable. Amnesiac characters are in danger, they cannot trust anyone, and they are deprived of reliable information about virtually everything. Indeed, some of them will struggle to hide the fact that they have no memories. They are also at the mercy of their own previous self and of the current effects of their past behavior. This shows just how much we take memory for granted, as well as the solid grounding in reality it offers and the sense of accountability it entails. A more specific consequence of these characters' predicament is that they have to learn to know themselves. Not only do they need to gather information from external sources, a sometimes unreliable and dangerous process, but they must be finely tuned to their inner feelings. Anne Perry's William Monk and Patrick Modiano's detective are good examples: at each step of their investigation, they experience spontaneous reactions that can only be explained by some forgotten episode. This can be a sudden shivering or arousal prompted by a voice or an object, an irrational sensation of distrust for someone, a strange sense of unexplainable familiarity with a scene or smell, etc. In short, it could be any type of the innumerable bodily sensations that nonamnesiacs experience on a daily basis and pass entirely unnoticed most of the time. This inner and hidden life of the organism is thus forcefully revealed by amnesia. The same applies to specific skills that amnesiacs can sometimes discover to their surprise. The detective William Monk, although he has no conscious recollection of his trade, can never be sure whether his obvious talent at his job depends, in his current state,

[1] As a side note, we point out that the role of physicians in amnesia stories is most often restricted to that of convenient lecturers. Besides providing a diagnosis, and perhaps performing some testing, oftentimes they would deliver a crash-course on the nature of amnesia relevant to both the protagonists and the readers, and they sometimes also offer some hapless recommendations in place of treatment. Their behavior varies across novels between ineptitude, arrogance, cynicism, and empathy.

on some preserved skills and habits, some intrinsic or innate reliance on instinct, or merely common sense.

Another important use of amnesia is to illustrate the notion that identity should not be confused with fate. Losing one's past, although a terrible event, can also have positive effects. Instead of painstakingly seeking to reconstruct their lost existence, some amnesiacs will indeed happily embrace the possibility of rebirth offered to them. These stories illustrate the destructive power of habits, tradition, and memory, all narrowing forces of the human potential for freedom.

This brings us from the individual to the social level. We have seen that authors frequently use amnesia to make a broader point about the importance of memory for culture, history, and society as a whole. Writers frequently mix the individual and collective conceptions of memory. For instance, in *The Mysterious Flame of Queen Loana* by Umberto Eco (2004), an erudite book antiquarian loses all personal memories due to a stroke (according to his doctor, involving the right orbitofrontal cortex). He can, however, access his vast store of semantic knowledge acquired through books. The novel thus allows the author to explore his own childhood during the fascist years in Italy, and to address the limits of rational thought and abstract erudition compared to personal experience and subjective recollections.

For all these reasons, isolated retrograde amnesia, especially of the purely autobiographical type, has been much more frequently exploited in fiction than the actually more usual condition of anterograde amnesia in real life. Indeed, the narrative and symbolic power of anterograde amnesia seems much more restricted than the purely retrograde pattern. The idea of being stuck in the present is certainly a most unsettling one, yet apart from that existential anguish – perhaps analogous to the antique fear of being buried alive – it simply seems impractical to conceive of a plot based on a character that cannot encode new information (although we have seen earlier that some writers have taken up the challenge). Also, as we will see below, anterograde amnesia seems too close to a generic notion of insanity to be used effectively as a *selective* literary ploy. Finally, whereas retrograde amnesia seems easy to digest for our interpretative systems, anterograde amnesia appears to require a considerable cognitive effort to process (as can indeed be experienced when watching the movie *Memento*).

### *Amnesia and the Imagination*

Clearly, real-life cases of amnesia have been important sources for many stories with amnesiac characters. As we have just seen, authors have then exploited the condition to explore different aspects of identity and society. Yet a different way to approach the relationships between literary and clinical depictions of amnesia is to ask how authors and readers intuitively conceive of memory and its impairment, and in turn what these intuitive conceptions tell us about the human mind and imagination. Such an approach often pertains to the field of cognitive anthropology and shares themes familiar to the study of folk psychology and social cognition.

As we have previously argued, intuitive conceptions of memory and its impairments do not have to perfectly match scientific knowledge. However, one should not entirely dismiss prima facie the importance of naïve representations for the advancement of scientific knowledge. Indeed, the prominent memory researcher Endel Tulving relied precisely on such an intuitive hunch to develop one of the most fruitful theoretical proposals in memory research. His distinction between the episodic and semantic systems of memory first came to him, in his own terms, as a 'pre-theoretical' (or 'armchair' [65]) argument: 'The idea of differentiable episodic and semantic memory systems, he wrote, in its most rudimentary form, is simply a hunch that there is something basically different about the way people remember their own past and how they store and retrieve general information about the world' [66, p. 308]. Of course, further experimental, clinical and neuroimaging evidence would eventually forcefully establish the validity of the idea. Yet Tulving was speaking of a common-sense hunch, not of some divinely infused counterintuitive and revolutionary idea, and in retrospect it would explain why the episodic/semantic distinction is clearly present in many (but not all) early fictional depictions of amnesia. In fact, one could argue that we intuitively feel the distinction between these two systems of memory precisely because we *have* these two systems of memory. The imagination of writers, like that of Tulving, cannot escape the constraints imposed by their own cognitive architecture (and that of their readers).

In this sense, we are all endowed with an intuitive system for memory-understanding, plausibly based on the *actual* mechanisms of memory in the brain (a general case for this approach is made in Sperber and Hirschfeld [67]). Yet our intuitive conceptions of memory and its disorders might very well be biased towards some salient features of the system – for instance the autobiographical store and the retrieval system, rather than the semantic store and the encoding processes. Under this hypothesis, the prominence of retrograde autobiographical amnesia – rather than semantic dementia or anterograde amnesia – in literature would make sense.

More research is needed to explore this idea, but a preliminary attempt to describe a cognitive system devoted to the understanding of amnesia has recently been proposed by Boyer [68] as part of a more general framework exploring beliefs and intuitions about 'what is construed as expected and aberrant behavior'. On his view, memory is widely (and naïvely) conceived as a store, on which events get copied and retrieved later, much in the same form in which they were experienced. This conception of memory would lead to the prediction that memory impairment is conceived as some form of leakage. An individual who fails to recall an event previously known to him would be seen as having lost this information from his store, not has having failed to retrieve or encode it. Although this idea is not explored further, it can serve as a useful starting point for further research. In addition to laboratory- and survey-based approaches, the cross-cultural study of literary amnesia would be an extremely useful asset in such a project. More than a simple leakage detection device, the intuitive understanding of memory impairment could turn out to rely on the perception of radical personality changes, out-of-character claims, behaviors incongruent with previous events, repetitive actions and utterings, or lack of emotional reactions to familiar items. Such a collection of systems might favor the recognition and ascription of one specific type of amnesia, namely retrograde autobiographical amnesia, over other types described in the clinical literature.

The human system for understanding memory impairments might itself be dynamically modulated by cultural factors. On this view, literature and culture at large could in turn induce a 'looping effect' on clinical manifestations and favor the emergence of previously inexistent or very rare conditions. As we have seen, such a proposal has actually been advanced for the very existence of dissociative amnesia [46]. Whether and how entirely new types of amnesia can be invented and spread through society, perhaps under the influence of fictional and artistic depictions, is an interesting question in our world of hyperfast and wide-scale communication.

## References


1 Bogousslavsky J: La mémoire de Proust. Vevey, Le Cadratin, 2009.
2 Dieguez S: Proust ou la mémoire involontaire; in Dieguez S: Maux d'artistes: ce que cachent les oeuvres. Paris, Pour la science, 2010, pp 35–41.
3 Bogousslavsky J, Walusinski O: Marcel Proust and Paul Sollier: the involuntary memory connection. Schweiz Arch Neurol Psychiat 2009;160:130–136.
4 Schacter DL: Seven Sins of Memory: How the Mind Forgets and Remembers. New York, Houghton Mifflin Company, 2001.
5 Tadié JY, Tadié M: Le sens de la mémoire. Paris, Gallimard, 1999.
6 Whitty CWM, Zangwill OL: Amnesia, ed 2. London, Butterworths, 1977.
7 Weinrich L: Lethe: the art and critique of forgetting. Ithaca, Cornell University Press, 2004.
8 Bouvier D: La mémoire et la mort dans l'épopée homérique. Kernos 1999;12:57–71.
9 Dieguez S: *Le chant des sirènes*, un piège mental universel. Cerveau Psycho 2012;51:84–89.
10 Baxendale S: Memories aren't made of these: amnesia at the movies. BMJ 2004;329:1480–1483.
11 Assal G: L'amnésie retrograde: une nébuleuse neuropsychiatrique; in Ansermet F, Innocenti G, Steck A, Steck B (eds): Psyché et Cerveau. Lausanne, Payot, 1993, pp 71–87.
12 Warehime M: Originality and narrative nostalgia: shadows in Modiano's *Rue des boutiques obscures*. French Forum 1987;12:335–345.
13 Hunkin NM, Parkin AJ, Bradley VA, Burrows EH, Aldrich FK, Jansari A, Burdon-Cooper C: Focal retrograde amnesia following closed head injury: a case study and theoretical account. Neuropsychologia 1995;33:509–523.
14 Sellal F, Manning L, Seegmuller C, Scheiber C, Schoenfelder F: Pure retrograde amnesia following a mild head trauma: a neuropsychological and metabolic study. Cortex 2002;38:499–509.
15 Berrios GE: Historical aspects of memory and its disorders; in Berrios GE, Hodges JR (eds): Memory Disorders in Psychiatric Practice. Cambridge, Cambridge University Press, 2000, pp 3–33.
16 Janet P: L'amnésie psychologique: le cas Emma Dutemple. Oeuvres choisies II. Paris, L'Harmattan, 2006.
17 Ribot T: Les maladies de la mémoire. Paris, Baillière, 1981.
18 Sollier P: Les troubles de la mémoire. Paris, Rueff, 1892.
19 Lamb DG, Prigatano GP: Malingering and feigned memory disorders; in Berrios GE, Hodges JR (eds): Memory disorders in psychiatric practice. Cambridge, Cambridge University Press, 2000, pp 456–478.
20 MacDonald K, MacDonald T: Peas, pleas: a case report and neuroscientific review of dissociative amnesia and fugue. J Trauma Dissociation 2009;10:420–435.
21 Schacter DL: Implicit memory: history and current status. J Exp Psychol Learn Mem Cogn 1987;13:501–518.

22 Roediger HL III: Implicit memory: retention without remembering. Am Psychol 1990;45:1043–1056.

23 Hennig-Fast K, Meister F, Frodl T, Beraldi A, Padberg F, Engel RR, Reiser M, Möller H-J, Meindl T: A case of persistent retrograde amnesia following a dissociative fugue: neuropsychological and neurofunctional underpinnings of loss of autobiographical memory and self-awareness. Neuropsychologia 2008;46:2993–3005.

24 Conway MA, Fthenaki A: Disruption and loss of autobiographical memory; in Cermak LS (ed): Handbook of Neuropsychology, ed 2: Memory and Its Disorders. Amsterdam, Elsevier, 2000, vol 2, pp 281–312.

25 Kapur N: Syndromes of retrograde amnesia: a conceptual and empirical synthesis. Psychol Bull 1999; 125:800–825.

26 Kopelman MD, Kapur N: The loss of episodic memories in retrograde amnesia: single-case and group studies. Phil Trans R Soc Lond B 2001;356: 1409–1421.

27 Schnider A: The Confabulating Mind: How the Brain Creates Reality. Oxford, Oxford University Press, 2008.

28 Corkin S: What's new with the amnesic patient H.M.? Nat Rev Neurosci 2002;3:153–160.

29 Pasini W: A propos d'un cas d'amnésie hystérique rendu célèbre par la presse internationale. Congrès de Psychiatrie et de Neurologie de langue française, 63ème session. Paris, Masson, 1966.

30 Morris S: Do you know this man? Mystery of the silent, talented piano player who lives for his music. The Guardian 2005. http://www.guardian.co.uk/uk/2005/may/16/stevenmorris.

31 Della Sala S, Freschi R, Lucchelli F: Retrograde amnesia: no past, new life; in Halligan PW, Marshall JC (eds): Method in Madness: Case Studies in Cognitive Neuropsychiatry. Hove, Psychology Press, 1996, pp 209–233.

32 Wallis L: The stroke had turned me gay. BBC News 2012. http://www.bbc.co.uk/news/magazine-17703018.

33 Dieguez S, Viollier S, Bogousslavsky J: The man who had a stroke and could not remember he was a woman (patient XY): thalamic amnesia in a male-to-female transsexual. XIVth European Stroke Conference, Bologna, 2005.

34 Mishra NK, Russmann H, Granziera C, Maeder P, Annoni J-M: Mutism and amnesia following high-voltage electrical injury: psychogenic symptomatology triggered by organic dysfunction? Eur Neurol 2011;66:229–234.

35 Glisky EL, Ryan L, Reminger S, Hardt O, Hayes SM, Hupbach A: A case of psychogenic fugue: I understand, aber ich verstehe nichts. Neuropsychologia 2004;42:1132–1147.

36 Lethem J: The Vintage Book of Amnesia: An Anthology of Writing on the Subject of Memory Loss. New York, Vintage, 2000.

37 Tatu L, Bogousslavsky J: La folie au front: la grande bataille des névroses de guerre (1914–1918). Paris, Imago, 2012.

38 Le Naour JY: Le soldat inconnu vivant. Paris, Hachette Littératures, 2002.

39 Pujol M, Kopelman MD: Psychogenic amnesia. Pract Neurol 2003;3:292–299.

40 Levine B, Black SE, Cabeza R, Sinden M, Mcintosh AR, Toth JP, Tulving E, Stuss DT: Episodic memory and the self in a case of isolated retrograde amnesia. Brain 1998;121:1951–1973.

41 Lucchelli F, Muggia S, Spinnler H: The 'petites madeleines' phenomenon in two amnesic patients: sudden recovery of forgotten memories. Brain 1995; 118:167–183.

42 Dieguez S, Le voyageur sans bagage: peut-on vivre sans passé? Cerveau Psycho 2012;53:82–89.

43 Molin de Teyssieu M-Y-G: Brusque retour des souvenirs dans une amnésie retrograde consecutive à un incident de guerre. Ann Méd-Psychol 1919;11: 422–427.

44 Thomas-Antérion C, Mazzola L, Laurent B: Autobiographical memory: phenomenological aspects, personal semantic knowledge, generic events and characters (one case of pure retrograde memory recovery). Clin Neurophysiol 2008;38:171–176.

45 Sciascia L: Le théâtre de la mémoire. Paris, Maurice Nadeau/Boréal Express, 1981.

46 Pope HG Jr, Poliakoff MB, Parker MP, Boynes M, Hudson JI: Is dissociative amnesia a culture-bound syndrome? Findings from a survey of historical literature. Psychol Med 2007;37:225–233.

47 Kopelman MD: Focal retrograde amnesia and the attribution of causality: an exceptionally critical review. Cogn Neuropsychology 2000;17:585–621.

48 Baird AD, McKay RT: Psychological factors in retrograde amnesia: self-deception and a broken heart. Neurocase 2008;14:400–413.

49 Pope HG Jr, Poliakoff MB, Parker MP, Boynes M, Hudson JI: Author's reply to Altshuler and Ramachandran. Psychol Med 2007;37:1067–1068.

50 Goldsmith RE, Cheit RE, Wood ME: Evidence of dissociative amnesia in science and literature: culture-bound approaches to trauma in Poe, Poliakoff, Parker, Boynes, and Hudson (2007). J Trauma Dissociation 2009;10:237–253.

51 Markowitsch HJ, Staniloiu A: The impairment of recollection in functional amnesic states. Cortex 2012, E-pub ahead of print.

52 Hacking I: Mad Travelers: Reflections on the Reality of Transient Mental Illnesses. Charlottesville, University of Virginia Press, 1998.

53 Merckelbach H, Merten T, Lilienfeld SO: A skeptical look at a remarkable case report of 'overnight' amnesia: extraordinary symptoms, weak evidence, and a breakdown in peer review. Skeptical Inquirer 2011;35:35–39.
54 Dieguez S: Sous le volcan: l'écriture alcoolique. Cerveau Psycho 2011;47:82–87.
55 Rascovsky K, Growdon ME, Pardo IR, Grossman S, Miller BL: 'The quicksand of forgetfulness': semantic dementia in One Hundred Years of Solitude. Brain 2009;132:2609–2616.
56 Showalter E: Hystories: Hysterical Epidemics and Modern Culture. New York, Columbia University Press, 1997.
57 Lewandowsky S, Ecker UKH, Seifert C, Schwarz N, Cook J: Misinformation and its correction: continued influence and successful debiasing. Psychol Sci Public Interest, in press.
58 Dieguez S: Jorge Luis Borges: Funes ou la mémoire sans limite. Cerveau Psycho 2010;37:82–87.
59 Luria AR: The Mind of a Mnemonist. Cambridge, Harvard University Press, 1987.
60 Parker ES, Cahill L, McGaugh JL: A case of unusual autobiographical remembering. Neurocase 2006;12: 35–49.
61 Ally BA, Hussey EP, Donahue MJ: A case of hyperthymesia: rethinking the role of the amygdala in autobiographical memory. Neurocase, in press.
62 Bodei R: La sensation de déjà vu. Paris, Seuil, 2007.
63 Sno HN, Linszen DH, De Jonghe F: Art imitates life: déjà-vu experiences in prose and poetry. Br J Psychiatry 1992;160:511–518.
64 Dieguez S: 'A man can be destroyed but not defeated': Ernest Hemingway's near-death experience and declining health. Front Neurol Neurosci 2010;27:174–206.
65 Klatzky RL: Armchair theorists have more fun. Behav Brain Sci 1984;7:244.
66 Tulving E: What kind of a hypothesis is the distinction between episodic and semantic memory? J Exp Psychol Learn Mem Cogn 1986;12:307–311.
67 Sperber D, Hirschfeld LA: The cognitive foundations of cultural stability and diversity. Trends Cogn Sci 2004;8:40–46.
68 Boyer P: Intuitive expectations and the detection of mental disorder: a cognitive background to folk-psychiatries. Philos Psychol 2011;24:95–118.

Sebastian Dieguez, PhD
Laboratory for Cognitive and Neurological Sciences, Unité de Neurologie
Département de Médecine, Université de Fribourg
PER 09 (salle 2.106), 5 chemin du Musée, CH–1700 Fribourg (Switzerland)
E-Mail sebastian.dieguez@unifr.ch

his terrific characters and best horror novels when, as he reported, the addiction to alcohol and cocaine was florid.

This general emphasis on the effects of alcohol has grown up around characters [e.g. Mickey Rourke and Matt Dillon as Henry Chinaski in *Barfly* (1987) and *Factotum* (2006), respectively; John Belushi as John Blutarsky in *Animal House* (1978); Larry Hagman as J.R. of the TV series *Dallas*] or from press reports on real writers (e.g. James Joyce, Ernest Hemingway, Truman Capote, Dylan Thomas, William Faulkner, Charles Bukowski, Herman Melville, Tennessee Williams, John Cheever, Jack Kerouac), painters (Jackson Pollock, Thomas Kinkade), actors (William Holden, Marilyn Monroe, John Belushi, Mickey Rourke, Larry Hagman, Nicolas Cage, Johnny Depp, Robert Downey Jr.), and musicians (e.g. Billie Holiday, Jimi Hendrix, Jim Morrison, Eric Clapton, Britney Spears, Amy Winehouse) who abused alcohol.

Narratives and movies of fictional alcoholics hold a strong grip over the general public for several reasons. The prevalence of alcohol dependence and disability is very high [1], is found throughout the world, and affects women and men of all ages and social classes [2]. There is a tragic or romantic fascination in the deep sense of personal failure that drinking is able to relieve. The fight to stop alcoholism is very difficult. Some alcoholics seem to drink themselves to death on purpose as exemplified by the movie *Leaving Las Vegas* with Nicolas Cage (1995; based on the autobiographic novel by J. O'Brien who committed suicide a few weeks after the film rights were sold).

All alcoholics have qualms of conscience concerning the medical consequences of alcohol abuse. However, it is difficult to stop even for alcohol-addicted doctors in both fiction (e.g. Astrov in the novel *Uncle Vanja* by A. Chekhov) and real life (cf. *The End of My Addiction* by Dr. Olivier Ameisen, 2009). Surveys of hospital trusts found that roughly between 33% and 10% of male junior doctors and almost one in five of their female peers made some use of alcohol, cannabis, ecstasy, cocaine, and/or other hallucinogenic drugs [3–6]. Thus, the expected stress-relieving effect of alcohol consumption is also appreciated by health care professionals, though the latters might be more aware of the dangers.

Another interesting aspect of some unforgettable fictional alcoholics is the somewhat dissonant coexistence of high professional skills with the negative aspects of alcohol abuse and personal solitude. In literature and screenplays, this prototype is exemplified by the cigarette chain-smoking detective Philip Marlowe, the private investigator Matt Scudder, the diabetic and coffee-addicted Kurt Wallander, the borderline alcoholic John McClane played by Bruce Willis in the *Die Hard* series, the lawyer Frank Galvin masterly interpreted by Paul Newman in the movie *The Verdict* (1982), the alcoholic cop Ben Shockley played by Clint Eastwood in the *Gauntlet* (1977), and John Creasy played by Denzel Washington in *Man on Fire* (2004). In general, all these 'strong' characters do not make self-conscious efforts to overcome alcohol addiction until they start solving crimes, defending the weak, and saving human lives.

Bogousslavsky J, Dieguez S (eds): Literary Medicine: Brain Disease and Doctors in Novels, Theater, and Film.
Front Neurol Neurosci. Basel, Karger, 2013, vol 31, pp 169–177 (DOI: 10.1159/000343259)

# Alcoholism between Fiction and Reality

Antonio Carota[a] · Pasquale Calabrese[b]

[a]GSMN Neurocenter, Genolier Clinic, Genolier, [b]Cognitive Psychology, Basel University, Basel, Switzerland

**Abstract**

Alcoholism has always been emphasized in literature, narratives, and theater as its prevalence and related disability are very high, is found throughout the world, and affects women and men of all ages and social classes. There is a tragic or romantic fascination in the deep sense of personal failure that drinking is able to relieve and in the uncontrollable inability to stop drinking. These aspects have been portrayed well by fictional alcoholics in movies and novels. It has become evident that biological traits together with a complex series of psychosocial factors (e.g. negative life events, depression, anxiety, and other psychiatric or personality disorders), which are also well represented in novels and movies, can lead to alcohol addiction. Behavioral (euphoria, disinhibiting behaviors, aggressiveness) and neurological changes (confusion, bradypsychism, slurred speech, ataxia, blackouts) related to alcohol intoxication are also well portrayed by fictional characters. Delirium tremens, epilepsy, alcohol dementia, and Wernicke-Korsakoff disease, however, find less representation in literature and on the stage and screen. The treatment of alcoholic dependence is very difficult (as often reported by fictional and real stories), but should never be considered hopeless. It should be initiated at any stage of the disease. The support offered by Alcoholics Anonymous has always had great appeal for the public. Fictional works can portray alcohol addiction superbly and show some dark sides of human nature (negative emotions and autodestructive thoughts and behaviors), and, at the same time, the severity and pervasiveness of mental illnesses. The psychiatric and psychosocial aspects of alcohol addiction in movies and novels could be an inspiring source for new psychological studies and rehabilitation programs.



Alcohol has been present in literature, narratives, and theater since the ancient Greek and Roman periods [e.g. the mythology of the Greek god Dionysus (the Roman god Bacchus), son of Zeus, god of winemaking and wine, but also of intoxication and ritual madness]. The positive and negative valence of alcohol was personified by Silenus, the most drunken of the satyrs of Dionysus, who when intoxicated had access to special knowledge and prophecy.

Alcohol abuse was a source of artistic inspiration for the 'maudit' poets (C. Baudelaire, P. Verlaine, A. Rimbaud, S. Mallarmé). In the 1980s, Stephen King created

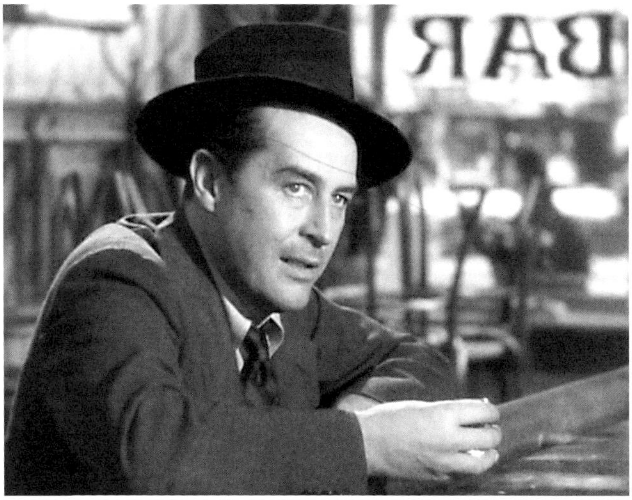


**Fig. 1.** Ray Milland playing in the movie, *The Lost Weekend* (1945). ©Paramount Pictures, Inc.

Another aspect of alcohol abuse that is often emphasized in works of fiction and movies is that it disrupts conjugal life, isolates from families and close friends, and leads to abandonment of one's profession [e.g. the failed alcoholic writer Don Birnam played by Ray Milland (fig. 1) in the movie *The Lost Weekend* (1945), which was directed by Billy Wilder and won four Oscars, and is probably the best-known film on alcoholism and its social and medical consequences].

Other examples are found in the movies *The Country Girl* (1952; starring Bing Crosby, Grace Kelly, and William Holden), *Days of Wine and Roses* (1962; with Jack Lemmon as the main protagonist), *Who's Afraid of Virginia Woolf?* (unconsciously offering Elisabeth Taylor and Richard Burton an artistic way to 'act out' their problematic relationship), and *When a Man Loves a Woman* (written by Al Franken and Ronald Bass and starring Andy Garcia and Meg Ryan).

Fictional alcoholics, generally men, are violent, hit their spouses or children, and end up in prison or attempt suicide. An example is the *Woman Who Walked into Doors* (1996) by Roddy Doile, a story set in a Dublin suburb and narrated by the wife of an alcoholic man remembering early times with her husband filled with joy and lust, and then, later, violence. She used the classic excuse for justifying her bruises: 'I walked into a door'.

A very dark example of how alcohol changes temper and induces violent acts is Edgar Allan Poe's novel *Black Cat* (1843). As a matter of fact, alcoholism is one of the leading causes of dysfunctional families. The movie *This Boy's Life* (1993, starring Leonardo di Caprio and Robert de Niro), which refers to the autobiography of the writer Tobias Wolff, tells the story of an alcoholic man who abuses both his wife and her son. Approximately 1 in 4 children younger than 18 years in the United States [7], and 1 in 7–10 children younger than 15 years in European countries [8] are exposed to parental alcohol abuse, which is a risk factor for future mental illness [9]. *The*

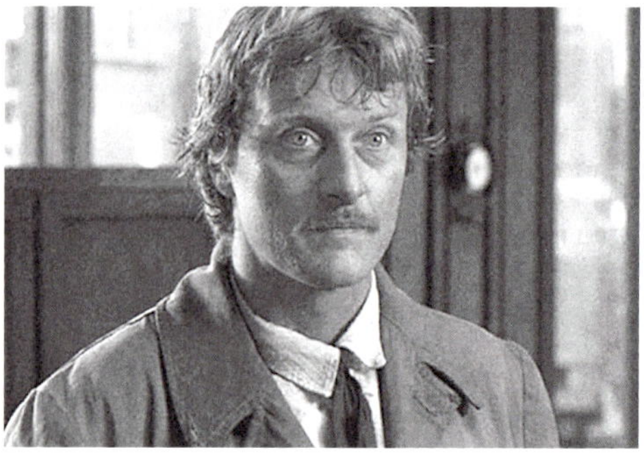

**Fig. 2.** Rutger Hauer starring in the film, *Legend of the Holy Drinker* (1988). ©Radiotelevisione Italiana (RAI), Cecchi Gori Group Tiger Cinematografica, Télémax, Aura Film.

*Affliction* (1999), with Nick Nolte and James Coburn, is an intensive elaboration of the impact of parental alcoholism on children's behaviors.

As a consequence of long-lasting heavy drinking, some alcoholics experience a decline in social standing, ultimately ending up as tramps on the streets. The award-winning movie *The Grass Arena* (1990) is based on the real story of John Healy, who was talented as both a boxer and chess player, but because of his addiction to alcohol, ended up living in a park with other alcoholics. When alcoholics end up as a 'street person', they usually seem to accept alcoholism as their destiny in life [see the award-winning film *Ironweed* (1987), based on the novel by W. Kennedy, directed by H. Babenco, and starring Jack Nicholson and Meryl Streep].

Romantic social perspectives on alcoholism have been expressed by a few fictional characters who have taken shelter in alcoholism to refuse the evils of the human nature. An example of this is *The Legend of the Holy Drinker* (1988), a film directed by E. Olmi and based on the 1939 autobiographic novel of the Austrian novelist Joseph Roth (fig. 2).

In the early stages, drinking might function as a shelter from problems, social inhibition, and anxiety, as well as act as a 'mood stabilizer'. As tolerance increases, the need of alcohol becomes more intense and early during the day. Relatives, coworkers, or neighbors begin to note that something is wrong. Hand tremors, hangovers, and gastritis appear, but are blamed on other factors. In later stages, drinking behavior gradually gets out of control. Abusers start to use 'eye-openers' to start the day, and drink to 'calm the nerves', lessen a hangover, or to 'quiet feelings'. At this stage, drinkers neglect personal hygiene, food and water intake, and experience serious financial, employment, legal, and relational problems. At later stages drinking is no longer a choice and alcohol is ingested in whatever form – wherever and whenever. In the final stages the most severe medical and neurologic complications emerge.

All the stages and conditions of alcoholism have been more than superbly portrayed by fictional alcoholics in movies and novels, including such works as *Come Back, Little Sheba* (1952), *Country Girl* (1954), *I Will Cry Tomorrow* (1955), *Voice in the Mirror* (1958), *A Long Day's Journey into Night* (1962), *Opening Night* (1977), *Only*

*When I Laugh* (1981), *Frances* (1982), *Under the Volcano* (1984), *The Razor's Edge* (1964 and 1984), *Talk Radio* (1988), *Clean and Sober* (1988), *Skin Deep* (1989), *Wired* (1989), *Postcards from the Edge* (1990), *Short Cuts* (1993), *28 Days* (2000), *Bad Santa* (2003), and *Sideways* (2008).

## The Multifaceted Etiology of Alcohol Addiction

Though an exact definition of alcoholism is difficult, it has become evident that biological traits [10] together with negative life events, cultural elements, depression, anxiety, and other psychiatric or personality disorders can lead to alcohol addiction. Thus, alcoholism should be considered a 'biopsychosocial' mental illness. However, it is of importance for healthcare professionals that addiction itself not be the only facet (this would be a stigmatization) of the intimate personality of alcoholics.

In this regard, the characters of the novel *Cannery Row* by the literature Nobel Prize winner J. Steinbeck and the 1982 movie directed by D.S. Ward (featuring Nick Nolte and Debra Winger) are exemplary. The protagonists of the story are the wretches of society and subject to every abuse, but Steinbeck was able to depict what makes them honorable and good-hearted people. On the contrary, in the dramatic, sweet, and pitiless movie *The Fire Within* (1963; directed by Louis Malle and starring Maurice Ronet), the protagonist is cured of alcoholism but commits suicide as the effect of depression and personal emptiness, which previously drove him to alcoholism.

## Alcohol Intoxication

Amazing examples of alcohol intoxication (euphoric behaviors, ataxia, slurred speech, hallucinations, delirium, and hangovers) were superbly interpreted by Johnny Depp and the cast of the movie *The Rum Diary* (2011; based on a novel by H.S. Thompson). Additionally, the opening scene of *Apocalypse Now* (1979; directed by Francis Ford Coppola) was recorded when Martin Sheen was drunk, which led to an incredible scene of alcoholic madness [11].

Only in the later stages does the chronic alcoholic develop tolerance and might show fewer behavioral changes even after consumption of large quantities of alcohol. In *The Three Musketeers* (written by Alexandre Dumas, 1844), Athos is described as having some gait imbalance only after a two-week binge of ten bottles a day, which leads us to believe that he was affected by chronic alcoholism.

The term 'blackout' indicates the amount of time of memory loss during severe intoxication, or perhaps with rapidly increasing high alcohol blood levels. One cannot remember events because alcohol intoxication interferes with memory storage mechanisms. There is not yet sufficient scientific evidence on factors that make some individuals vulnerable to this phenomenon in comparison to others, even at similar blood alcohol concentrations. It is probable that biological differences in memory mechanisms among individuals play a role [12, 13].

Though alcoholic blackouts might be strategically advocated by legal defense in court cases [14], it has to be noted that the efforts themselves in reconstructing the events of the blackout could induce false memories or beliefs [15] and might thus compromise the defense. Examples of alcohol blackouts are found in the 1997 movie *The Blackout* (directed by A. Ferrara, starring Matthew Modine, Claudia Schiffer, and Béatrice Dalle). Another example is *The Hangover* (2009; directed by T. Philips). This exhilarating comedy set in Las Vegas portrays the adventures of some buddies after a blackout due to the combination of alcohol and a benzodiazepine. After waking up, they find their hotel suite upside down, a tiger in the bathroom, a baby in the closet, and a chicken scratching around. One of them has a missing tooth, another one has a hospital bracelet, and one is missing. They have no clue what happened the night before. Although the characters have impaired retrieval of recent memories, they still have intact reasoning which allows them to investigate the events of the night.

## Withdrawal Syndrome

Withdrawal syndrome presents in about 5–10% of heavy chronic addicts [16] after one or two weeks of relative or absolute abstinence (e.g. after admission into the hospital for an unrelated illness), and its manifestations (singularly or in combination) are tremulousness, visual (usually animals, i.e. zoopsia) or auditory (usually human voices of known persons discussing in third person) hallucinosis or hallucinations, seizures ('rum fits'), and delirium tremens. In the semiautobiographical novel *Big Sur*, J. Kerouac, as Jack Duluoz, battles all the withdrawal symptoms and delirium tremens, together with depression and paranoia.

Delirium tremens is the most severe form of withdrawal and manifests with deep confusion, slurred speech, uninhibited behavior, staggering gait, delusions, vivid hallucinations, sleeplessness, and increased autonomic activity (fever, tachycardia, perspiration), and can even lead to stupor, coma, and death (often because of cardiac arrhythmia and respiratory failure). It seldom occurs until the abuser has been drinking heavily for at least the past ten years. The syndrome follows within a few days (until a maximum of two weeks) after stopping drinking. The mortality rate for delirium tremens improved from the last century from 37% to 2–7% of patients with the disorder [17] due to advances in intensive care medicine. The etiology of delirium tremens is related to functional changes in the GABA neurotransmitter and NMDA receptors, which lead to unbalanced effects of excitatory transmitters. One of the best descriptions of this in literature was given by Charles Jackson in the novel *The Lost Weekend* (1944), and Mark Twain gave a superb description of the disease with the alcoholic and abusive father in *Huckleberry Finn*. Edgar Allan Poe probably died because of delirium tremens (even if there is some controversy on this issue), calling out the name Reynolds (perhaps the explorer Jeremiah N. Reynolds) and repeating for hours 'Lord help my poor soul'.

### Alcoholic Nutritional Diseases

The clinical description of Wernicke's disease (nystagmus, abducens nerve and conjugate gaze palsy, gait ataxia, and mental confusion) and Korsakoff psychosis (a pervasive cognitive and behavioral disorder where episodic anterograde memory is disproportionately affected compared to all other cognitive functions) has been around since the end of the 19th century. The two conditions can manifest together (the Wernicke-Korsakoff disease), generally over few days, and are related to severe malnutrition and consequent vitamin $B_1$ (thiamine) depletion since these patients get their entire caloric intake from alcohol. Confabulation is a frequent feature of the disease and consists of the narration of false events that the patient reports as real against all odds. The Wernicke-Korsakoff syndrome usually follows many years of chronic alcoholism or malnutrition and is seldom seen among people younger than 20 years of age. E. Einhorn, an American novelist and director known for a series of plays on neurological disorders, based the novel *Strangers* (2005) on the Korsakoff syndrome. In the novel *Now Wait for Last Year* by Philip K. Dick (1966), the main character's wife is diagnosed with the syndrome after years of drug and alcohol abuse. Another example can be seen in the television series *House, M.D.*, in which a diagnosis of Wernicke-Korsakoff disease and confabulations is delivered by Dr. House to surprised students in the first season series (episode 'Histories'). Dr. House told them to put the patient on thiamine and give her some food.

### Treatment of Alcohol Addiction

The main force underlying chronic alcoholism is the deep and uncontrolled inability to stop drinking. The treatment of alcoholic dependence is very difficult, but should never be considered hopeless. Treatment should be attempted at any stage of the disease, by either a doctor or specialist approaching the patient. The attitude should be empathetic but straightforward. The patient is gently driven to full awareness by removing his denial. The objective is the total abstinence from alcohol since it is unrealistic to realize only moderate drinking. The autobiographic book *Drinking: A Love Story* (2002) by Caroline Knapp is the real story of her 20-year battle against alcoholism – a story of hunger, need, horror, sadness, degradation, and despair.

The patient is the only one to take the final responsibility of the medical treatment. This could be the admission to rehabilitation hospitals (as an inpatient) and/or to mental health programs and self-help support groups like Alcoholics Anonymous (as an outpatient). Some patients could benefit from the use of disulfiram.

Support by Alcoholics Anonymous has proven to be one of the most effective forces in the psychosocial rehabilitation of alcoholic patients. The (somewhat sanctifying) novels and movies *My Name is Bill W.* (1989; directed by Daniel Petrie) and *When Love Is Not Enough* (2010; interpreted by Winona Ryder and directed by Terry Gould) depict the early history of Bill Wilson, the cofounder of AA. Admission to the Alcoholics Anonymous fellowship association requires that the individual, in front of the other members, admits his/her alcoholism and recognizes the difficulty to quit drinking without peer support.

Alcoholism is very frequently associated with psychiatric diseases (depression, anxiety, mania), the so-called 'dual diagnosis', which requires specific long-term treatment.

## Conclusions

It has become evident that besides persistent excessive drinking, there are other biological (genetic) as well as psychological and social factors which might predispose an individual to become a 'drinker'. The complex psychological, behavioral, medical, and social changes related to alcohol consumption and dependence might explain why alcohol-related themes have always been a privileged scenario in literature and movies to represent dark sides of human nature (reflected in negative emotions and autodestructive thoughts and behaviors) and, at the same time, the severity and pervasiveness of mental illnesses.

The psychiatric and psychosocial aspects, more so than the neurological aspects, of alcohol addiction have been extremely well represented and summarized in movies and novels, and therefore might be a strong inspiring source for new psychological studies and rehabilitation programs.

## References


1 Hasin DS, Stinson FS, Ogburn E, Grant BF: Prevalence, correlates, disability, and comorbidity of DSM-IV alcohol abuse and dependence in the United States: results from the National Epidemiologic Survey on Alcohol and Related Conditions. Arch Gen Psychiatry 2007;64:830–842.

2 Global Status Report on Alcohol and Health. Geneva, WHO, 2011.

3 Fowlie DG: The misuse of alcohol and other drugs by doctors: a UK report and one region's response. Alcohol Alcohol 1991;34:666–671.

4 Brooke D, Edwards G, Andrews T: Doctors and substance misuse: types of doctors, types of problems. Addiction 1993;88:655–663.

5 Bissell L, Skorina JK: One hundred alcoholic women in medicine. An interview study. JAMA 1987;257:2939–2944.

6 Bohigian GM, Bondurant R, Croughan J: The impaired and disruptive physician: the Missouri Physicians' Health Program – an update (1995–2002). J Addict Dis 2005;24:13–23.

7 Grant BF: Estimates of US children exposed to alcohol abuse and dependence in the family. Am J Public Health 2000;90:112–115.
8 McNeill A: Alcohol problems in the family. A report to the European Union. London, Eurocare (European Alcohol Policy Alliance) and COFACE (Confederation of Family Organisations in the EU), 1998.
9 Rognmo K, Torvik FA, Ask H, Røysamb E, Tambs K: Paternal and maternal alcohol abuse and offspring mental distress in the general population: the Nord-Trondelag Health Study. BMC Public Health 2012;12:448.
10 Hillemacher T: Biological mechanisms in alcohol dependence – new perspectives. Alcohol Alcohol 2011;46:224–230.
11 The Way: Interview with Martin Sheen and Emilio Estevez. The Telegraph By Craig McLean, March 2011.
12 Wetherill RR, Fromme K: Acute alcohol effects on narrative recall and contextual memory: an examination of fragmentary blackouts. Addict Behav 2001;8:886–889.
13 Wetherill RR, Schnyer DM, Fromme K: Acute alcohol effects on contextual memory BOLD response: differences based on fragmentary blackout history. Alcohol Clin Exp Res 2012;36:607–617.
14 Van Oorsouw K, Merckelbach H, Ravelli D, Nijman H, Mekking-Pompen I: Alcoholic blackout for criminally relevant behavior. J Am Acad Psychiatry Law 2004;32:364–370.
15 Nash RA, Takarangi MKT: Reconstructing alcohol-induced memory blackouts. Memory 2011;19:566–573.
16 Saitz R, O'Malley SS: Pharmacotherapies for alcohol abuse. Withdrawal and treatment. Med Clin North Am 1997;81:881–907.
17 Monte R, et al: Analysis of the factors determining survival of alcoholic withdrawal syndrome patients in a general hospital. Alcohol Alcohol 2010;45: 151–158.

Dr. Antonio Carota
Clinique de Genolier
Route du Muids 3 – CP 100
CH–1272 Genolier (Switzerland)
E-Mail acarota@genolier.net

Bogousslavsky J, Dieguez S (eds): Literary Medicine: Brain Disease and Doctors in Novels, Theater, and Film.
Front Neurol Neurosci. Basel, Karger, 2013, vol 31, pp 178–187 (DOI: 10.1159/000343237)

# Protagonists with Parkinson's Disease

Joost Haan

Department of Neurology, Rijnland Hospital and Leiden University Medical Centre,
Leiderdorp/Leiden, The Netherlands

**Abstract**

Parkinson's disease is a complex disorder with many fascinating features. Its onset is creeping, the progression is slow but inevitable. There are motor symptoms, such as a tremor, rigidity, bradykinesia, mask-like facial expression, and postural abnormalities, but also hallucinations, cognitive deterioration, and depression. In many novels, fictive patients with Parkinson's disease play a role. It seems that authors have used many aspects of the disease to emphasize their messages. Their narratives include themes such as rigidity, petrifaction, confusion, dementia, and hallucinations. In this chapter, as examples, several protagonists with Parkinson's disease will be described from works of John Updike, Jonathan Franzen, Sue Miller, J.M. Coetzee, and John Harding, among others.



The many faces of Parkinson's disease have fascinated writers of novels for a long time. Protagonists with the disease can already be found in the novels of Charles Dickens [1] and William Shakespeare [2, 3], but also in many contemporary works of fiction [4]. In this chapter, some of the many possible examples will be described, with emphasis on the kaleidoscope of metaphors the disease offers.

## Parkinson Matters

Rohinton Mistry was born in India but lives in Canada. In his novel *Family Matters*, on the one hand there are *family* matters, important – but not always nice – things that take place in families, while on the other hand the family *matters*, having a special place in the heart [5].

The 79-year-old Nariman Vakeel is a retired professor of literature. He lives with his stepdaughter Coomey and stepson Jal in a large but neglected apartment. His daughter Roxana lives with her husband Yezad and sons Jehangir and Murad not far away in a small but luxurious house. Nariman has Parkinson's disease. Because of this, he falls regularly.

Nariman sat, trying to maintain a dignified silence. His hands were shaking wretchedly, defying all the effort of his will to keep them steady in his leap. The tremor in his legs was growing too, making his knees bounce like some pervert jiggling his thighs. He tried to remember: had he taken his medication after lunch?

Nariman has a tremor which has altered his handwriting. He speaks in a soft voice, walks unstable, and has a stooped posture. He is treated with L-Dopa, but this has not prevented his falls. One day he breaks his ankle and is brought home, unable to walk. Coomey and Jal have to nurse him, but this turns out to be more problematic than they had thought. They suddenly realize that they do not love him very much. Nariman has never been very nice to their mother, he even had a girlfriend. Now they have to take care of his excrements, have to wash him, and wrestle with his pyjamas, chamber pot, pillows, and smells.

They continued to cope, poorly, with the excretions and secretions of their stepfather's body, moving from revulsion to pity to anger, and back to revulsion. They were bewildered, and indignant, that a human creature of blood and bone, so efficient in good health, could suddenly become so messy. Neither Nariman's age nor his previous illnesses had served to warn them. Sometimes they took it personally, as though their stepfather had reduced himself to this state to harass them.

Jal and Coomey decide that they cannot handle the situation. Nariman is – without previous notice – put on transport to Roxana and her family. There, amazingly, he is very welcome. Nariman is nursed well and is allowed to sleep on the sofa. The apartment is very small, so Murad has to sleep on the balcony under a piece of plastic.

Being immobile makes Nariman depressive. Unfortunately, when he tries to walk after a period of rehabilitation, he breaks his ankle again. After this setback, he needs even more care and becomes more depressive and confused. One year after breaking his ankle, Nariman dies, nursed to the end by the loving part of his family.

### Parkinson Holiday

I'm worried about Dad. He just isn't well. It seems crazy to say that because of course he isn't well. How could you possibly call a man who cannot walk or talk, who dribbles, snorts and snuffles, is blind, covered in eczema, dandruff-dusted, has one hand frozen into a claw, cannot pee when he wants to, is constipated and so confused he doesn't know what day or perhaps even what decade he is in, well? And yet there is a kind of level of illness in Dad to which we've all grown accustomed, which changes so imperceptibly from day to day we hardly notice the deterioration each year brings. . .

These words are from Nick Taylor, the narrator of the novel *What We Did on Our Holiday* by John Harding [6]. Nick has had the idea to take his father with Parkinson's disease and mother with adiposity (120 kg) to Malta, as a birthday present. It turns out that father already was on Malta shortly after the war. He 'left a little piece of himself' there, and thus Nick realizes that the holiday also will be a search for his unknown half-brother.

The flight to Malta turns out to be a 'Parkinson adventure'. Father has to pee and with much effort he is guided out of his chair to the toilet. There, Nick has to take his father's penis in his hand. When father accidentally turns down the light, Nick hears urine clattering against the wall. Back in their seats, he ignores the large wet spot in father's trousers and the drops on his shoes. Other passengers now seem to avoid the toilet. The stewardesses are on their knees to clean the floor.

Mother Lil is proud that her husband does not have the 'shaking type' of Parkinson. Unfortunately, he does have all other serious symptoms: unintelligible speech, a mask-like expression, excessive drooling, hesitation, akinesia, orthostatic hypotension, postural instability, and cognitive deterioration with loss of decorum. Bedsores on his buttocks have to be rubbed with ointment every day, and to make things worse, the medication causes eczema, constipation, and hallucinations.

On Malta, they manage to trace the presumed half-brother, Anthony, who looks like Omar Sharif and is very nice. Anthony has some problems with the new situation. 'You say that this is my father? This man? But, he is. . . so old.' His mother died many years ago, he was raised as an orphan. In the end it becomes clear that Anthony is not Anthony. Nick's real half-brother was killed a couple of years ago. The present Anthony is an impostor. The holiday is a disaster as everything goes wrong.

And then father asks Nick to swim with him in the sea.

> 'Nick. *Don't let me go! Don't let me go!'*
> 'It's OK, I've got you Dad. Trust me. I won't let you go.'
> 'No! No!' He screams.
> 'It's all right, Dad,' I say firmly. 'I won't let you go.'
> He bares his teeth in a smile of frustration.
> He lifts his head out of the water in an effort to emphasise what he's saying, making his whole body rock.
> 'No, Nick, I'm not saying that. I'm saying, *Let me go! Let me go!'*
> I look into his dead, watery eyes and perhaps by some trick of the bright light, I could almost swear they are smiling at me.

Nick takes a step back. Father waves, drifts away. Nick goes ashore with tears in his eyes. End of the story.

*What We Did on Our Holiday* combines deep insight into the impact of Parkinson's disease with very funny and compassionate scenes. Every Parkinson patient would like to have a son like Nick.

## Parkinson Short

Amy Bloom's collection of short stories *A Blind Man Can See How Much I Love You* has been called a masterpiece [7]. The story *The Gates Are Closing* begins with double-meaning.

> Help me.
>
> I slid my hands up the legs of Jack's shorts to stroke the top of his thigh, and he lost his grip on the paint roller. A hundred tiny drops flew through the air at me. Thoroughly speckled, squinting to keep the paint out of my eyes, I stroked higher under his boxers, right up the neat, furry juncture of his crotch.
>
> 'Jesus,' he said. 'It's not like I have any balance anyway.' Which is true. He has Parkinson's, and no sensible group of people would have him painting their synagogue.

The 'I', Andrea, is in love with Jack, who is married to Naomi. Jack has Parkinson's disease.

> His face so often shows only a tender, masked expressiveness, I covet the tiny rips and leaks of affect in the corner of his mouth, in the middle of his forehead. His hand shook. He shakes. Mostly at rest. Mostly when he is making an effort to relax. And sometimes, after we've made love, which he does in a wonderfully unremarkable, athletic way, his whole right side trembles and his arm flutters wildly, as if we've set it free.

Then Jack's Parkinson gets worse and he asks Andrea to help him with a 'self-chosen death.' Andrea is shocked and in doubt. If her answer is negative, Jack will not see her anymore; if positive, she will lose the person she loves.

The reader of the story does not get to know her decision. The story ends with the words: 'I am waiting. I have cleaned my house. I paint. I listen.'

## Parkinson Redux

John Updike has written a number of masterpieces. Connoisseurs consider *The Rabbit Omnibus* as his best work [8]. The Rabbit books span four decades and consist of *Rabbit, Run* (1960), *Rabbit Redux* (1971), *Rabbit Is Rich* (1981), *Rabbit at Rest* (1990), and *Rabbit Remembered* (2000). In all of these novels, Updike gives a perfect description of the spirit of the ages. The life-story of the antihero Harry 'Rabbit' Angstrom can be seen as a 'moral' history of modern America. In *Rabbit, Run*, Harry is 26 years old. He works as a salesman of kitchen equipment and is married to Janice. Their son Nelson is two years old. Harry is not satisfied with his life. In high school he was a successful basketball player, but now he is a middle-class workman without prospects and his wife is addicted to alcohol. Harry starts a relation with Ruth, a hooker. When his second child – a daughter – is born, Harry returns to Janice. He starts to work at the Toyota garage of Janice's father.

Unfortunately, Janice lets their daughter drown in the bathtub, and Harry returns to Ruth, who appears to be pregnant. In *Rabbit Redux,* Harry is back with Janice. He works in a printing shop. Janice has a relation with an employee of her father's garage and leaves home. Harry starts a sort of 'commune' in his house and lives with two drug addicts, Jill and Skeeter. Unfortunately, the 'free sex' takes place under the attention of Nelson, Harry's son. In a fire, Jill is killed. Finally, Janice returns to Harry and her son Nelson, as her boyfriend had an affair with another woman (Harry's sister). In *Rabbit Is Rich,* Harry is rich. He has inherited the Toyota garage of his father-in-law. To be rich, however, does not mean to be happy. Janice is still an alcoholic, Nelson a 'good-for-nothing'. Even partner-swapping does not improve Harry's mood. He decides to search for Ruth, and meets his daughter. In *Rabbit at Rest* Nelson has taken over the Toyota garage, but makes a mess of it. Harry mainly lives in Florida, bored and overweight. He has an affair with his daughter-in-law and for this is abandoned by his family. Then he has his fatal heart attack.

In *Rabbit Redux*, Harry's mother Mary suffers from Parkinson's disease. He discusses her disease with his father:

> Ritually, he asks his father how his mother is.
>
> But his father declines to make a ritual answer. Usually he says, 'As good as can be hoped.' Today he sidles a conspiratorial inch closer at the bar and says, 'Not as good as could be hoped, Harry.'
>
> She has had Parkinson's Disease for years now. Harry's mind slides away from picturing her, the way she has become, the loosely fluttering knobbed hands, the shuffling sheepish walk, the eyes that study him with vacant amazement though the doctor says her mind is as good as ever in there, and the mouth that wanders open and forgets to close until saliva reminds it.

Mary gets the 'usual' pills. A pill to sleep, and green pills to stay calm. Later she also gets the wonder drug L-Dopa, but unfortunately this does not help her very much. She develops a lot of side-effects including hypersexuality. In the course of the story, Mary becomes increasingly immobile. She lies in bed all the time. To communicate, she uses the phone or taps with her walking stick on the floor. Every time Harry visits her, he smells a remarkable odor; for him it is the smell of dying. Indeed, in *Rabbit Redux,* Mary finds her rest.

### Parkinson Corrected

Alfred Lambert has Parkinson's disease. His hands shake and flutter through the air. He speaks in a flat tone. His face is mask-like, he shuffles when he walks, hesitates, falls. When he sits in his chair, he sleeps. On top of all that, he is very self-willed and confused.

Alfred is a protagonist in *The Corrections*, a wonderful and complex novel written by Jonathan Franzen [9]. Although the novel contains many other characters, Alfred and his disease form a central theme in the narrative.

He closed his eyes and thanked her. As if waiting for a break in a downpour so that he could run from his car into a grocery store, he waited for a lull in his tremor so that he could reach out and safely eat what she'd brought him.

His affliction offended his sense of ownership. These shaking hands belonged to nobody but him, and yet they refused to obey him. They were like bad children. Unreasoning two-year-olds in a tantrum of selfish misery. The more sternly he gave orders, the less they listened and the more miserable and out of control they got. He'd always been vulnerable to a child's recalcitrance and refusal to behave like an adult. Irresponsibility and undiscipline were the bane of his existence, and it was another instance of that Devil's logic that his own untimely affliction should consist of his body's refusal to obey him.

If thy right hand offend thee, Jesus said, cut it off.

Alfred used to be a hardworking employee of the Midland Pacific Railroad. He is married to Enid, and they have three children, Gary, Chip, and Denise. Alfred's handicap and stubbornness turn life into a guerrilla with Enid as the enemy; she is popping up from all corners to correct him. The story line of *The Corrections* is rather simple. Alfred and Enid go on a cruise. On board, Alfred becomes more confused and disoriented. He climbs on the railing to answer nature's call and falls overboard, but, amazingly, survives. Enid's main concern is the Christmas dinner with the family, as this could be the last opportunity they will all be together. Although this is the whole story, the book is voluminous (>500 pages). All characters are worked-out in detail, their history, thoughts, motivations. In addition, the perspective changes, so that occurrences are described from different standpoints.

Son Chip has failed as a university professor, and now tries unsuccessfully to earn his money as a scriptwriter. Daughter Denise is a top cook, earns a lot of money, but is unhappy in her relations (with men and women). Gary is a successful banker, but very depressive. He has some Parkinson's disease symptoms himself.

Mother Enid indeed succeeds in bringing her family together for Christmas. It is the climax of the book.

The old man pushed his chair away from the table and turned once more to Chip. He said, 'You can see it's not without its difficulties.'

As he stood up, his leg buckled and he pitched to the floor, dragging his plate and mat and coffee cup and saucer along with him. The crash might have been the last bar of a symphony. He lay on his side amid the ruins like a wounded gladiator, a fallen horse.

Chip knelt down and helped him into a sitting position while Denise hurried to the kitchen.

'It's quarter to eleven,' Gary said as if nothing unusual had happened. 'Before I leave, here's a summary. Dad is demented and incontinent. Mom can't have him in this house without a lot of help, which she says she doesn't want even if she could afford it.'

[. . .]

Alfred rested his shaking hands on Chip's shoulders and gazed in wonder at the room's furnishings. Despite his agitation, he was smiling.

'My question,' he said, 'is who owns this house? Who takes care of all of this?'

'You own it, Dad.'

Alfred shook his head as if this didn't square with the facts as he understood them.

Not long after Christmas, Alfred is admitted to a nursing home, waiting for the end.

Alfred lasted longer after that than everyone expected. He was a lion to the end. His blood pressure was barely measurable when Denise and Gary flew into town, and he still lived another week. He lay curled up on the bed and barely breathed. He moved for nothing and responded to nothing except to shake his head emphatically, once, when Enid tried to put an ice chip in his mouth. The one thing he never forgot was how to refuse. All her corrections had been for naught. He was as stubborn as the day she'd met him.

### Parkinson Masked

Lily will take all morning to eat the cereal. This is what it's come to. Parkinson's. Worst so far in her face, which is frozen in blank, childish expectancy; and in her throat, so that swallowing is a slow, consciously controlled activity. She has been taking the evening meal with Gaby and Alan, but she eats almost nothing, preferring to wait until she's alone again to struggle with solid food (though Gaby, seeing how little Lily manages to get down even then, has recently begun to put her dinner into the blender before she brings it in to Lily). She can drink more easily, and she does, and several times has wound up a little tipsy by the end of the meal.

Lily Roberts Maynard is a famous writer of essays, an autobiography and a novel. She is now over eighty and unable to write any more, as she has advanced Parkinson's disease. Lily lives with her son Alan and Gaby her daughter in law. She is unable to care for herself. Waiting for a free place in a nursing home she uses her excess of free time to arrange her memories of the past. She rereads and destroys letters from her mother and her husband.

She could get up by herself – at home she had to and she did – but it is a struggle, and she'd just as soon wait. Simply to be *waiting*, though, makes her aware, abruptly, of the tension in her body, of its wish – she sees her illness this way, as having its *own* will – to turn to stone, to become utterly rigid. She is dying, she is freezing, she feels it acutely, and stills, her eyes open. Time stops. She thinks to reach for the bell again. But doesn't. Or call. Or move.

In the description of her protagonist Lily in *The Distinguished Guest*, Sue Miller repeatedly emphasizes the mask-like face, more than any other feature of Parkinson's disease [10]. One of the most important themes is what hides behind the mask. Lily's stay with her son's family has a great impact. She continuously tries to manipulate him. For this, Alan spends as much time as possible outdoors. Another guest in Alan's house is Linnett Baird, a journalist who interviews Lily to write an article on her life. Linnett discovers that behind her mask Lily uses her disease to get what she wants. Confused when she needs to be and naughty in another situation, Lily plays a role in the theater. She offends her family, but blames her Parkinson's disease. In fact, her whole life was full of conflicts, with her father, her husband, and her children, as she always wanted to be the center of attention. In the end of the book, she accidentally commits suicide, as she is convinced that someone will find and rescue her after she takes her pills.

> She stirred, her hands fluttered on the coverlet. She struggled back to near consciousness.
> And then the center of the storm passed over her, and there was a great, hollow stillness. Lily had recovered just enough of herself to know what this was: the eye.
> The *I*, she thought. *Lily.*
> And was amused at this joke. Her joke. God's joke. A nearly invisible smile twitched on her face.

**Parkinson Various**

There are many more novels that contain descriptions of Parkinson's disease [4]. It is virtually impossible to give a complete list. Below, short summaries of a couple of remarkable examples follow.

> Six years ago my father was injured when he fell off a ladder. He was working on a sculpture that the city had commissioned him to do in Carl Schurz Park. He hit his head on the base of the sculpture and knocked himself out. The doctor told him he was lucky to have only a concussion but to keep an eye out for lingering problems. When my father's left hand started to shake a few months later, he chalked it up to the accident, figuring it wasn't a big deal and that it would go away on its own. But two months later it was still shaking. My mom finally forced him back to the doctor, who sent him to a neurologist. About a thousand tests later the whole family was called in to hear his diagnosis: Parkinson's disease, or PD, as the neurologist affectionately called it.

This citation is from Daphne Grab's novel *Alive and Well in Prague, New York* [11]. Sixteen-year-old Matisse tells about her dad.

> But the doctor, who my dad sarcastically dubbed 'the Genius,' ended up being wrong. The drugs, which subdued all my dad's symptoms at first, became less effective after only three years, leaving him with longer 'off' periods when the symptoms could not be masked. He moved slowly, which made things like getting dressed take ages; he had tremors; and at times his arms and legs got so rigid that he couldn't move them. His face, once always relaxed and animated, became stiffer, and even during an 'on' period it never looked like it used to. For longer and longer blocks of time, my dad was subservient to the disease; PD had taken over.

Because of dad's Parkinson disease, the family moves from New York to Prague. There, Matisse has problems to adjust herself, but finally manages to find her place and accept her father's disease.

In *Une belle mort* (A Good Death) written by the Canadian Gil Courtemanche, a large family celebrates Christmas. At a first glance, everybody seems to have a pleasant time. They have lively conversations, they eat and drink wine. But appearances are deceptive. The narrator, 60-year-old André Lévesque, thinks of his unpleasant youth and the many troubled relations in the family. The main cause of all problems is his father, Anatole Lévesque. He was a tyrant, but now is powerless, as he suffers from Parkinson's disease.

Anatole hangs in his chair, mumbles incomprehensibly, eats with his hands, cries when he hears sentimental music, drinks a mix of white and red wine, tries to get up, falls, and returns half naked to continue his dinner. He is a 'fallen dictator'. As a matter of fact, his family hates him so that they do not want to help him. But André realizes that his father is a dying old man and decides to help him. But death does not come quickly. André and his mother are no advocates of euthanasia, as they do not want to become 'murderers'. They let father eat and drink in large amounts everything he likes, hoping that this will somehow bring his life to an end. Anatole is very happy with this 'solution' and stuffs himself with food and wine. In contrast to what is hoped, his health improves. Then another solution is sought for. André takes father and mother on a fishing trip. As expected, father drowns in the grey water. Mother asks André to give her a push also.

*Diary of a Bad Year*, written by the Nobel prize winner J.M. Coetzee, is a very peculiar book. The pages are divided in two or three parts by horizontal lines. In the upper part are erudite essays on themes such as Machiavelli, Tolstoj, Tony Blair, bird-flu, or Al-Qaida. These texts are dictated by Señor C, a South African writer who now lives in Australia, to Anya, who he has met in the laundry room of the building. The two or three texts under the horizontal lines form first-person narratives of Señor C and Anya. Señor C has Parkinson's disease. His handwriting has become illegible, so he needs Anya's help to write his essays. Señor C considers Anya as 'a woman with a derrière so near perfect as to be angelic'. Anya on her part at first strongly dislikes Señor C. The novel is said to deal with 'the mind-body conflict'. Indeed, Señor C is mainly 'mind' (but has a body with Parkinson's disease) and Anya is 'body' (but also an angel).

In *Le désert de l'amour* (Desert of Love), written by François Mauriac, another Nobel prize winner (in 1952), Dr. Paul Courrèges, a successful physician, has a midlife crisis [12]. He thinks of breaking with his wife, and taking a mistress. Early in the novel, he loses contact with Raymond, his 17-year old son. Many years later the two meet again. Dr. Courrèges now has a severe form of Parkinson's disease. He has become a shadow, motionless, unable to sit upright. The son is especially shocked by the tortured face, the stiffening, and the mask of stone.

Joseph O'Loughlin is a clinical psychologist. He is the main character in Michael Robotham's *The Suspect* (2004) and plays a minor role in *Lost* (2005). O'Loughlin has a beautiful wife, a nice daughter, and a flourishing practice; in short, he should be a happy man. Unfortunately, he suffers from Parkinson's disease. For example, he has to shave with two hands and still cuts himself. His legs do not react to his will, his face is like a mask. In the story, he is suspected of murdering one of his patients. He has to fly, his calm life changes to hell, and he has to be a detective. Thus, *The Suspect* contains three intriguing stories: an exciting thriller, the description of a psychologist and his patients, and – most fascinating – the case-report of a patient with Parkinson's disease.

## References


1 Schoffer KL, O'Sullivan JD: Charles Dickens: the man, medicine, and movement disorders. J Clin Neurosci 2006;13:898–901.
2 Fogan L: The neurology in Shakespeare. Arch Neurol 1989;46:922–924.
3 Stien R: Shakespeare on Parkinsonism. Mov Dis 2005;20:768–769.
4 Haan J, Meulenberg F: De trillende Tuinman en andere Parkinsonbeelden. Houten, Springer, 2009.
5 Mistry R: Family Matters. London, Faber and Faber, 2002.
6 Harding J: What We Did on Our Holiday. London, Black Swan Books, 2000.
7 Bloom A: A Blind Man Can See How Much I Love You. New York, Random House, 2000.
8 Updike J: A Rabbit Omnibus. New York, Penguin Books, New York, 1991.
9 Franzen J: The Corrections. New York, Picador, 2001.
10 Miller S: The Distinguished Guest. London, Bloomsbury, 1995.
11 Grab D: Alive and Well in Prague, New York. New York, HarperCollins Publishers, 2008.
12 Posen S: The Doctor in Literature. Volume 2. Private Life. Oxford, Radcliffe Publishing Ltd., 2006.



Joost Haan, MD, PhD
Department of Neurology
Rijnland Hospital
NL–2353 GA Leiderdorp (The Netherlands)
E-Mail jhaan@rijnland.nl

Bogousslavsky J, Dieguez S (eds): Literary Medicine: Brain Disease and Doctors in Novels, Theater, and Film.
Front Neurol Neurosci. Basel, Karger, 2013, vol 31, pp 188–194 (DOI: 10.1159/000343239)

# Some Movement Disorders

G.D. Perkin

Charing Cross Hospital, London, UK

**Abstract**

As with my previous writings on the neurology of literature, all the references used have been personally read. Indeed, I should hasten to stress that the prime motive in my reading has been a love of literature, a secondary gain being an insight into the way in which a variety of writers has viewed neurological disease. Some of the descriptions leave no doubt as to the condition being described: in other descriptions, I have used a degree of imagination! All the references to foreign texts have been read in translation.


## Hemifacial Spasm

It might seem perverse to begin this chapter with a collection of descriptions of hemifacial spasm. The condition is perhaps not considered a movement disorder, though it is certainly a disorder of movement. The extracts quoted do not antedate descriptions of the disorder in the neurological literature, but they largely excel in their powers of observation and, in one case, amuse by their assumption as to the natural history of the disorder.

The public prosecutor with his very black, thick eyebrows and with his left eye that kept winking slightly, . . . winking with his left eye and flicking his beard with his handkerchief to brush the snuff from it [1].

It would have seemed good natured were it not for the expression of the eyes, which had a watery, glassy gleam under the lids with nearly white eyelashes, which twitched almost as though he were continually winking.

Again he suddenly seemed to wink at him with his left eye, and laughed noiselessly – exactly as before [2].

There was something strange about his eyes. The lid of the left eye twitched; it fell down and snapped up; it was exactly as though the lid of the eye were a window shade and someone stood inside the doctor's head playing with the cord [3].

There was once a man who got run in for winking at girls in the street, so he said it was a permanent affliction and he winked all through his trial and got off, but the sad thing is that now he can't stop and he's been winking ever since [4].

One side of his cheek was drawn up in a sort of tic, the corner of the mouth as well, and the eye winked in sympathy [5].

The French officer returned his salute – a drained-out figure with a twitch in the left eyelid [6].

They were a few metres apart when the left side of the man's face was suddenly contorted by a sort of spasm. It happened again just as they were passing one another. It was only a twitch, a quiver, rapid as the clicking of a camera shutter, but obviously habitual [7].

Since his dental practice has ceased growing, Irv had developed a tic in his right cheek that often gave him the appearance of smiling inexplicably [8].

Most unexpectedly his right eye flickers, in the ghost of a wink. . .and again his right eye flickers, almost as if it is a tic, outside his control. . .and once again she sees that tic in his right eye. . .and then again there comes that minute spasm of his eyelid. . .she receives one last tic of his right eyelid, and then he is gone [9].

## Tremor

Though the characteristic feature of the essential tremor syndrome is an upper limb tremor, other sites can be involved, either concurrently or independently, leading to a tremor of the head or the voice. An isolated head tremor can be of the yes/yes or no/no variety.

She had that peculiar trembling of the head which, in ladies of her excitable nature, may be taken as a sure indication of their breaking out again very shortly [10].

The effort at concealment was the beginning of the tremulous motion of head and hands which I have seen ever since in Miss Matty [11].

He wears a hare-skin on his chest, and has a trembling in his talk [12].

Miss Gailey flushed slightly, with the characteristic movement of the head. . . 'Oh! My poor dear!' Sarah Gailey moaned feebly, her head bobbing with its unconscious nervous movements [13].

It was this posture also which helped to steady an incipient shaking of the head, gave him his look of being sternly reined up, and caused him to support his chin on his neckcloth in the manner so congenial to little Hans Castorp's taste. . . Young Hans Castorp noticed that the ancestral tremor brought on by his ill-advised walk continued to trouble him – he found it rather an embarrassment when in the dining room. Almost as a regular thing now, his head would begin shaking at table; he found this impossible to prevent and hard to dissemble. He tried various devices to disguise the weakness, for he could not continually support his chin on his collar; he would keep his head in action, turning to the right and left in conversation, or bear hard against the table with the left forearm when he carried a spoonful of soup to his mouth, and support his head with his hand [14].

## Dystonia

Dystonia may be generalized, affect adjacent segments (segmental dystonia), or be confined to a particular body part (focal dystonia). My examples are largely confined to the last named.

Focal dystonias include spasmodic torticollis, writer's cramp, occupational cramps (for example in a violinist), blepharospasm, oromandibular dystonia, and laryngeal dystonia.

*Spasmodic Torticollis*
'Ah! Kostya!' he said suddenly, recognizing his brother, and his eyes lit up with joy. But at the same time he turned to look at the young man and convulsively jerked his head and neck as if his necktie were strangling him, . . . [15].

*Writer's Cramp*
I had no longer reason to lament the want of business; for he furnished me with so much, that in half a year I almost write myself blind. I likewise contracted a distemper by my sedentary life, in which no part of my body was exercised but my right arm, which rendered me incapable of writing for a long time [16].

*Violinist's Cramp*
Morel was suffering at the time from violent cramp in the hand, and found himself obliged to contemplate the possibility of having to give up the violin [17].

*Blepharospasm*
Mr. Bates was further distinguished from the common herd by a perpetual blinking of the eyes; and this, together with the red-rose tint of his complexion, and a way he had of hanging his head forward, and rolling it from side to side as he walked, gave him the air of a Bacchus in a blue apron, . . . [18].

*Laryngeal Dystonia*
Mr. Pilgrim generally spoke with an intermittent kind of splutter; indeed, one of his patients had observed that it was a pity such a clever man had a 'pediment' in his speech. . .

Mr. Pilgrim was not a man to sit quiet under a sarcasm, nature having endowed him with a considerable share of self-defensive wit. In his most sober moments he had an impediment in his speech, and as copious gin-and-water stimulated not the speech but the impediment, he had time to make his retort sufficiently bitter [18].

## Generalized Dystonia

It is perhaps being over-imaginative to describe Dick Ostler as having a generalized dystonia.

When Dick had looked at the paper, he winked with one eye, extended his grotesque mouth from ear to ear, like a navigable canal. . . 'Why, then,' said Dick, giving the head-band of his breeches a knowing hoist with one hand, and kicking out one foot behind him to accommodate the adjustment of that important habiliment . . . he ducked with his head and shoulders, scraped with his more advanced hoof, bolted the alcohol, to use the learned phrase, and withdrew to his own domain [19].

## Sydenham's Chorea

Sydenham's chorea (St. Vitus's dance) was first described by Sydenham in 1686. Once common, it is now relatively rare, and typically follows an episode of rheumatic fever. Antibodies are believed to react with epitopes in the basal ganglia and can be detected in affected cases. Most cases occur in mid-childhood and typically embrace behavioral phenomena, including agitation, irritability, and in some cases a confusional state, coupled with chorea which is typically generalized but may sometimes be unilateral.

All of the references I have encountered are somewhat oblique, and make no reference to the behavioral issues.

> This spectacle restoring her to a sense of the proprieties, she stood for some few moments silent, with her mouth wide open: and then, posting off to the bed on which the baby lay asleep, danced in a weird, Saint Vitus manner on the floor, . . . [20].
>
> For anybody 'ud think you'd got the St Vitus's dance, to see the things you've throwed down [21].
>
> In answering them, he incidentally disclosed the fact that he really had been away a long time from Russia – over four years – that he had been sent abroad for reasons of health, because of some strange nervous disease, something in the nature of epilepsy or St Vitus's dance, some kind of convulsive spasms and twitchings [22].

### Involuntary Movements of Uncertain Nature

My failure to identify the exact movement disorder in the following extracts probably owes more to my lack of expertise than a failure in the author's description.

> He jerked himself about, after this compliment, in such an intolerable manner, that my aunt, who had sat looking straight at him, lost all patience.
>
> 'Deuce take the man!' said my aunt, sternly, 'What's he about? Don't be galvanic, sir!!'
>
> 'I ask your pardon, Miss Trotwood,' returned Uriah; 'I'm aware you're nervous.'
>
> 'Go along with you, sir!!' said my aunt, anything but appeased. 'Don't presume to say so! I am nothing of the sort. If you're an eel, sir, conduct yourself like one. If you're a man, control your limbs, sir! Good God!' said my aunt with great indignation, 'I am not going to be serpentined and corkscrewed out of my senses!' [23].

Uriah Heep writhes through the whole of David Copperfield. Charles Keeping's depiction of him, of necessity a static image, shows, interestingly, a dystonic quality to the posture of the right hand, though admittedly it has just been struck by Mr. Micawber wielding a ruler (fig. 1)! I suspect Uriah Heep was not athetoid, and that Dickens' depiction is to illustrate his serpentine and manipulative nature.

> They sat side by side at the table, Lily turning over the pages. Constance, for all her vast bulk, continually made little nervous movements. Occasionally she would sniff and occasionally a mysterious noise would occur in her chest; she always pretended that this noise was a cough, and would support the pretence by emitting a real cough immediately after it [24].

This is the only reference to Constance's involuntary movements in Bennett's novel, and it appears towards the end. There is a suggestion of multiple tics here, but surely not appearing towards the end of life. Constance certainly does not have Tourette's. Indeed I have found only one example which might fulfill the criteria for that diagnosis.

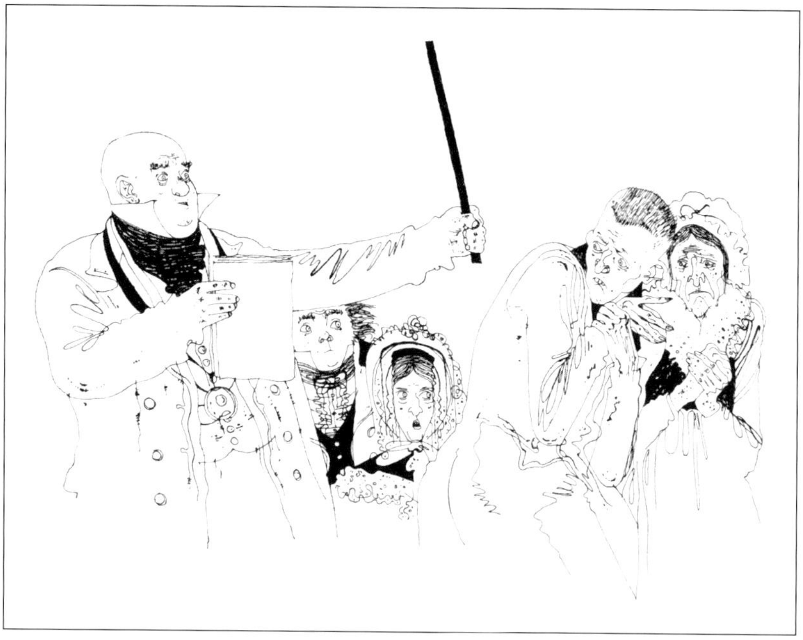

**Fig. 1.** From *David Copperfield*, C. Dickens. The Folio Society, 1983, with kind permission.

'I cannot help myself at all, for so he uses all my limbs and organs, my neck, my tongue, and my lungs, whenever he pleases, causing me to speak or to cry out; and I hear the words as if they were spoken by myself, but I am altogether unable to restrain them; and when I try to engage in prayer he attacks me more violently, thrusting out my tongue' [25].

The poor wretch in question believed he was possessed by the Devil. The issue of movement disorders being attributed to the Devil, acting through witchcraft, is one which I shall discuss briefly at the end of this chapter.

*Myoclonus*

She lay half sitting, supported by pillows, and seemed very restless; she laughed incessantly, struggling the while for breath: a high, purling, silver laughter, as though her plight excited or amused her. She was amused too, very likely, by the Hofrat's turns of phrase in introducing the visitor, and called out repeated thanks and good-byes as he went off; waved her hand at his departing back, sighed melodiously, with runs of silver merriment, and pressed her hand against her heaving breast under the batiste night-gown. Her legs, it seemed, were never still [14].

The lady in question had been treated with an artificial pneumothorax for her tuberculosis. When her pneumothorax was topped up by an incompetent physician, 'he filled her too full' and she suffered from 'cardiac depression'. I wonder if Mann is describing postanoxic myoclonus?

Examples of myoclonus have proved hard to come by, at least in the confines of my reading.

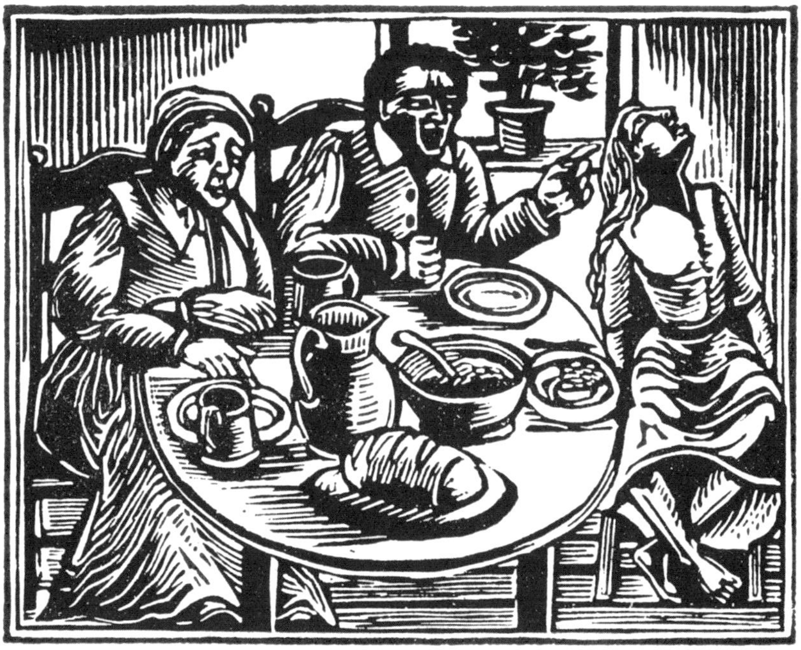

**Fig. 2.** Illustration by Clare Melinsky from the Folio Society edition of *The Witches of Salem*, a documentary narrative edited by Roger Thompson, 1982, with kind permission.

Palatal myoclonus is certainly audible with a stethoscope. Is it sometimes sufficiently loud to modify speech?

> It evoked a strong desire to mock and ape, and produced in his throat a cough of singular scornfulness, more particularly when Mr Rusper also assisted with an assumed unconsciousness that was all his own...
>
> '(Kik) jer doing?' he said at last.
>
> 'Tin mantraps!' said Mr Polly.
>
> 'Jer (kik) doing?'...
>
> 'Put it (kik) all (kik) back (kik).' [26].

### The Witches of Salem

On a final note, what was the underlying mechanism of the movement disorders displayed by the witches of Salem?

> And then her eyes were presently pulled into her head, so farr, that one might have fear'd she would never have us'd them more [27] (fig. 2).

One trusts few would now believe that the affected were possessed by the Devil. They clearly had oculogyric crises and abnormal neck posturing. Oculogyric crises can be part of a conversion disorder, at least according to Bramwell [28]. Though, in epidemic encephalitis, the ocular symptoms are usually late, it has been reported that they can appear in the acute stages of the disease [29]. Could the witches of Salem have been the victims of an epidemic of encephalitis?

## References


1 Gogol N: Dead Souls. Moscow, Moscow University Press, 1842.
2 Dostoevsky F: Crime and Punishment. Moscow, The Russian Messenger, 1866.
3 Anderson S: Winesburg, Ohio. New York, B.W. Huebsch, 1919.
4 Waugh E: Black Mischief. London, Chapman & Hall, 1932.
5 Mann T: Doktor Faustus. Stockholm, Bermann Fischer, 1947.
6 Greene G: The Heart of the Matter. London, Heinemann, 1948.
7 Orwell G: 1984. London, Secker & Warburg, 1949.
8 Heller J: Good as Gold. New York, Simon & Schuster, 1979.
9 Fowles J: A Maggot. London, Cape, 1985.
10 Dickens C: Martin Chuzzlewit. London, Chapman & Hall, 1844.
11 Gaskell E: Cranford. London, Smith Elder & Co., 1864.
12 Eliot G: The Mill on the Floss. Edinburgh, William Blackwood & Sons, 1860.
13 Bennett A: Hilda Lessways. London, Methuen & Co., 1911.
14 Mann T: The Magic Mountain. Berlin, S. Fischer, 1924.
15 Tolstoy L: Anna Karenina. Moscow, The Russian Messenger, 1877.
16 Fielding H: Joseph Andrews. London, A. Miller, 1742.
17 Proust M: Remembrance of Things Past, The Captive. Paris, Gallimard, 1923.
18 Eliot G: Scenes of Clerical Life. Edinburgh, William Blackwood & Sons, 1858.
19 Scott W: The Heart of Midlothian. Edinburgh, Archibald Constable, 1818.
20 Dickens C: The Cricket on the Hearth. London, Bradbury & Evans, 1846.
21 Eliot G: Adam Bede. Edinburgh, William Blackwood & Sons, 1859.
22 Dostoyevsky F: The Idiot. Moscow, Russian Herald, 1869.
23 Dickens C: David Copperfield. London, Bradbury & Evans, 1850.
24 Bennett A: The Old Wives' Tale. London, Chapman & Hall, 1908.
25 Sprenger J, Kramer H: Malleus Maleficarum. 1486. Translated by Summers M. London, The Folio Society, 1968.
26 Wells HG: The History of Mr. Polly. London, Thomas Nelson & Sons, 1910.
27 Thompson R (ed): The Witches of Salem. London, The Folio Society, 1982.
28 Bramwell E: The upward movements of the eyes. Brain 1928;51:1–37.
29 Stengel E: Zur Klinik und Pathophysiologie des Postenzephalitischen Blickkrampfes. Monat P.U.N. 1928;70:305



G.D. Perkin
Emeritus Consultant Neurologist
Charing Cross Hospital, Fulham Palace Road
London W6 8RF (UK)
E-Mail d.perkin@ic.ac.uk

Bogousslavsky J, Dieguez S (eds): Literary Medicine: Brain Disease and Doctors in Novels, Theater, and Film.
Front Neurol Neurosci. Basel, Karger, 2013, vol 31, pp 195–214 (DOI: 10.1159/000343236)

# Epilepsy in Dostoevsky's Novels

Piet H.A. Voskuil

Hans Berger Clinic for Epilepsy, Oosterhout, The Netherlands

**Abstract**

Fyodor Mikhailovich Dostoevsky (1821–1881) suffered from epilepsy. Some type of psychopathology can be found in about 25% of the characters of his novels. Some of them have seizures. In at least five of them Dostoevsky clearly intends them to have epilepsy. Others are more likely to be created as people with hysteria or sometimes, for instance, possession. In this essay an inventory is given by more or less comprehensive quotes of different types of seizures in five novels. The seizures are named in the novels with a varying vocabulary based on the concepts of nosology in the 19th century, the knowledge of Dostoevsky of these concepts, his own experiences, and problems in translation and transliteration. In the discussion, analysis of the role these factors played in the understanding of what Dostoevsky really expressed is given attention. Special attention is given to the so-called ecstatic aura. This element of focal epileptic seizures is so rare that in the past the description of it raised doubts on its existence as such and therefore the embellishment by Dostoevsky, describing his own experience and/or that of his epileptic characters Kirillov and Myshkin. The consequence of this analytic approach, however, should not be losing one's amazement of the genius polyphonic creativity of Dostoevsky to integrate so many profound aspects of the human and especially the Russian soul in the characters of his novels.



Fyodor Mikhailovich Dostoevsky (1821–1881) suffered from epilepsy. His medical history is documented in excellent biographies [1–7] based on good sources such as notebooks, letters, and recollections. In articles from the medical literature his seizures are classified by a majority of authors as focal, mostly secondary generalizing [8–12]. Gastaut [13] revised his original hypothesis of primary generalized epilepsy [14] in an eclectic conjecture wherein both etiologies are associated. Hughes [15] and Seneviratne [16] more or less do the same: the first stressing the idiosyncratic aspects, and the latter stressing the focal aspects. There were some doubts, however, as a so-called 'ecstatic aura' (indicating a partial limbic onset), as described by Dostoevsky, was seen as an embellishment of his own experience in some of the characters in his novels. In Dostoevsky's case, however, complex partial seizures with other semiology were seen as well. Seneviratne [16] extensively analyzed the seizure semiology of Dostoevsky and the characters in many of his novels.

In this chapter, I will describe the role seizures played in Dostoevsky's novels. To begin with, the stories of the novels are told as guided by the seizure-related quotes. In a discussion, I will elaborate on the interpretation of these quotes in the complex interrelationship of Dostoevsky's own experience, his medical knowledge, the concept of epilepsy and related disorders of personality in the 19th century, and transliteration and translation of the vocabulary based on these concepts. I will also look at characters in the stories and briefly mention other persons with attacks of a different kind: Murin, Ordynov, and Katerina in *The Landlady* (Hozyajka), 1847; Nellie (Elena, Lenotchka) and Natasha in *Humiliated and Insulted* (Unizhennye I oskorblennye), 1861; Myshkin in *The Idiot* (Idiot), 1869; Kirillov in *Demons* (Besy), 1872; and Smerdyakov in *The Brothers Karamazov* (Brat'ya Karamazovy), 1880.

## *The Landlady*

In this short novel, the protagonist Ordynov is an unworldly scholar looking for a place to stay. He finds a humble room let by Ilya Murin. Murin is an old man living in an adjacent room with a beautiful young woman named Katerina. She is under the psychological sway of Murin who is depicted as a clairvoyant with a Mephistopheles-like character. Katerina and Ordynov develop an emotional relationship. When emotions run high, all of them tend to have physical complaints in which their states of consciousness are disturbed.

### *Murin's Seizures*

In Murin's case epilepsy is mentioned: 'Murin was on the ground, his body writhed in spasms, his face was contorted in pain and the foam stood on his compressed lips. Ordynov understood that the unfortunate was heaviest hit by an *attack of epilepsy*' (I, 365).[1] Murin reveals to Ordynov: 'Who could know that you too are visited by an ugly disease? But in my case *it happens repeatedly*' and 'Also, I put a knife in the chest last almost . . . he murmured, nodding his head in Katerina's direction, I'm a sick man, *from time to time I have seizures*' (I 397). This refers to an earlier passage where Murin threatens Katerina with a knife.

[1] Numbers in parenthesis indicate volume and page of the quote from Dostoevsky's completed work, compilated in 10 volumes in the Dutch 'Russische Bibliotheek' [Russian Library] edited by G.A. van Oorschot, Amsterdam. English translations in all of the discussed novels are by Constance Garnett (e-text www.online-literature.com/dostoevsky.), with one exception: in *The Idiot,* translations are taken from Eva Martin in the 2001 Gutenbergproject http://books.rakeshv.org/html/idiot10/idiot10.html. Vocabulary related to epilepsy is by Djoeke Leistra matched with the Russian text from: Gosudarstvennoe izdatel'stvo cudozhestvennoy literatyry, Moskva, 1956.

*Ordynov's Seizures*

In Ordynov's case there is only one occasion that is suspicious of an epileptic event, but it could also be an emotional reaction or pseudoepileptic seizure. There is no mentioning of recurrent seizures.

But to his own astonishment he gradually got into a strange state: He had to be seated on a sofa and felt to fall asleep. Intermittently he came to oneself again and noticed that his sleep was no real sleep but more a kind of grievous state of oblivion. . .

He arose and fancied that he walked already to them, but stumbled and fell. . .

Now he lost his reflection totally and when he opened his eyes after a long, long time he noticed full of surprise that he still lay dressed on the same sofa. . .

But his arms were heavy as lead, he wasn't able to move; his tongue seems like paralyzed and he only felt, his blood rushing in his vessels as trying to lift him from his bed. Somebody provided him some water. Finally he lost his consciousness (I, 356).

*Katerina's Seizure*

Katerina is described as having just one attack. An epileptic nature is possible, but in the novel no previous or recurrent seizures are noted.

Katerina sat there deathly pale. She stared motionless in the air, her lips were blue, like in a dead body and her eyes veiled by a dull harassing grief.

She rose slowly, made two steps and fell with a screech in front of the icon. . . falteringly and incoherent words escaped from her chest. She became unconscious (I, 380).

### *Humiliated and Insulted*

The character with epilepsy is Elena (Netochka). Her deceased mother called her Nellie, the name which is most used. Nellie is 12 or 13 years of age and the granddaughter of Smith (fig. 1). A few weeks after the death of his daughter, Nellie's mother, a period which he suffered numbed senses, Smith dies. Nellie herself has a heart ailment.

But especially the strange heart beating struck me. It started to beat always louder, so loud that it could be heard on two, three steps distance, like suffering from an aneurysma (III, 447).

Yes she will die soon. She has an organic heart defect. . . (III, 606).

*Nellie's Seizures*

But at that instant we heard a piercing, inhuman shriek. I looked. Elena, who had been standing as though unconscious, uttering a strange, unnatural scream, fell with a thud on the ground, writhing in awful convulsions, her face, was working. *She was in an epileptic fit* (III, 453).

She sobbed till she became *hysterical* (III, 502).

'She has *epileptic fits*,' I answered (III, 562).

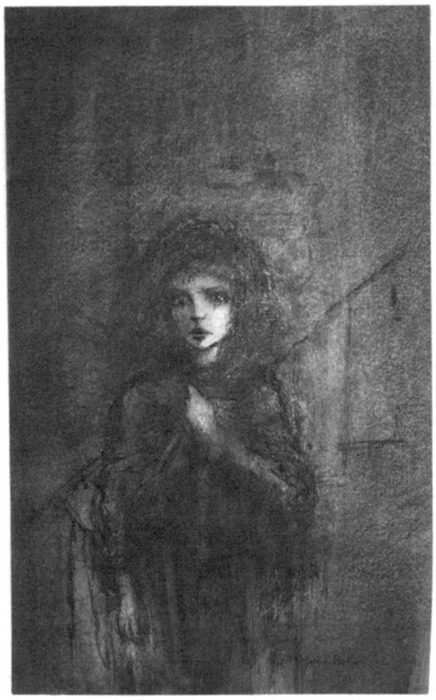

**Fig. 1.** Nellie. Nadezhda Vereschagina-Rozanova. *Humiliated and Insulted.* 1930. With kind permission from Dostoevsky Museum St. Petersburg, Russia.

She nestled up to me tremulously as though she was afraid of something, said something, rapidly and impetuously, as though she had only been waiting for me to come to tell me it. But her words were strange and incoherent; I could understand nothing. She was in *delirium* (III, 603).

At last something like a thought was apparent in her face. After a violent *epileptic fit* she was usually for some time unable to collect her thoughts or to articulate distinctly. And so it was now. After making an immense effort to say something to me and realizing that I did not understand, she held out her little hand and began to wipe away my tears, and then put her arm round my neck, drew me down to her and kissed me. It was clear that she had had *a fit* in my absence, and it had taken place at the moment when she had been standing at the door. Probably on recovery she had been for a long time unable to come to herself. At such times reality is mixed up with delirium and she had certainly imagined something awful, some horror.

. . .so she must have been meaning to go out, and had probably been already unlocking the door when she was suddenly struck down by the fit. Where could she have been meaning to go? Was she already in *delirium*? Meanwhile the fever did not leave her, and she soon sank into *delirium and unconsciousness*. She had twice already had a fit in my flat, but it had always passed off harmlessly; now, however, she seemed in a high fever.

. . .she was pale; her lips were parched with fever and stained with blood, probably from the fall (III, 604).

But she bent on him with a strange, long gaze. 'Mother, where's mother?' she brought out, as though in delirium. 'Where is my mother?' she cried once more, stretching out her trembling hands to us. And suddenly a fearful, unearthly shriek broke from her bosom; her face worked convulsively, and she fell on the floor in a terrible fit (III 673).

But at last Nellie felt faint, and she was carried indoors. Nikolay Sergeyitch was much alarmed and vexed that we had let her talk so much. She had a sort of attack or *fainting-fit*. She had had such attacks several times (III 690).

### *Nellie's Death*

She died a fortnight later. In that fortnight of her last agony she never quite came to herself, or escaped from her strange fantasies. Her intellect was, as it were, clouded (III, 701).

### *Natasha's Seizure*

Natasha, another main character in the novel, lost her consciousness on one occasion.

I caught her up and carried her into the room. She was *fainting*! 'What shall I do?' I thought. 'She'll have brain-fever for certain!'

Natasha told me that for the first minute she was not even surprised to see the prince. 'My brain was in a whirl' she said.

When I ran back into the room I saw the doctor was supporting Natasha, who was writhing and struggling out of his arms as though in *convulsions*. For a long time we could not soothe her; at last we succeeded in getting her to bed; she seemed to be in the *delirium of brain-fever*.

'Doctor, what's the matter with her?' I asked with a sinking heart.

'Wait a little,' he answered, 'I must watch the attack more closely and then form my conclusions... but speaking generally things are very bad. It may even end in brain-fever'... (III 648).

We can conclude from Nellie's medical history that she is supposed to have different types of seizures (the quotes on this and previous page are by the present author, indicated in italics): epileptic, hysterical, and syncopal. However, we must be aware of problems in translation (see Discussion). In Natasha's case, the attack has more the characteristics of a psychogenic pseudoepileptic seizure.

## The Idiot

The protagonist of the novel is *Prince Lev Nikolaevich Myshkin*, who is:

...of about twenty-six or twenty-seven years of age, slightly above the middle height, very fair, with a thin, pointed and very light coloured beard; his eyes were large and blue, and had an intent look about them, yet that heavy expression which some people affirm to be a peculiarity, as well as evidence, of an *epileptic subject*.

...He had been sent abroad for his health; he had suffered from some strange nervous malady – *a kind of epilepsy, with convulsive spasms*. His interlocutor burst out laughing several times at his answers; and more than ever, when to the question, 'whether he had been cured?' the patient replied: 'No, they did not cure me' (VI 10).

...He was very absent; he would appear to listen-and heard nothing; and he would laugh of a sudden, evidently with no idea of what he was laughing about (VI 13).

His fits were so frequent then, that they made almost an idiot of him (the prince used the expression 'idiot' himself; VI 37).

The name of the treating Swiss doctor is Schneider.

Although he had not quite cured him, he had greatly improved his condition (VI 38).

'Fits?' asked the prince, slightly surprised. 'I very seldom have fits nowadays. I don't know how it may be here, though; they say the climate may be bad for me' (VI 70).

'This was after a long series of fits. I always used to fall into a sort of torpid condition after such a series, and lost my memory almost entirely; and though I was not altogether without reason at such times, yet I had no logical power of thought. This would continue for three or four days, and then I would recover myself again. I remember my melancholy was intolerable' (VI 72).

The previous lines appear almost autobiographical for Dostoevsky. And what about the following?

'I once heard the story of a man who lived twelve years in a prison – I heard it from the man himself. He was one of the persons under treatment with my professor; he had fits, and attacks of melancholy, then he would weep, and once he tried to commit suicide. This man had once been brought to the scaffold in company with several others, and had had the sentence of death by shooting passed upon him for some political crime. Twenty minutes later he had been reprieved and some other punishment substituted' (VI 77).

Myshkin experiences preictal alterations in his mental state and consciousness.

'Because when I jumped out of the train this morning, two eyes glared at me just as yours did a moment since.'

'Ha! And whose eyes may they have been?' said Rogojin [who is Myshkin's important counterpart in the novel] suspiciously. It seemed to the prince that he was trembling.

'I don't know; I thought it was a hallucination. I often have hallucinations nowadays. I feel just as I did five years ago when my fits were about to come on.'

He had absently taken up the knife a second time, and again Rogojin snatched it from his hand, and threw it down on the table (VI 256).

He remembered that the last time he had been engaged in looking around him for the unknown something, he was standing before a cutler's shop, in the window of which were exposed certain goods for sale. He was extremely anxious now to discover whether this shop and these goods really existed, or whether the whole thing had been a hallucination.

He felt in a very curious condition today, a condition similar to that which had preceded his fits in bygone years.

He remembered that at such times he had been particularly absentminded, and could not discriminate between objects and persons unless he concentrated special attention upon them.

He remembered seeing something in the window marked at sixty copecks. Therefore, if the shop existed and if this object were really in the window, it would prove that he had been able to concentrate his attention on this article at a moment when, as a general rule, his absence of mind would have been too great to admit of any such concentration; in fact, very shortly after he had left the railway station in such a state of agitation (VI 278-279).

*Myshkin's Ecstatic Aura*

This must be thought out; it was clear that there had been no hallucination at the station then, either; something had actually happened to him, on both occasions; there was no doubt of it. But again a loathing for all mental exertion overmastered him; he would not think it out now, he would put it off and think of something else. He remembered that during his epileptic fits, or rather immediately preceding them, he had always experienced a moment or two when his whole heart, and mind, and body seemed to wake up to vigour and light; when he became filled with joy and hope, and all his anxieties seemed to be swept away for ever; these moments were but presentiments, as it were, of the one final second (it was never more than a second) in which the fit came upon him. That second, of course, was inexpressible. When his attack was over, and the prince reflected on his symptoms, he used to say to himself: 'These moments, short as they are, when I feel such extreme consciousness of myself, and consequently more of life than at other times, are due only to the disease – to the sudden rupture of normal conditions. Therefore they are not really a higher kind of life, but a lower.' This reasoning, however, seemed to end in a paradox, and lead to the further consideration: 'What matter though it be only disease, an abnormal tension of the brain, if when I recall and analyze the moment, it seems to have been one of harmony and beauty in the highest degree – an instant of deepest sensation, overflowing with unbounded joy and rapture, ecstatic devotion, and completest life?' Vague though this sounds, it was perfectly comprehensible to Myshkin, though he knew that it was but a feeble expression of his sensations.

That there was, indeed, beauty and harmony in those abnormal moments, that they really contained the highest synthesis of life, he could not doubt, nor even admit the possibility of doubt. He felt that they were not analogous to the fantastic and unreal dreams due to intoxication by hashish, opium or wine. Of that he could judge, when the attack was over. These instants were characterised – to define it in a word – by an intense quickening of the sense of personality. Since, in the last conscious moment preceding the attack, he could say to himself, with full understanding of his words: 'I would give my whole life for this one instant,' then doubtless to him it really was worth a lifetime. For the rest, he thought the dialectical part of his argument of little worth; he saw only too clearly that the result of these ecstatic moments was stupefaction, mental darkness, idiocy. No argument was possible on that point. His conclusion, his estimate of the 'moment,' doubtless contained some error, yet the reality of the sensation troubled him. What's more unanswerable than a fact? And this fact had occurred. The prince had confessed unreservedly to himself that the feeling of intense beatitude in that crowded moment made the moment worth a lifetime. 'I feel then,' he said one day to Rogojin in Moscow, 'I feel then as if I understood those amazing words – 'There shall be no more time.' And he added with a smile: 'No doubt the epileptic Mahomet refers to that same moment when he says that he visited all the dwellings of Allah, in less time than was needed to empty his pitcher of water' (VI 279–281).

During this whole period there is a further threat looming.

He was seized all at once by a violent desire, almost a temptation, against which he strove in vain.

He tried to take an interest in all he saw; in the sky, in the Neva. He spoke to some children he met. He felt his epileptic condition becoming more and more developed (VI 282).

During an attempted murder by Parfen Rogojin, Myshkin's seizure develops into secondary generalization.

Rogojin's eyes flashed, and a smile of insanity distorted his countenance. His right hand was raised, and something glittered in it. The prince did not think of trying to stop it. All he could remember afterwards was that he seemed to have called out:

'Parfen! I won't believe it' (fig. 2).

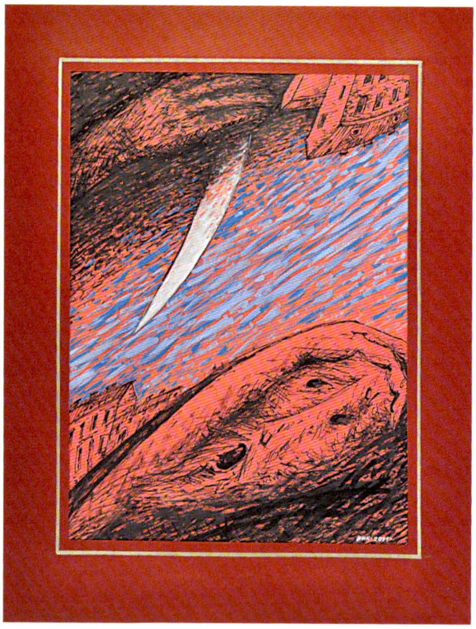

**Fig. 2.** Prince Myshkin. Vyacheslav Zabelin. 'Parfyon! I won't believe it.' Illustration to *The Idiot*. 2011. With kind permission from Dostoevsky Museum St. Petersburg, Russia.

Next moment something appeared to burst open before him: a wonderful inner light illuminated his soul. This lasted perhaps half a second, yet he distinctly remembered hearing the beginning of the wail, the strange, dreadful wail, which burst from his lips of its own accord.

Next moment he was absolutely unconscious; black darkness blotted out everything. . . . He had fallen in an epileptic fit.

As is well known, these fits occur instantaneously. The face, especially the eyes, become terribly disfigured, convulsions seize the limbs, a terrible cry breaks from the sufferer, a wail from which everything human seems to be blotted out, so that it is impossible to believe that the man who has just fallen is the same who emitted the dreadful cry. It seems more as though some other being, inside the stricken one, had cried. Many people have borne witness to this impression; and many cannot behold an epileptic fit without a feeling of mysterious terror and dread.

The prince's body slipped convulsively down the steps till it rested at the bottom. Very soon, in five minutes or so, he was discovered, and a crowd collected around him.

A pool of blood on the steps near his head gave rise to grave fears. Was it a case of accident, or had there been a crime? It was, however, soon recognised as a case of epilepsy, and identification and proper measures for restoration followed one another, owing to a fortunate circumstance. The sufferer was immediately taken to his room, and though he partially regained consciousness, he lay long in a semi-dazed condition.

The doctor stated that there was no danger to be apprehended from the wound on the head (VI 291).

The prince was in a fever all night. It was strange, but he had suffered from fever for several nights in succession. On this particular night, while in semi-delirium, he had an idea: what if on the morrow he was to have a fit before everybody? (VI 646).

This premonition becomes reality when Myshkin accidentally breaks a Chinese vase.

But one very curious fact was that all the shame and vexation and mortification which he felt over the accident were less powerful than the deep impression of the almost supernatural truth of his premonition. He stood still in alarm – in almost superstitious alarm – for a moment; then all mists seemed to clear away from his eyes; he was conscious of nothing but light and joy and ecstasy; his breath came and went; but the moment passed. Thank God it was not that! He drew a long breath and looked around (VI 671).

But shortly thereafter, he had risen, and was speaking standing up. The old gentleman was looking at him now in unconcealed alarm. Lizabetha Prokofievna wrung her hands. 'Oh, my God!' she cried. She had guessed the state of the case before anyone else. Aglaya rushed quickly up to him, and was just in time to receive him in her arms, and to hear with dread and horror that awful, wild cry as he fell writhing to the ground. There he lay on the carpet, and someone quickly placed a cushion under his head (VI 678).

His attack of yesterday had been a slight one. Excepting some little heaviness in the head and pain in the limbs, he did not feel any particular effects. His brain worked all right, though his soul was heavy within him (VI 680).

After this seizure, in an only vaguely specified space of time, the condition of the prince deteriorates. The doctor from Switzerland who previously treated him comes to see him.

If Schneider himself had arrived then and seen his former pupil and patient, remembering the prince's condition during the first year in Switzerland, he would have flung up his hands, despairingly, and cried, as he did then: 'An idiot!' (VI 748).

Evgénie Pávlovitch took the deepest interest in the fate of the unfortunate 'idiot', and, thanks to his influence, the prince found himself once more with Dr. Schneider, in Switzerland.

But Dr. Schneider frowns ever more and more and shakes his head; he hints that the brain is fatally injured; he does not as yet declare that his patient is incurable, but he allows himself to express the gravest fears (VI 749).

Lizabeta Prokofievna said:

'At all events, I've had a good Russian cry over this poor fellow,' she added, pointing to the prince, who had not recognised her in the slightest degree (VI 752).

### *Demons* (The Possessed)

The title alludes to the exorcism of demons as in Lucas 8:32–36 of the Bible. At the core of the story is a group of dissidents, headed by Pjotr Stepanowich. They are trying to create social unrest. The group is composed of a handful young people, one of whom is a civil engineer named *Alexei Nilych Kirillov*.

He was a young man, about twenty-seven, decently dressed, well made, slender and dark, with a pale, rather muddy-coloured face and black lustreless eyes. He seemed rather thoughtful and absent-minded, spoke jerkily and ungrammatically, transposing words in rather a strange way, and getting muddled if he attempted a sentence of any length (VII 96).

He has returned to Russia after 4 years in America and hopes to get appointed for a railway project. In the course of the story he loses his belief in the rebel movement and, in line with his philosophy of life, becomes suicidal.

With his immanent suicide in mind, he promises (VII 569) his revolutionary group that he will leave a suicide note behind in which he confesses his supposed guilt for everything they dictate, most particularly the murder of Shatov, another member of the group. In America, Kirillov and Shatov travelled together in order to experience the lifestyle of the American laborer under extremely difficult circumstances, but he came back completely exhausted. He lives next door to Lebyadkin and his crippled sister Maria Timofeevna, who is mentally handicapped. 'His sister has fits of some sort every day, she shrieks and he "keeps her in order" with the whip' (VII 102).

The often cited description of Kirillov's possible epileptic aura is depicted only once in the novel near the end of his life.

> He [Shatov] found Kirillov still pacing up and down his room so preoccupied that he had forgotten the arrival of Shatov's wife, and heard what he said without understanding him.
>
> 'Oh, yes!' he recollected suddenly, as though tearing himself with an effort and only for an instant from some absorbing idea, 'yes. . . an old woman. . . . A wife or an old woman? Stay a minute: a wife and an old woman, is that it? I remember. I've been, the old woman will come, only not just now. Take the pillow. Is there anything else? Yes. . . . Stay, do you have moments of the eternal harmony, Shatov?'
>
> 'You know, Kirillov, you mustn't go on staying up every night.'
>
> Kirillov came out of his reverie and, strange to say, spoke far more coherently than he usually did; it was clear that he had formulated it long ago and perhaps written it down.
>
> *'There are seconds – they come five or six at a time – when you suddenly feel the presence of the eternal harmony perfectly attained. It's something not earthly – I don't mean in the sense that it's heavenly – but in that sense that man cannot endure it in his earthly aspect. He must be physically changed or die. This feeling is clear and unmistakable; it's as though you apprehend all nature and suddenly say, 'Yes, that's right.' God, when He created the world, said at the end of each day of creation, 'Yes, it's right, it's good.' It. . . it's not being deeply moved, but simply joy. You don't forgive anything because there is no more need of forgiveness. It's not that you love – oh, there's something in it higher than love – what's most awful is that it's terribly clear and such joy. If it lasted more than five seconds, the soul could not endure it and must perish. In those five seconds I live through a lifetime, and I'd give my whole life for them, because they are worth it.'*
>
> 'To endure ten seconds one must be physically changed. I think man ought to give up having children – what's the use of children, what's the use of evolution when the goal has been attained? In the gospel it is written that there will be no child-bearing in the resurrection, but that men will be like the angels of the Lord. That's a hint. Is your wife bearing a child?'
>
> 'Kirillov, does this often happen?'
>
> 'Once in three days, or once a week.'
>
> 'Don't you have fits, perhaps?'
>
> 'No.'
>
> 'Well, you will. Be careful, Kirillov. I've heard that's just how fits begin. An epileptic described exactly that sensation before a fit, word for word as you've done. *He mentioned five seconds, too, and said that more could not be endured. Remember Mahomet's pitcher from which no drop of water was spilt while he circled Paradise on his horse. That was a case of five seconds too; that's too much like your eternal harmony, and Mahomet was an epileptic.* Be careful, Kirillov, its epilepsy!'
>
> 'It won't have time,' Kirillov smiled gently (VII 611, 612).

This last answer refers to his intention to commit suicide (VII 643–649).Thus, the fictitious character Kirillov does not think he has epilepsy, but through Shatov, Dostoevsky explains that Kirillov's symptoms might originate from epilepsy ('an epileptic described exactly. . .', etc.). The dialogue between Shatov and Kirillov shows that Dostoevsky is familiar with the fact that in a person's medical history a period of only aura symptoms can exist without secondary generalized seizures starting later on in life.

### *The Brothers Karamazov*

The character with epilepsy in this novel is Pavel Fyodorovitch Smerdyakov. He is the lackey of Fyodor Pavlovitch Karamazov.

Fyodor Pavlovitch is the father of three brothers. Smerdjakov is his illegitimate son from his relationship with Lizaveta Smerdyashtchaya. Three other sons are from two marriages: Dmitry (Mitya) from his first marriage with Adelaida, and Ivan and Alexey (Alyosha) from his second wife, Sofya.

Sofya's seizures are referred to with different words on different occasions.

> . . . and this unhappy young woman, kept in terror from her childhood, fell into that kind of nervous disease which is most frequently found in peasant women who are said to be *'possessed by devils'*. At times after terrible *fits of hysterics* she even lost her reason. Yet she bore Fyodor Pavlovich two sons, Ivan and Alexey, the eldest in the first year of marriage and the second three years later (IX 19).

> 'Do you know', he used often to say, looking at Alyosha, 'that you are like her, *"the crazy woman"* – that was what he used to call his dead wife, Alyosha's mother.' (IX 30).

> 'I knew her attacks always used to begin like that. The next day she would begin shrieking hysterically. . .'
> 'Alyosha, I never insulted the poor *crazy* girl!' (IX 172).

*Alyosha's Seizure*

Precisely what he was describing in the *crazy* woman was suddenly repeated with Alyosha. He jumped up from his seat exactly as his mother was said to have done, wrung his hands, hid his face in them, and fell back in his chair, shaking all over in an hysterical paroxysm of sudden violent, silent weeping. His extraordinary resemblance to his mother particularly impressed the old man (IX 172).

Before going to the main epileptic character in this novel (Smerdyakov), two other women in this novel who have attacks will be briefly discussed. Their attacks seem to be randomly named. They are related to possession and hysteria, and are detailed below.

*The Possessed Woman's Seizure*

She has no name. She is attending a sermon by Father (The Starets) Zosima who 'began blessing the women who thronged about him. One *crazy* woman was led up to him. As soon as she caught sight of the elder she began shrieking and writhing as though in the pains of childbirth.'

'I do not know how it may be now, but in my childhood I often happened to see and hear these *"possessed"* women in the villages and monasteries. They used to be brought to Mass; they would squeal and bark like a dog so that they were heard all over the church. But when the sacrament was carried in and they were led up to it, at once the "possession" ceased, and the sick women were always soothed for a time. I was greatly impressed and amazed at this as a child; but then I heard from country neighbours and from my town teachers that the whole illness was *simulated* to avoid work, and that it could always be cured by suitable severity; various anecdotes were told to confirm this. But later on I learnt with astonishment from medical specialists that there is no pretence about it, that it is a terrible illness to which women are subject, especially prevalent among us in Russia, and that it is due to the hard lot of the peasant women. It is a disease, I was told, arising from exhausting toil too soon after hard, abnormal and unassisted labour in childbirth, and from the hopeless misery, from beatings, and so on, which some women were not able to endure like others. The strange and instant healing of the frantic and struggling woman as soon as she was led up to the holy sacrament, which had been explained to me as due to *malingering* and the trickery of the "clericals," arose probably in the most natural manner. Both the women who supported her and the invalid herself fully believed as a truth beyond question that the evil spirit in possession of her could not hold if the sick woman were brought to the sacrament and made to bow down before it. And so, with a nervous and psychically deranged woman, a *sort of convulsion* of the whole organism always took place, and was bound to take place, at the moment of bowing down to the sacrament, aroused by the expectation of the miracle of healing and the implicit belief that it would come to pass; and it did come to pass, though only for a moment. It was exactly the same now as soon as the elder touched the sick woman with the stole' (IX 60, 61). [italics by P.V.].

### *The Seizures of Katerina Ivanovna*

Through Katerina Ivanovna, one of the main characters in the novel, Dostoevsky expresses some knowledge on hysteria.

Katerina Ivanovna went into a fit of hysterics. She sobbed, and was shaken with convulsions (IX 191).

Alyosha told him [Ivan] she had been hysterical, and that she was now, he heard, unconscious and delirious.

Nobody dies of hysterics, though. They don't matter. God gave woman hysterics as a relief. I won't go to her at all (IX 288).

### *Lise*

Lise is Katerina Ivanovna's daughter and is said to have had 3 hysterical seizures that are not described (IX 700).

### *Smerdyakov*

Smerdyakov is a key character in this novel (fig. 3).

[He is a] young man of about four and twenty, remarkably unsociable and taciturn'. Not that he was shy or bashful. On the contrary, he was conceited and seemed to despise everybody. He was

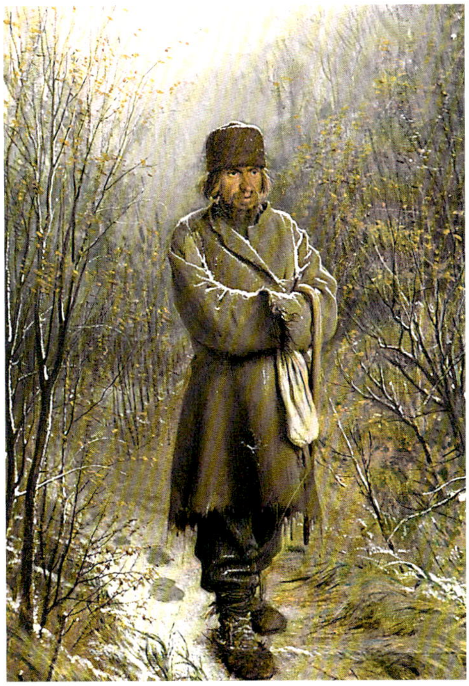

**Fig. 3.** The painting *A Contemplator* by Ivan Kramskoy (1876). Reproduced with permission from The Museum of Russian Art in Kiev, Ukraine.
In *The Brothers Karamazov* it reads: ‚There is a remarkable picture by the painter Kramskoy, called *Contemplation*. There is a forest in winter, and on a roadway through the forest, in absolute solitude, stands a peasant in a torn kaftan and bark shoes. He stands, as it were, lost in thought. Yet he is not thinking; he is ‚contemplating.' (...) There are a good many ‚contemplatives' among the peasantry. Well, Smerdyakov was probably one of them, and he probably was greedily hoarding up his impressions, hardly knowing why (IX 158-159).

brought up by Grigory and Marfa, but the boy grew up 'with no sense of gratitude', as Grigory expressed it: he was an unfriendly boy and seemed to look at the world mistrustfully. In his childhood he was very fond of hanging cats, and burying them with great ceremony. He used to dress up in a sheet as though it were a surplice, and sang, and waved some object over the dead cat as though it were a censer.

All this he did on the sly, with the greatest secrecy. Grigory caught him once at this diversion and gave him a sound beating. He shrank into a corner and sulked there for a week. 'He doesn't care for you or me, the monster', Grigory used to say to Marfa, 'and he doesn't care for anyone. Are you a human being?' he said, addressing the boy directly. 'You're not a human being. You grew from the mildew in the bath-house. That's what you are.'

The boy looked sarcastically at his teacher. There was something positively condescending in his expression. Grigori could not restrain himself. 'I'll show you where!' he cried, and gave the boy a violent slap on the cheek. The boy took the slap without a word, but withdrew into his corner again for some days. A week later he had his first attack of the disease to which he was subject all the rest of his life – epilepsy. . .

'But as soon as he [Fyodor Pavlovich] heard of his illness, he showed an active interest in him, sent for a doctor, and tried remedies, but the disease turned out to be incurable. The fits occurred, on an average, once a month, but at various intervals. The fits varied too, in violence: some were light and some were very severe (IX 155, 156).

His fits were becoming more frequent, and on the days he was ill Marfa cooked, which did not suit Fyodor Pavlovich at all.

Why are your fits getting worse?' asked Fyodor Pavlovich (IX 158).

*Smerdyakov's Seizures*

Only one seizure of Smerdyakov is described in detail, but by several people. It is the one that plays an important role in the plot because it happens on the day Fyodor Pavlovich is murdered. For that reason the question arises as to whether the seizure is faked.

This seizure is described by five different persons in the novel. The first description comes from Smerdyakov himself. He predicts his seizure the day before it actually occurs (i.e. the day he murdered father Karamazov). He tells Ivan:

> 'I feel certain, sir, that I shall have a long fit to-morrow.'
>
> 'What do you mean by "a long fit"?'
>
> 'A long fit, lasting a long time – several hours, or perhaps a day or two. Once it went on for three days. I fell from the garret that time. The struggling ceased and then began again, and for three days I couldn't come back to my senses. Fyodor Pavlovich sent for Herzenstube, the doctor here, and he put ice on my head and tried another remedy, too. . . . I might have died.'
>
> 'But they say one can't tell with epilepsy when a fit is coming. What makes you say you will have one to-morrow?' Ivan inquired, with a peculiar, irritable curiosity.
>
> 'That's just so. You can't tell beforehand.'
>
> 'Do you mean to pretend to be ill to-morrow for three days, eh?'
>
> Smerdyakov, who was looking at the ground again, and playing with the toe of his right foot, set the foot down, moved the left one forward, and, grinning, articulated: 'If I were able to play such a trick, that is, pretend to have a fit – and it would not be difficult for a man accustomed to them – I should have a perfect right to use such a means to save myself from death' (IX 333, 334).

After the murder, Ivan visits Smerdyakov three times. The first visit was in the hospital where Smerdyakov was admitted after his prolonged seizure. Smerdyakov tells:

> 'As I was going down to the cellar, I was in terrible dread and doubt. What frightened me most was losing you and being left without defence in all the world. So I went down into the cellar thinking "Here, it'll come on directly, it'll strike me down directly, shall I fall!" And it was through this fear that I suddenly felt the spasm that always comes. . . and so I went flying.'
>
> 'And did you tell them that you can sham fits, as you boasted then?'
>
> 'No, I didn't tell them that either' (IX 734).

Smerdyakov recounts his seizure a third time when he is released from the hospital. On that occasion he confesses to Ivan that he murdered father Karamazov.

> 'Aren't you tired of it? Here we are face to face; what's the use of going on keeping up a farce to each other? Are you still trying to throw it all on me, to my face? You murdered him; you are the real murderer, I was only your instrument, your faithful servant, and it was following your words I did it' (IX 754).

Shortly afterwards he describes his seizure again. Ivan asks:

> 'In a fit or in a sham one?'

'A sham one, naturally. I shammed it all. I went quietly down the steps to the very bottom and lay down quietly, and as I lay down I gave a scream, and struggled, till they carried me out.'

'Stay! And were you shamming all along, afterwards, and in the hospital?'

'No, not at all. Next day, in the morning, before they took me to the hospital, I had a real attack and a more violent one than I've had for years. For two days I was quite unconscious' (IX 757).

Shortly before the final hearing in the murder trial Alyosha tells Ivan: 'An hour ago Smerdyakov hanged himself' (IX 788).

Fyodor Pavlovich also tells of Smedyakov's seizure.

'Smerdyakov went to the cellar for something and fell down from the top of the steps. Fortunately, Marfa Ignatyevna was in the yard and heard him in time. She did not see the fall, but heard his scream – the strange, peculiar scream, long familiar to her – the scream of the epileptic falling in a fit. They could not tell whether the fit had come on him at the moment he was decending the steps, so that he must have fallen unconscious, or whether it was the fall and the shock that had caused the fit in Smerdyakov, who was known to be liable to them. They found him at the bottom of the cellar steps, writhing in convulsions and foaming at the mouth. It was thought at first that he must have broken something – an arm or a leg – and hurt himself, but 'God had preserved him'.

The sick man did not regain consciousness; the convulsions ceased for a time, but then began again, and everyone concluded that the same thing would happen, as had happened a year before, when he accidently fell from the garret (IX 346, 347).

Marfa Ignatyevna is also one of the characters who talks about Smerdyakov's seizure after she hears a scream when Smerdjakow is taken out of the cellar and put in the room next to hers.

That scream always preceded his fits, and always terrified and upset Marfa Ignatyevna. She could never get accustomed to it. She jumped up and ran half-awake to Smerdyakov's room. But it was dark there, and she could only hear the invalid beginning to gasp and struggle (IX 555).

They lighted a candle and saw that Smerdyakov was no better, that he was writhing in convulsions, his eyes fixed in a squint, and that foam was flowing from his lips (IX 556).

The police doctor gives his rendition of the seizure as well.

But he was particularly interested in the condition of the servant, Smerdyakov.

'Such violent and protracted epileptic fits, recurring continually for twenty-four hours, are rarely to be met with, and are of interest to science,' he declared enthusiastically to his companions (IX 558).

The prosecutor, Ippolit Kirilovich, also gives an account of the seizure.

'We found the servant Smerdjakow, concerning whom you inquire, lying unconscious in his bed, in an epileptic fit of extreme severity, that had recurred, possibly, ten times. The doctor who was with us told us, after seeing him, that he may possibly not outlive the night' (IX 581).

'. . . and within an hour of his young master's departure Smerdyakov was taken with an epileptic fit. But that's perfectly intelligible. Here I must mention that Smerdyakov, oppressed by terror and despair of a sort, had felt during those last few days that one of the fits from which he had suffered before at moments of strain, might be coming upon him again. The day and hour of such an attack cannot, of course, be foreseen, but every epileptic can feel beforehand that he is likely to have one. So the doctors tell us. And so, as soon as Ivan Fyodorovitch had driven out of the yard, Smerdyakov, depressed by his lonely and unprotected position, went to the cellar. He went down the stairs wondering if he would have a fit or not, and what if it were to come upon him at once. And that very apprehension, that very wonder, brought on the spasm in his throat that always precedes such attacks, and he fell unconscious into the cellar. And in this perfectly natural occurrence people try to detect a suspicion, a hint that he was shamming an attack on purpose. But, if it were on purpose, the question arises at once, what was his motive? What was he reckoning on? What was he aiming at? I say nothing about medicine: science, I am told, may go astray: the doctors were not able to discriminate between the counterfeit and the real' (IX 859).

The prosecutor describes the personality of Smerdyakov ('who had cut short his life in a fit of insanity')

'as a man of weak intellect, with a smattering of education, who had been thrown off his balance by philosophical ideas above his level and certain modern theories of duty' (IX 857).

Finally, the defending counsel, Fetyoekovitch, gives his account of the seizure.

'The talented prosecutor, with extraordinary subtlety, sketched for us all the arguments for and against the hypothesis of Smerdyakov's guilt, and asked us in particular what motive he had in feigning a fit. But he may not have been feigning at all, the fit may have happened quite naturally, but it may have passed off quite naturally, and the sick man may have recovered, not completely perhaps, but still regaining consciousness, as happens with epileptics.'

'The prosecutor asks at what moment Smerdyakov could have committed the murder. But it is very easy to point out that moment. He might have waked up from deep sleep (for he was only asleep – an epileptic fit is always followed by a deep sleep)' (IX 898).

## Discussion

### *Concepts of Epilepsy in Dostoevsky's Knowledge*

In the middle of June 1863, Dostoevsky secured permission from the police and the Tsar to travel abroad for a consultation with Romberg in Berlin and Trousseau and Herpin in Paris [2]. He obtained a medical testimonial about his epilepsy from Dr. V. Beier, a professor at the Imperial Surgical Academy. According to this petition he had also consulted Doctors V.V. Besser, I.M. Barch, and Rozenberg in Petersburg.

In a letter to Turgenev (June 17, 1867) he wrote that because of contradictory advice from the Petersburg physicians he 'had absolutely lost faith in them'. There is no documentation confirming any consultation having occurred with any of the specialists abroad.

The person who contributed most to Dostoevsky's knowledge of epilepsy was probably Dr. Stepan Dmitrievich Janovsky (1817–1897). He was his close friend and physician already before Dostoevsky was sentenced to prison in Siberia (1849).

Dostoevsky borrowed books from Dr. Janovsky's library and met with him for 3 years at least thrice weekly according to a fixed schedule for discussions. Only a few works he read are known with certainty, but most probably he read writings from Esquirol, Trousseau, and Romberg on Janovsky's recommendation and probably borrowed from his library [2].

*Esquirol.* In 1847 excerpts from his work were published in journals for the Russian general public. Symptoms described by Esquirol as postictal psychosis and depression were recognized by Dostoevsky as 'mystical experiences' incapacitating days with fear and anxiety.

*Trousseau.* Dostoevsky learned of Trousseau's reputation from an abridged account of an essay on epilepsy in an official periodical from the Medical Department of the Ministry of War. Trousseau noted the diversity of forms of epilepsy and the possible combination of epilepsy and hysteria. Pre- and postictal symptoms were listed, several of which were familiar to Dostoevsky and recorded in the seizure logs that he began to keep that same year (1862). Several cases were reported and sometimes the epileptic aura was the only manifestation. Esquirol's opinion that attacks continuing for years have harmful effects on the mental capabilities was confirmed by Trousseau.

*Herpin.* According to Rice [2], Dostoevsky was undoubtedly familiar with the work of Herpin and we may be sure that Herpin's posthumous volume, *Des accès incomplets d'épilepsie* (Paris 1867) would have caught the attention of Dostoevsky. Herpin, who was a corresponding member of the Academy in St. Petersburg, worked for 30 years in Geneva. During Dostoevsky's residence in Geneva in the last months of 1867, the memory of Herpin was still promoted by the booksellers. Rice concludes that Dostoevsy was reading this study while making the first draft of *The Idiot*.

*Romberg.* In his reports of premonitory symptoms, calling them 'auras' and including 'rarely – an extraordinary euphoria, lasting from a few minutes to a couple of hours (1843)', Dostoevsky would have read about phenomena which he later recognised in himself as the so-called ecstatic aura.

*Interpretion of Illness in Dostoevski's Characters in the Light of Later Medical Knowledge*

The psychiatrist Vladimir Chizh [2, p. 201] wrote a monograph entitled *Dostoevsky: A Psychopathologist* (1884, 1885). He attempted to compile a full inventory on the cases of mental illness in Dostoevsky's novels and estimated that out of 100, 25% were clearly cases of psychopathology, a frequency unparalleled in literature.

Vladimir Mikhailovich Bechterev [2, p. 226] concluded in lectures and papers (1914, 1921, 1924) that Dostoevsky 'experienced much in pathological states which he portrayed for us in artistic images and at the same time was a good observer of pathology in the living environment from which he gathered his material.' Thus, nearly a hundred years later the question as to whether the ecstatic auras of Myshkin and Kirillov were based on Dostoevski's own experience can be answered in line with this statement.

In many of the recent papers, speculative interpretations on changes in the behavior of characters are forced to fit in possibilities of an epileptic origin. Seneviratne [16] expresses his doubts on epilepsy in the case of Golyadkin's autoscopy in *The Double* (1846), but not enough in the Semjon Ivanovich case in Mr. Prokharchin (1846), who is more likely to have prolonged states of pseudoepileptic seizures, or Dolgoruky in *A Raw Youth* (1875), who's experience indeed is suggestive of jamais vu, but without any other indication for (temporal lobe) epilepsy. Ivan Ilyich's 'strange sensations' in *A Disgraceful Affair* (A Nasty Anecdote, 1862) do not occur after 'a glass of vodka'. He seldom drank, but this time he was dead drunk (IV, 39) after five glasses of wine, two bottles of champagne, and a glass of vodka.

There is an increasing number of well-substantiated papers describing patients with an ecstatic aura. In comments and case reports of so called 'Doestoevsky's epilepsy', one should not forget to define the semiology of an ecstatic aura. Feelings of mere 'ictal pleasant sensations' should be further analyzed as is properly done by Stefan et al. [17]. Hansen and Brodtkorb [18] in a nice paper following Penfield's terminology of 'experiential seizures', defined ecstatic seizures as ictal sensations of intense pleasure, joy, and contentment. Cognitive and spiritual experiences may occur as components. The sensations as told by their first (of eleven) patients should be 'outside the spectrum of what the patient ever experienced outside a seizure', and they were 'fully absorbed by them'. They must be distinguished from joy, pleasure, or happiness that can occur as pleasure-seeking behavior by self-induction in photosensitive generalized epilepsy.

There is growing agreement that, though an ecstatic aura is very rare, patients can sometimes experience being 'totally pervaded by a feeling of total bliss'. This might occur in persons with unique personal religious or artistic emotions if epileptic discharges deeply affect their limbic system.

Often patients find these sensations indescribable. Dostoevsky, more eloquently than in his personal recollections, tries to express his experiential seizures using his preferred tool, depicting the characters of Myshkin and Kirillov.

## Problems with Transliteration and Translation

Dostoevsky told three friends (Wrangel [2, 19], Strakhov [2], and Kovalevskaja [2]) about his ecstatic experience.

Shortly after his release from prison, Dostoevsky described his epileptic aura to Alexander Jegorovitch Wrangel (referring to the period 1854–1856) as: 'an indescribable sense of well-being' [19], an 'inexpressible feeling of voluptuousness (okhvatyvaet . . . chuvstvo sladostrastiia)' (Rice [2, p. 69]), and an 'inexpressible feeling of sensuousness (sladostrastie: fleshly passion) (Rice [2, p. 83].

Nikolay Nikolayevich Strakhov (1828–1896) [2, p. 83] wrote in his biography that Dostoevsky experienced '. . . happiness that is impossible in an ordinary state . . .. I feel a full harmony in myself and in the world. . . a few seconds of such bliss.'

To Sófja Kovalevskaja (1850–1891) [2, p. 84], Dostoevsky said 'I felt that heaven descended to earth and swallowed me. I really attained God and was imbued with him. . . all the joys life can give I would not take in exchange for it'.

Both Strakhov and Kovalevskaja mention this seizure on the day before Easter, but nowhere in Dostoevsky's own memoires is there mention of a seizure at this time. Maybe Kovalevskaja (1887) in her memoires was already influenced by reading Strakhov's biography (1883).

On the discussion of fact and fiction I agree with Rice (1938–2011), Professor of Russian and Comparative Literature at the University of Oregon in Eugene, that 'clearly, creative fiction emerges directly from the symptomatic experience and description depends on subjectivity and memory of the biographer'. But one should add: on the memory of Dostoevsky as well! As is known, Dostoevsky had severe memory disturbances himself. As he said to Soloviev [20]: 'Everything that happened after the first attack I very often forget. . . when I was finishing *The Devils* I had to read everything from the beginning, because I had even forgotten the names of the characters.'

Other problems with vocabulary are sometimes related to translation and sometimes to differences in concepts of nosology in the 19th century. There are several examples from *The Brothers Karamazov* (IX 19, 30, 60, 61, 172). In the Russian text, the word 'Klikusjetsku' (meaning hysteria) is found where the English translation (Constance Garnett) more or less randomly uses 'hysterical', 'crazy', or 'possessed', and for Alosha and his mother's seizure even the word 'epileptisch' (epileptic) is found in the Dutch translation (Jan van der Eng).

In cases where epilepsy is most evident, as in the characters of Nellie, Murin, and Myshkin, where Dostoevsky used his experience and knowledge of epilepsy and showed his familiarity with the concept of hysteria, we find less problems in vocabulary and translation of:

- 'Pripadke padushchey bolezni' = 'seizures of falling sickness' (Murin I, 365)
- 'Paduchaja bolezn'; 'posle sil'nogo pripadka padushchey bolezni' = 'falling sickness' 'epileptic fits'; 'after a severe attack of falling sickness', 'violent epileptic fits' (Nellie, III 562, 604)
- 'Pripadok epilepsii' = by epileptic seizure (Myshkin, VI 291)

In cases where other epileptic seizure types in Dostoevsky's vocabulary are lesser known in translators' knowledge, translating '*S nej byl kakoj to pripadok, vrode obmiranija*' with 'fainting' (Nellie III 690) seems to be incorrect. It would be better to translate it with 'a kind of seizure in which stiffening of the body occurs'.

## Conclusion

Dostoevsky's novels are an inexhaustible source for scholars of philology, ethics, law, sociology, art history, religion, and philosophy. However, his epilepsy and the influence of that illness on the characters in his novels will long continue to intrigue and interest physicians reading his works, especially concerning developing medical knowledge.

## Acknowledgements

We would like to thank Djoeke Leistra, Master Slavonic Languages, for transliteration and transcription.

## References

1 Catteau J: La creation literaire chez Dostoïevski. Paris, Institut d'Etudes Slaves, 1978.
2 Rice JL: Dostoevsky and the Healing Art: An Essay in Literary and Medical History. Ann Arbor, Ardis, 1985.
3 Frank J: Dostoevsky: The Seeds of Revolt 1821–1849. Princeton, Princeton University Press, 1976, vol 1.
4 Frank J: Dostoevsky: The Years of Ordeal, 1850–1859. Princeton, Princeton University Press, 1983, vol 2.
5 Frank J: Dostoevsky: The Stir of Liberation, 1860–1865. Princeton, Princeton University Press, 1986, vol 3.
6 Frank J: Dostoevsky: The Miraculous Years, 1865–1871. Princeton, Princeton University Press, 1995, vol 4.
7 Frank J: Dostoevsky: The Mantle of the Prophet, 1871–1881. Princeton, Princeton University Press, 1983, vol 5.
8 Alajouanine T: Dostoiewski's epilepsy. Brain 1963; 86:209–218.
9 Alajouanine T: Littérature et épilepsie. Léxpression littéraire de l éxtase dans les romans de Dostoievski et dans les poems de Saint Jean de la croix; in: Dostoievski. Paris, Cahier de l'Herne, 1973, vol 24, pp 309–324.
10 Voskuil PHA: The epilepsy of F.M. Dostoevsky. Epilepsia 1983;24:658–667.
11 Baumann CR, Novikov VPI, Regard M, Siegel AM: Did F.M. Dostoevsky suffer from mesial temporal lobe epilepsy? Seizure 2005;14:324–330.
12 Iniesta I: Dostoevsky's epilepsy: a contemporary 'paleodiagnosis' (letter to the editor). Seizure 2007; 16:283–285.
13 Gastaut H: New comments on the epilepsy of Fyodor Dostoevsky. Epilepsia 1984;25:408–411.
14 Gastaut H: F.M. Dostoevsky's involuntary contribution to the symptomatology and prognosis of epilepsy. Epilepsia 1978;19:186–201.
15 Hughes JR: The idiosyncratic aspects of the epilepsy of Fyodor Dostoevsky. Epilepsy Behav 2005;7: 531–538.
16 Seneviratne U: Fyodor Dostoevsky and his falling sickness: a critical analysis of seizure semiology. Epilepsy Behav 2010;18:424–430.
17 Stefan H, et al: Ictal pleasant sensations: cerebral localization and lateralization. Epilepsia 2004;45: 35–40.
18 Hansen BA, Brodtkorb E: Partial epilepsy with 'ecstatic' seizures. Epilepsy Behav 2003;4:667–673.
19 Baron Alexander Wrangel (1854–1865), recollections of Dostoevsky; in: Letters of Fyodor Michailovitch Dostoevsky to His Family and Friends, ed 1 (transl Mayne EG). New York, The Macmillan Company, 1914, pp 272.
20 Soloviev E: Dostoievsky, his life and literary activity. A biographical sketch. London, George Allen and Unwin Ltd., 1916.

Piet H.A. Voskuil MD
Neurologist
Torendreef 14
NL–4851 BH Ulvenhout (The Netherlands)
E-Mail p.voskuil@wxs.nl

Bogousslavsky J, Dieguez S (eds): Literary Medicine: Brain Disease and Doctors in Novels, Theater, and Film.
Front Neurol Neurosci. Basel, Karger, 2013, vol 31, pp 215–224 (DOI: 10.1159/000343266)

# Theater in Professor Charcot's Galaxy

Jacques Poirier[a] · Jacques Philippon[b]

Medical Doctors, [a]Paris, and [b]Lamorlaye, France

**Abstract**

Jean-Martin Charcot, famous professor of the Chair of Clinic for Diseases of the Nervous System at Salpêtrière Hospital in Paris, was himself an artist, surrounded by artists, and adored the theater. His close colleague Charles Brown-Séquard was ridiculed by Georges Feydeau in a brief freakish monologue recited by Coquelin Cadet, from the Comédie-Française, concerning his claims to rejuvenate himself and others with animal testicle extracts. His friend and patient Alphonse Daudet had written many novels, short stories, and plays. Léon Daudet, Alphonse Daudet's son (and friend of Jean-Baptiste Charcot, the son of the professor), after having abandoned his medical studies, became a writer whose novel *Les morticoles* was a cruel satire of the medical profession. Among Charcot's pupils, Alfred Binet, Gilbert Ballet, Édouard Brissaud, and Joseph Babinski were particularly involved in the theater. Gilbert Ballet wrote the foreword to *La folie au théâtre* (Madness in Theatre) by André de Latour. Édouard Brissaud wrote a satiric play *Le chèque* (The Check), and Joseph Babinski, under the pseudonym of Olaf, was the coauthor with Palau of the drama *Les détraquées* (The Deranged Women). However, when all is said and done, perhaps the greatest actor in his entourage was Charcot himself.


During the 20th century, literature, poetry, and the theater went hand in hand with physicians. Many doctors were duty physicians in theaters. In their spare time some of them, especially neurologists, primarily those orbiting in professor Charcot's galaxy, wrote plays and many nonphysician authors wrote plays featuring doctors, medicine, alienation, or hysteria, sometimes with the collaboration of physicians or psychologists.

## Jean-Martin Charcot (1825–1893)

Jean-Martin Charcot [1], Professor of the Chair of Clinic for Diseases of the Nervous System, was considered as the founder of French neurology. However, Charcot's celebrity came especially from his work on hysteria (fig. 1) carried out

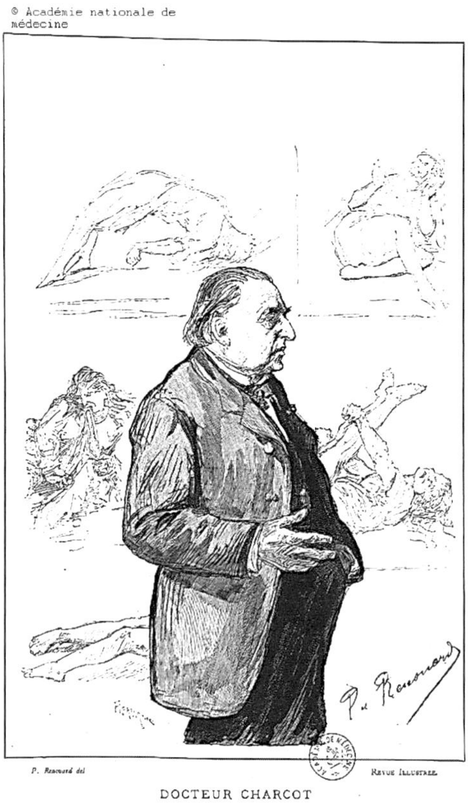


**Fig. 1.** Charcot by Renouard, Académie nationale de Médecine, with kind permission.

at Salpêtrière Hospital for around twenty years from 1870 until his death. In his lessons, attended by the 'tout-Paris', hysteric patients were theatrically exhibited and hypnotized in public by the 'master' [2] (fig. 2). Charcot was an artist: 'he was not only a fine expert, erudite and wise critic; he wielded pencil and paintbrush with true skilfulness' [3]. He loved artists and was surrounded by them; his wife painted, sculpted, and created objects of style. With Paul Richer (1849–1933), a former Charcot resident, talented sculptor, and professor of artistic anatomy at the École nationale des Beaux Arts (National School of Fine Arts), he wrote *Les démoniaques dans l'art* (Demoniacs in Art) [4] and *Les difformes et les maladies dans l'art* (Deformed People and Diseases in Art) [5]. Henry Meige (1866–1940), Charcot's former temporary resident, was Édouard Brissaud's (1852–1909) favorite pupil and close friend [6]. Guided by Paul Richer, he developed his artistic capacities, especially through the *Nouvelle iconographie de la Salpêtrière* (The New Salpêtrière's Iconography) and became Richer's successor as Professor of Artistic Anatomy at the École des Beaux Arts. In the book he devoted to Charcot as an artist, Henry Meige highlighted the strong interest that Charcot had for the theater:

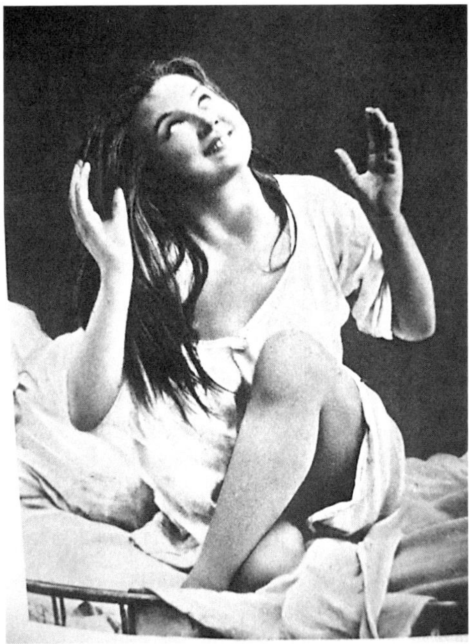

**Fig. 2.** Attitudes passionnelles, Extase (Passionate Attitudes, Trance), *Iconographie photographique de la Salpêtrière* (Salpêtrière Photographic Iconography) (Service de M. Charcot), by Bourneville and P. Regnard, Paris, Aux bureaux du Progrès Médical, 1878, pl. XXIII (personal collection).

We know with what devotion he honoured Shakespeare, who he has read, read again, and annotated himself. The philosophy of the English playwright was particularly dear to him, inasmuch as it was based on a careful study of nature. In the works of Shakespeare, Charcot saw a model for analysing feelings and passions. He found in it that strict observation of the human race he applied himself at the clinic. And, in the actor, he enjoyed the sincere naturalism of sallies and witty remarks. So Charcot's humor was eminently 'Shakespearean' [3].

On St. Martin's Day – the Christian name of Charcot was Jean-Martin – in his private townhouse in Faubourg Saint-Germain, his children and pupils would put on plays, for example *Macbeth* in 1887, with his son and daughter, often his chief-resident Joseph Babinski (1857–1932), and his pupils Henry Meige and Paul Berbez comprising the actors [7]. Despite his passion for the theater, Charcot himself never wrote a play.

## Charcot's Friends

### *Charles Brown-Séquard (1817–1894)*

Charles Brown-Séquard [8], though slightly older than Charcot, was a close colleague, but probably not a close friend. Georges Feydeau (1862–1921) made fun of Brown-Séquard and his rejuvenating injections, which used pulverized rabbit testicles, in *Tout à Brown-Séquard !. . .* with a brief freakish monologue recited by Alexandre Honoré Ernest Coquelin, who went by the name Coquelin Cadet (1848–1909), from the Comédie-Française:

> Brown-Séquard, he is greater than the Eiffel Tower, which is fated to age. . . whereas he, he is made to rejuvenate. . .to rejuvenate others if you, please ! [. . .] I have met several old men who were treated, like me, by Brown-Séquard. They were true kids! I found them playing marbles! There were even some of them who sucked. They was just like those who were in childhood. It was charming, a true spring! [. . .] [9].

*Alphonse Daudet (1840–1897) and His Son Léon (1867–1942)*
Alphonse Daudet [1] was Charcot's close friend and also his patient. He wrote many novels, tales, short stories, and plays, such as *La dernière idole* (1862), *Les absents* (1864), *L'oeillet blanc* (1865) in collaboration with Ernest L'Épine (1826–1893) and *L'arlésienne* (1872) with music by Georges Bizet (1838–1875). His son Léon Daudet [1] was a regular at the Charcot receptions and a friend of his son Jean-Baptiste (1867–1936). After his medical studies and his failure in 1891 at the 'concours de l'internat' (selective examination for residency), he became a theater critic, writer, and polemicist. His novel *Les morticoles*, published in 1894, was a cruel satire of the medical institution, especially of the hospital, and its patronal hierarchy ('patrons'), implicating Charcot, under the pseudonym Fontage. He never wrote plays.

## Charcot's Pupils

*Jules Clarétie (1840–1913)*
Although not a medical student, the writer and playwright Jules Clarétie [10] can certainly be considered as a Charcot pupil. He attended Charcot's classes at Salpêtrière and was represented on the famous canvas by André Brouillet (1857–1914), *Une leçon de Charcot à la Salpêtrière,* exhibited at the 1887 salon. From 1885 to 1913, Clarétie was a theater critic and general administrator of the Comédie Française. He wrote many novels, in particular *Les amours d'un interne* (The Loves of a Resident) and *Profils de théâtre* (1902), as well as several plays, including *Les muscadins* (1874), *Le régiment de Champagne* (1877), *Les Mirabeau* (1879), and *Monsieur le ministre* (1883). He also wrote the lyrics for three operas (music by Jules Massenet): *La Navarraise* (1894), *Thérèse* (1907), and *Amadis* (completed posthumously in 1922).

*Alfred Binet (1857–1911)*
After having qualified as a lawyer, Alfred Binet began to study medicine, which he did not finish, and then turned to psychology. Introduced at La Salpêtrière by Joseph Babinski (1857–1932) and Charles Féré (1852–1907), Binet attended Charcot's lectures and carried out several studies on hysteria and hypnosis under the supervision of Charcot. He rejected Charcot's theories in 1890 and devoted himself to research on cognition. The Binet-Simon Intelligence Scale made him famous. On the other hand, he worked, as a scientific collaborator, with André Latour, comte de Lorde (1869–1942), author of some 150 plays, especially dramas, for the well-known Parisian

horror and terror theater Grand-Guignol. Binet became a friend of de Lorde and mainly contributed when the topic of the play was of a medical nature, especially when it concerned hysteria or other mental diseases, such as *L'obsession* (Obsession; 1905), *L'horrible expérience* (Horrible Experience; 1909), and *L'homme mystérieux* (The Mysterious Man; 1910). One of the most famous plays by de Lorde, *Une leçon à la Salpêtrière* (A Lesson at the Salpêtrière; 1908), was dedicated to Alfred Binet and was also probably written with his collaboration.

*Gilbert Ballet (1853–1916)*
In 1913, Gilbert Ballet, another of Charcot's former residents, Professor of the Chair of the Clinic of Mental and Brain Diseases at the Paris Faculty of Medicine, wrote the foreword to a book by André de Lorde (1869–1942), *La folie au théâtre* (Madness in the Theatre) [11].

*Édouard Brissaud (1852–1909)*
Charcot's favorite pupil, Édouard Brissaud [6], physician in the Paris hospital system and a professor at the Faculty of Medicine, was a distinguished neurologist. His works are innumerable and very diverse, covering all fields of neurology, neuropathology, and psychiatry. In his childhood, Brissaud had been an actor. Within his family circle, he played comedies with his sisters and his cousins. Comedian to the core, he loved to put on a show, using the mask of a cheerful impulsive joker to hide a natural anxiety and depression. The students loved his lessons, full of 'bons mots' and theatrical expressions. He was surrounded by writers, poets, painters, and several comedians, and grew up in a large family full of artists, painters, musicians, and above all actors and singers. The most well-known was his great-grandfather Jacques-Marie Boutet de Monvel (1745–1812), nicknamed 'Le Grand Monvel' (The Great Monvel) [6]. He started his career at the Comédie-Française, then became director of the Théâtre Français (French Theatre) in Stockholm, under the protection of the King of Sweden Gustav III (1746–1792). When he came back to Paris, Monvel was appointed professor at the Conservatoire d'Art Dramatique de Paris (Paris Conservatory of Dramatic Art). With François-Joseph Talma (1763–1826), he founded the Théâtre de la République, which became a rival of the Comédie-Française. He wrote several plays which met with some success, especially *Les victimes cloîtrées* (Cloistered Victims; 1791), one of the most famous and most performed dramas at that time.

Brissaud wrote a humorous play, *Le chèque* (The Check; the manuscript, kept in the familial archives of Dr. Pierre Chauveau, Édouard Brissaud's great-grandson, was first published in 2010 [12]), where a medical disciple and his master discuss the interim of the Chair of the Clinic for the Study of the Nervous System, a position that Brissaud held in 1893–1894 after the death of Charcot (fig. 3). *Le chèque* has never been performed. On the other hand, Brissaud liked to organize performances of theater at home, with his children, friends, and pupils as actors (fig. 4, 5).

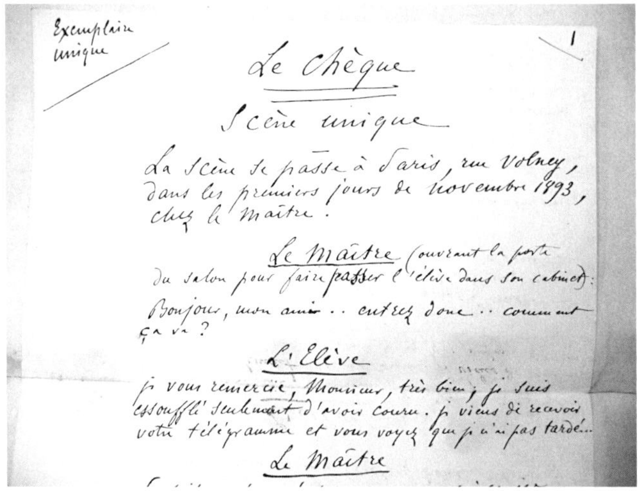
Exemplaire unique

1

Le Chèque

Scène unique

La scène se passe à Paris, rue Volney, dans les premiers jours de novembre 1893, chez le maître.

Le Maître (ouvrant la porte du salon pour faire passer l'élève dans son cabinet):

Bonjour, mon ami.. entrez donc.. comment ça va?

L'Élève

Je vous remercie, Monsieur, très bien, je suis essoufflé seulement d'avoir couru. Je viens de recevoir votre télégramme et vous voyez que je n'ai pas tardé...

Le Maître

**Fig. 3.** First page of the autographed manuscript of the Édouard Brissaud's play *Le chèque* (courtesy of Dr. Pierre Chauveau, Édouard Brissaud's great-grandson).

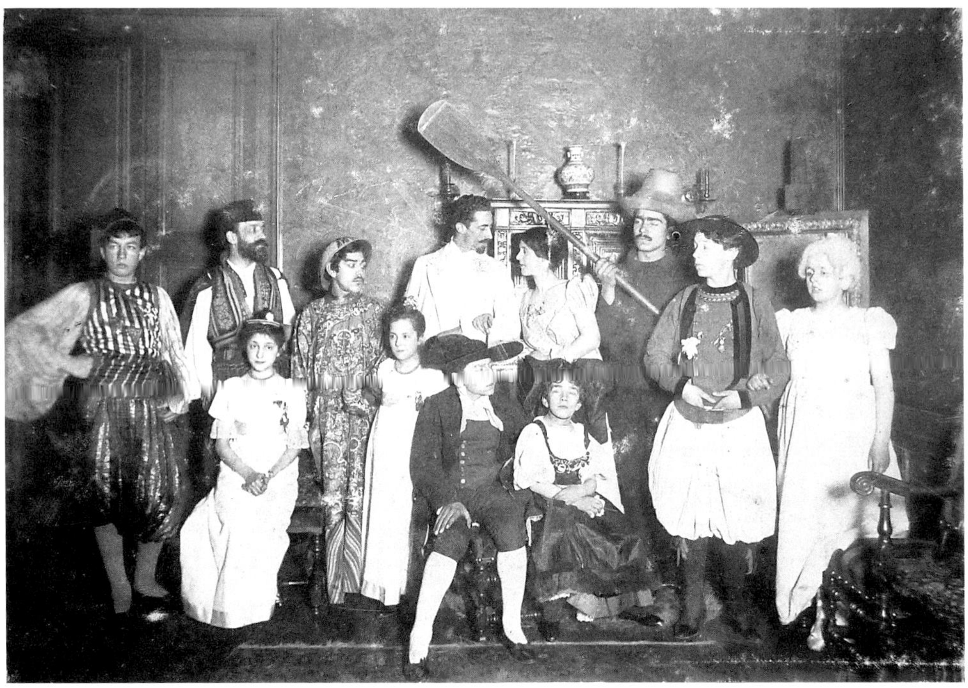

**Fig. 4.** Theater at Parisian Brissaud's home (courtesy of Mrs. Olivier Chauveau, Édouard Brissaud's granddaughter).

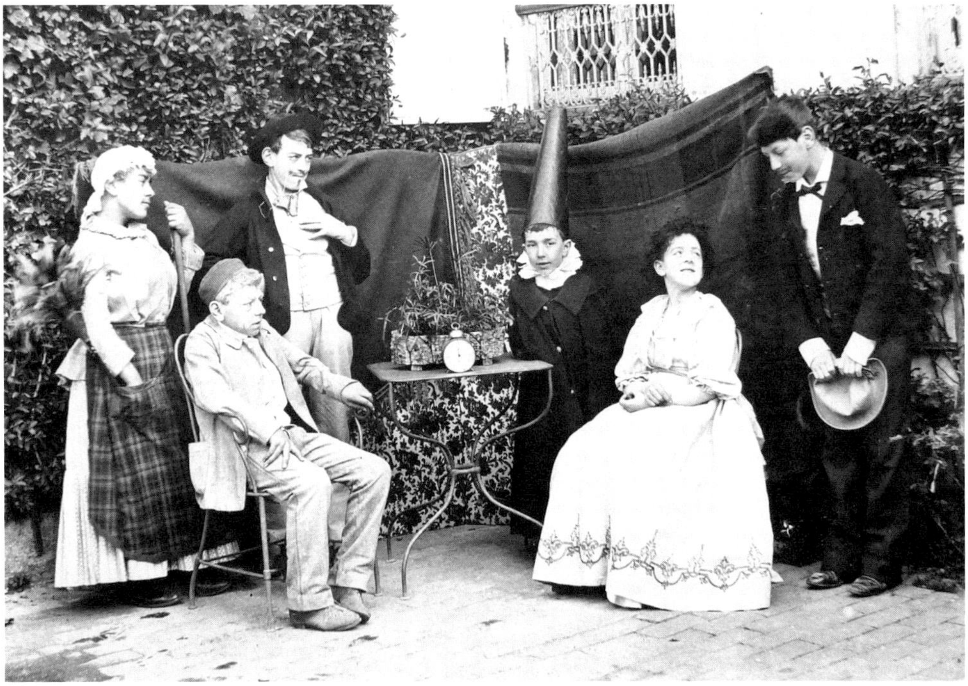

**Fig. 5.** Theater at Nemours Brissaud's country house (courtesy of Mrs. Olivier Chauveau, Édouard Brissaud's granddaughter).

*Joseph Babinski (1857–1932)*

A French neurologist of Polish origin, Joseph Babinski [13, 14] was a physician in the Paris hospital system and member of the Academy of Medicine. Early in his career, he worked as an anatomopathologist and histologist. After his chief-residency under Charcot (1885–1887), Babinski abandoned his previous interests and became increasingly involved with hysteria. He thus became a semiologist, eager to detect objective neurological signs that would allow the clinician to distinguish between organic (due to a lesion) and functional (hysterical) illnesses. He is well known for the discovery of the sign (the toes phenomenon) which bears his name. Beyond this, his semiological work in the field of neurology is also important.

Some years after Charcot's death, he criticized the Charcot conception of hysteria and created the concept of pithiatism, which refers to symptoms produced by suggestion and cured by persuasion. Joseph Babinski was fond of literature, poetry, music, and paintings, and he made the most of his permanent access pass to the Musée du Louvre (Louvre Museum). He and his beloved elder brother Henri Babinski, both bachelors, lived together and were inseparable. Under the pen name Ali-Bab, Henri wrote *Gastronomie pratique*, a monumental cookbook which received tremendous recognition.

*Les détraquées* (The Deranged Women) was a drama written by Olaf and Palau [15]. The play, in two acts, was presented for the first time at the Théâtre des Deux-Masques

(Two Masks Theatre) on February 15, 1921. The drama took place in a private girls' boarding school. At the end of the year, Madame de Challens, head teacher, regularly called to her office Mademoiselle Solange, Professor of Dance; both of them, obviously lesbian, subjected a young pupil to their cruel perverted tastes, leading to the death of the poor girl. At the end of December 2011, *Les détraquées* was still being played in Paris! Pierre Palau (1885–1966) was an actor, author of drama and comedies, film director, and TV series producer. The identity of Olaf was disclosed by André Breton (1896–1966) in the first issue of his review *Le surréalisme, même* [16]: behind the pseudonym of Olaf was hidden Dr. Babinski. In fact, to carry out his project, Palau needed a physician specialized in nervous diseases; the surgeon Paul Thiéry put him in touch with Babinski, who agreed to collaborate [17]. Fascinated by mental pathology and attracted by the intensity of attacks in the press against *Les détraquées*, André Breton went to see the play. He was captivated by the actress Blanche Derval (1885–1973), saying that he had been deeply moved and that it was one of the greatest theatrical experiences of his life. In 1928, Breton discussed it at length in *Nadja* [18]. The relationship of André Breton with medicine and especially with psychiatry is unclear and ambivalent, associating simultaneously admiration (especially for Babinski), fascination for mental disease, and perversions and denigration of psychiatric practices, particularly in mental hospitals.

Why did Babinski choose 'Olaf' as a pseudonym? The answer to this is a speculative one. Contrary to the assertions of Léon Babinski [19], and repeated by Gazecki and Hachinski [20], we know [21] that – as already suspected by Richard Kalil [22] – in 1905, after the death of Henri Parinaud (1844–1905) and his wife, Joseph Babinski, as per Parinaud's will [23], became the tutor of his friend's three orphaned daughters, Ebba (1893–1967), Ellen (1897–1981), and Karen (1903–1975), who were 12, 8, and 2 years of age, respectively [personal communication of Martine Briand, Henri Parinaud's great-granddaughter] (fig. 6). Before her marriage, Parinaud's wife was a Danish citizen and Olaf was the name of several kings of Denmark. Thus, the purpose of the choice of this pseudonym by Babinski would be to give a nod to Parinaud's wife.

## Conclusion

Charcot's 'lessons' were in reality a theatrical production where patients, assistants, and the audience all had a role to play under the direction of the esteemed professor. The public entered an unlit amphitheater and waited in the dark while they heard the 'scene' being set up. Suddenly a light focuses on the patient and Charcot enters on stage to begin his demonstration. What an example of the theatrical art to align selected patients bearing plumed head dresses to show the difference in tremor between healthy and parkinsonian subjects, clearly seen even from the back of the room. Perhaps when all is said and done, the greatest actor in his entourage was Charcot himself.

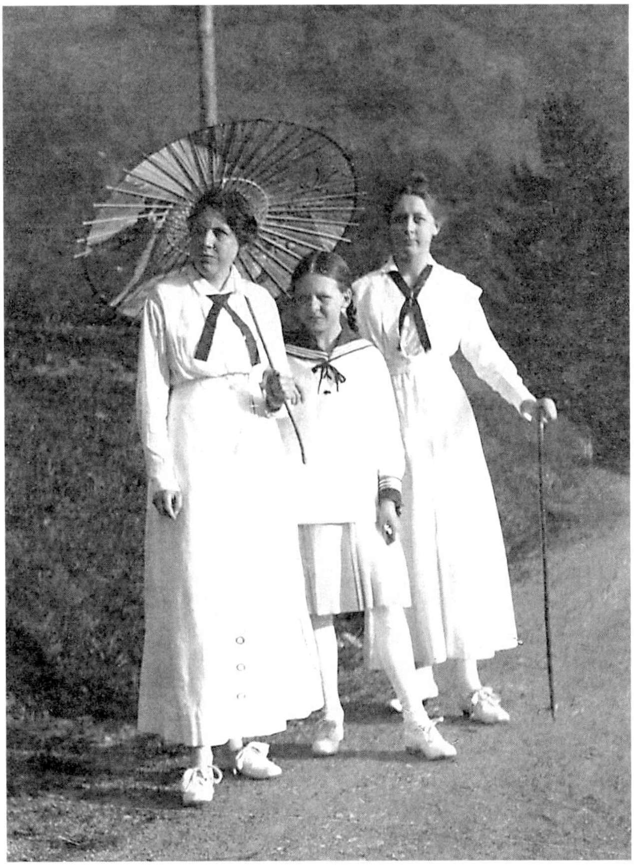

**Fig. 6.** The three girls of Parinaud, Ebba, Helen and Karen, who Babinski tutored (courtesy of Mrs. Martine Briand, Dr. Henri Parinaud's great-granddaughter).


## Acknowledgments

We are greatly indebted to Véronique Leroux-Hugon (chief curator of the Charcot Library at La Salpêtrière Hospital), Laurence Camous (chief curator of the Library of the Académie nationale de Médecine), Martine Briand (great-granddaughter of Henri Parinaud, for kindly providing familial pictures and personal communications), Mrs. Olivier Chauveau (granddaughter of Edouard Brissaud) and Dr. Pierre Chauveau (great-grandson of Edouard Brissaud), as well as Nathalie Philippon-Tulloch (for supervision of the English language).


## References


1 Goetz CG, Bonduelle M, Gelfand T: Charcot: Constructing Neurology. New York, Oxford University Press, 1996.
2 Edelman N: Les métamorphoses de l'hystérique, du début du XIXe siècle à la Grande Guerre. Paris, La Découverte, 2003.
3 Meige H: Charcot artiste. Paris, Masson et Cie, 1925.
4 Charcot JM, Richer P: Les démoniaques dans l'art. Paris, Delahaye et Lecrosnier, 1887.
5 Charcot JM, Richer P: Les difformes et les malades dans l'art. Paris, Lecrosnier et Babé, 1889.
6 Poirier J: Édouard Brissaud, un neurologue d'exception. Paris, Hermann, 2010.

7 Walusinski O: Jean-Martin Charcot's house officers at La Salpêtrière; in Bogousslavsky J (ed): Following Charcot: A Forgotten History of Neurology and Psychiatry. Front Neurol Neurosci. Basel, Karger, 2011, vol 29, pp 9–35.
8 Bonduelle M: History of neurology. Charles-Édouard Brown-Séquard. Rev Neurol (Paris) 2001; 157:234–238.
9 Feydeau G: Tout à Brown-Séquard. Paris, Ollendorf, 1890.
10 Grappe G: Jules Clarétie. Paris, E. Sansot et Cie, 1906.
11 de Lorde A: La folie au théâtre. L'homme mystérieux. La petite Roque. Les invisibles. Paris, Fontemoing et Cie éditeur, 1913.
12 Poirier J: Édouard Brissaud, neurologue méconnu et comédien dans l'âme (Édouard Brissaud, a neglected neurologist and an artist at heart). Bull Acad Natl Méd 2010;194:163–175.
13 Philippon J, Poirier J: Joseph Babinski: A Biography. New York, Oxford University Press, 2009.
14 Poirier J, Philippon J: Renewing the fire: Joseph Babinski; in Bogousslavsky J: Following Charcot: A Forgotten History of Neurology and Psychiatry. Front Neurol Neurosci. Basel, Karger, 2011, vol 29, pp 91–104.
15 Olaf, Palau: Les Détraquées; in: Le Grand Guignol, le théâtre des peurs de la Belle Époque (préface et notices par Agnès Pierron). Paris, Robert Laffont, 1995, pp 808–839.
16 Breton A: Le surréalisme même, No. 1 (Octobre). Paris, Pauvert, 1956.
17 Le Grand Guignol, le théâtre des peurs de la Belle Époque (foreword and notices by Agnès Pierron). Paris, Robert Laffont, 1995, pp 808–809.
18 Breton A: Nadja. Paris, Gallimard, 1928, pp 47–62.
19 Babinski L: Sylwetka Jozefa Babinskiego na tle jego zycia codziennego (Babinski in his everyday life), Neurol Neurochir Pol 1969;III:543–546.
20 Gasecki A, Hachinski V: On the names of Babinski. Can J Neurol Sci 1996;23:76–79.
21 Poirier J: Henri Parinaud (1844–1905), pionnier de l'ophtalmologie française (Henri Parinaud (1844–1905), Pioneer of French Opthalmology), Pratiques Ophtalmologie 2011;5:2–7.
22 Khalil R: Vie et œuvre de Babinski (Babinski's Life and Works); in: Conférences lyonnaises d'histoire de la neurologie et de la psychiatrie. Lyon, Documentation Médicale Oberval, 1982, pp 255–280.
23 Poirier J: Le testament de Joseph Babinski (The Will of Joseph Babinski). Neurologies 2011;14:4–8.

Jacques Poirier, MD, PhD
40 rue d'Alleray
FR–75015 Paris (France)
E-Mail poirierpaulin@aol.com

the development of the sciences, secondly from the large number of famous doctors practicing at the time, and finally from the conception Balzac had of depicting reality in his work.

## Medicine and the Sciences in the 19th Century

The sciences developed considerably in France in the first part of the nineteenth century, in both physics and chemistry (e.g. Fresnel, Ampère, Arago, etc.), and especially in natural sciences with Cuvier (*Règne animal* in 1816 and *Histoire des sciences naturelles* in 1828) and Geoffroy Saint-Hilaire (*Philosophie anatomique* in 1818). In physiology, significant work was carried out by individuals such as Beclard (*Eléments d'anatomie générale* in 1832), Cruveilhier (pathology), Magendie (studies on morphine, veratrine, strychnine, etc.), and Flourens (embryology, 1836). Famous doctors of the time include Bouillaud, who studied brain inflammation and heart disease, Bretonneau, who published work on diphtheria in 1826, and Trousseau, who wrote a treatise on laryngeal phthisis. Doctors such as Vicq d'Azyr, Baudelocque, Lebert, Chaufferd, and Grisolle also practised at time. Surgeons such as Dupuytren, Percy, Pelletan, and Larrey all flourished during this period, with Dupuytren, the first surgeon of Charles X, being the most famous. The atmosphere was saturated with everything scientific. It would cause a veritable revolution in thinking. This is the environment in which Balzac lived [1].

Balzac's scientific curiosity and love of medical essays, which can be found at any point in his magnum opus, *La comédie humaine*, are thus all the more understandable. Following the example of the great naturalists, Balzac wanted to describe social species just as scientists had described zoological species. Balzac named himself a 'doctor of social sciences'. These considerations on the environment in which Balzac lived are all the more legitimate in that that the great novelist made it a principle never to separate the study of a human being from the study of his or her environment. Applying his method to himself was indispensable.

## Balzac's Life and Personal Experiences

Balzac was born in the century in which a profound change in medical thinking occurred. Medicine was soon ubiquitous in society. It penetrated all backgrounds, and medical knowledge was fashionable in the rising bourgeoisie and aristocratic world. Several contradictory schools of thought were developed in the eighteenth and early nineteenth centuries – some more promising and popular than others. This is what interested Balzac more than anything else. Even early on in life, during his studies at Vendôme, he was interested in the relationship between man's physical and moral aspects. During his schooling, one of his teachers, Dessaignes, author of *Études*

Bogousslavsky J, Dieguez S (eds): Literary Medicine: Brain Disease and Doctors in Novels, Theater, and Film.
Front Neurol Neurosci. Basel, Karger, 2013, vol 31, pp 225–235 (DOI: 10.1159/000343671)

# Doctors in Balzac's Work

Thierry Moulin

Service de Neurologie, CHU de Besançon, Hôpital Jean Minjoz, Besançon, France

**Abstract**

Balzac wrote his novels during a time of great literary and scientific change. Romanticism gave way to the school of realism, of which Balzac could be considered the founder. It was via realism, where both the positive and negative aspects of life were depicted, that doctors naturally gained a much more active role in novels. In conjunction with this was the development of science and medicine, which fascinated Balzac, also leading to the significant and prevalent role of doctors in his works. His fascination with the sciences led to him to gain many acquaintances and much knowledge in the medical domain, especially in neuropsychiatry and physiology. His fictional doctors, such as Desplein and Bianchon, thus demonstrate considerable knowledge of pathology, physiology, and neuropsychiatry. The doctors in Balzac's novels can be grouped into four categories: provincial doctors, Parisian doctors, country doctors, and military doctors. They were most often fictitious representations of real individuals (e.g. Guillaume Dupuytren), and often symbolize schools of thought which were in vogue at the time. In addition to the accurate scientific depiction of doctors, it must be noted that his doctors not only played an active role in clinically assessing their patients, but also had a sociological role in assessing society; it is through his doctors that Balzac gave his opinion of the world in which he lived.


The majority of Balzac's literary work developed between 1829 and 1850, a significant period in the history of French literature. It was during this time that romanticism developed into realism, a new movement of which Balzac could be considered the founder. Romanticism depicts an ideal or idealized world where all so-called vulgar elements concerning everyday life are removed. As such, neither medicine nor doctors featured and if by chance a doctor did appear, it was hardly ever in a medical role. He was rather a philosopher conveying the ideas of the author [1].

The first work which brought Balzac to light, *La peau de chagrin*, breaks with the romantic genre and the aforementioned representation of doctors. In his works which followed, Balzac would greatly change the medical profession and, most importantly, give it an important place in his work. This literary shift seems to result firstly from *de l'homme moral fondées sur les rapports de ses facultés avec son organisation*, was like many others enthralled by mesmerism and Gall's theories, and had an impact on Balzac. Balzac was fascinated by the new emerging hospital medicine, especially Parisian medicine. In conjunction with this official medicine, he was also interested in magnetism, hypnotism, and phrenology.

### *Family*

His father, who had acquired numerous medical contacts during his ten years as administrator of Tours Hospice, had a large influence on his work. His stories, readings, personal studies, and booklets on sociomedical subjects were a great resource for Balzac. His mother, despite her lack of affection and physical presence, greatly influenced him concerning all pseudoreligious schools of thought, particularly the occult.

### *Friendships*

It was especially through his friends that Balzac drew most of his medical knowledge. He had links to many great scholars of his time, such as Dupuytren, Broussais, Cuvier, and Geoffroy Saint-Hilaire, to whom he dedicated *Le père Goriot* and the foreword in *La comédie humaine*. Some served as models for some doctors in *La comédie humaine*. Dr. Regnault, who he met in Paris in 1831 at the end of his medical studies, Dr. Menière, and Dr. Chapelain in particular were a great influence on him. He also met Dr. Origet, a family friend and doctor of Tours Hospice, who is often quoted in family conversations [2].

He had a lasting correspondence with Dr. Moreau of Tours, a family friend. Moreau was an organicist convinced of the relationship between the physical and moral aspects of man, whose ideas could only but appeal to Balzac. He studied the effects of hashish, the etiology of epilepsy (1854), and neuropathic madness (1869), among others. His influence on Balzac appears in his work through the descriptions of psychosomatic diseases, neuroses, and many mental illnesses, as well as that he used these more frequently in his portraits of women.

However, Balzac's closest acquaintance throughout his life was Dr. Jean-Baptiste Nacquart, a loyal friend and confidant who was present at his death. Balzac dedicated *Le lys dans la vallée* to him. Nacquart was interested in phrenology; in 1808 he published *Traité sur la nouvelle physiologie du cerveau, ou exposition de la doctrine de Gall*. The surprising presence of phrenology and physiognomy in *La comédie humaine* is essentially due to Nacquart's influence, largely inspired by Cabanis' theories on the relationship between the physical and moral aspects of man. Furthermore, Nacquart introduced Balzac to Lavaterm, whose writings deal with physiognomy, which he used in order to create and describe many of his characters. Nacquart's election to the Academy of Medicine in 1823, and presidency of it in subsequent years enabled Balzac to also meet many great names in medicine.

### *Balzac as a Physiologist*

Balzac prided himself on being a physiologist and does not conceal the fact that he is well informed on this subject. Thus, the medical professionals in *La comédie humaine*, *César Birotteau,* and *Le lys dans la vallée,* such as Vauquelin and de Mortsauf, converse like authentic pathologists. Balzac quite remarkably understands the physiology of all his characters: Birotteau's gout, Mortsauf's neurosis, Frasier's skin disease, Louis Lambert's catalepsy, etc. [3]. Many, not knowing the author of the book, believed him to be a doctor. At the time, Balzac is often described as 'the Dupuytren manuscript museum', 'the Molière doctor' [4].

Magnetism and somnambulism fascinated Balzac. He was obsessed by these inexplicable phenomena and they had considerable importance in his works. In *Ursule Mirouët* he recounts the history of mesmerism and describes swedenborgist Dr. Mironet as a strong supporter of Mesmer's theories. Magnetism and occultism are central to this novel. Balzac defends Mesmer against the Faculty of Medicine of Paris, all while condemning his financial conceit and lack of genius. He condemns the persecution against mesmerists such as Dr. Bouvard.

### *Balzac as a Neuropsychiatrist*

Balzac himself was a scientific precursor because, as a writer, he was interested in issues other than literature in the beginning of the nineteenth century. And he approached these issues in the manner of a scientist. He guessed the relevance of direct observation before the naturalists. He glimpsed the influence of the environment on the development of the individual. Perhaps he also sensed the influence of family background on himself and his desire and passion to write monumental work. Work, in terms of studying psychological structures, was perhaps the therapy he unconsciously created so as not to sink completely into madness; hence, the many allusions and descriptions taken from nascent nineteenth century psychiatry. Balzac is constantly fascinated by psychiatry as a science of thought, the functioning of the brain and of thought. He had access to a great many resources in this matter, including the *Dictionnaire des sciences médicales* by Esquirol, which contained many articles on delirium, dementia, monomania, erotomania, madness, anger, idiocy, hallucinations, melancholia, manias, and suicide. Balzac was especially attracted by brain physiology. He believed the brain to be 'the alembic to which the Animal conveys what each of its organizations, in proportion to the strength of that vessel, can absorb of that Substance, which returns it transformed into Will' [5].

## Description of Doctors

Other than his personal tastes for everything related to medicine, Balzac's realism is the most significant reason why doctors have such an important role in his novels. Society comes to life in the writings of Balzac, but it is a new society, stripped of its old forms: the priest is no longer the soul of the modern social state; the doctor has replaced him. Whether his novels recount the story of the rich or the poor in the country, provinces, or Paris, the doctor always has a role to fulfill. The doctor's presence is noticeable everywhere, and *La comédie humaine*, by copying society in all its aspects, captures all types of medicine.

### *Provincial Doctors*

The most prominent type of doctor in depictions of provincial life is Dr. Martener de Provins described in *Pierrette*. Balzac describes provincial life as divided by the governing party and the Liberal party. This is picture of petty rivalry between two doctors in the province. Just as one is capable of unscrupulous infamy to serve his party, the other, Dr. Martener, is a gentle soul who knows how to go without. It is via this humble practitioner, living modestly in a modest town, that Balzac developed his ideal of the medical profession.

More mixed is the description of Dr. Rouget, another type of provincial doctor in *La rabouilleuse*. Extremely miserly, he marries a rich and sickly woman, who he soon hopes to mourn.

### *Parisian Doctors*

Parisian in manners and mind, Balzac preferred studying all types of Parisian doctors. If his provincial doctors were modest, the Parisian doctors were his favorites, 'the princes of science'. Balzac rubbed shoulders with them and knew them so well that his portraits were sometimes the copy of the original.

The archetype of this local district doctor is Dr. Poulain from *Les parents pauvres*, a distinguished former intern, who is now a cautious and experienced practitioner. However, despite the grandeur and beauty of these functions, he only has a small number of patients, and barely enough to live on. He knows when to be generous. In reality, however, his pity and dedication to his patients are in direct proportion to their pecuniary resources. Despite this poverty, Dr. Poulain is ambitious. Regardless of means or cost, he wants to leave the obscurity in which he finds himself. He knowingly uses the vile lies of a patient who pretends to have a serious illness. He administers so-called 'remedies' and imagines a naturally very successful fantastic operation so as to be well known in the district. Finally, he aids a group of disreputable people in pursuit of an inheritance since he hopes to be appointed chief physician of a hospital or royal college as a reward for his cooperation.

This is in great contrast to the brilliant fame and fortune of these great Parisian surgeons or doctors who Balzac likes to describe in detail. It is worth discussing in depth the principal doctors: Desplein, 'one of the most illustrious, greatest geniuses of our time, a phenomenon in science, the greatest surgeon of ancient and modern times'; and Bianchon, 'the great and famous physician. . . one of the leading lights at the School of Paris.'

*Dr. Desplein*

He is the fictional version of Dupuytren and practices surgery in *La comédie humaine.* His history is found in *La messe de l'athée,* where the great surgeon tells his own story. He has a difficult start to life. Like Dupuytren, Desplein comes from a poor provincial family and goes to Paris at the end of the eighteenth century to study medicine. He is about to give up his studies due to a lack of resources when a poor water carrier from Saint-Flour takes a great liking to him, finances his exams and books, assures him all the material side of existence, and finally becomes his servant and father. Thanks to him, Desplein becomes an intern at Hôtel-Dieu and later a surgeon, making him famous and consequently opening the doors of the Academy of Sciences; hence, the mass given four times a year, in recognition of the latter. This story also recalls the disease that bears his name, fixed flexion contracture of the hand, which Dupuytren observed in water carriers.

Balzac described Desplein as a genius: '[He] had a godlike eye; he saw into the sufferer and his malady by an intuition, natural or acquired, which enabled him to grasp the diagnostics peculiar to the individual, to determine the very time, the hour, the minute when an operation should be performed' [6]. He is also a skilled ophthalmic surgeon and helps Modeste Mignon regain her sight [7]. Balzac does not give Desplein's diagnosis, but it is very likely that this is a cataract operation, Dupuytren's field of expertise. He also trepans Pierrette, who is suffering from a head injury, resulting in a subdural hematoma; however, despite the care, Pierrette dies. The genius is not infallible.

Balzac also portrays some repugnant character traits. He presents Desplein as an avaricious man: solitary and misanthropic, but loving honor [6]. For Balzac, the practice of medicine requires total unselfishness. He condemns gratification by decorations of which many are proud, as they only reinforce the idea that one can be useful to the nation and expect a reward in return. Having a strange sense of humor, and being irascible and irritable, Desplein also has many enemies who are envious of bringing about his fall and whose hatred and calumny isolates him in the most bitter and hard selfishness. How Balzac could accurately guess a part of Dupuytren's personality is made clearer by the rumor that Balzac became Caroline Marbouty's lover, who had also been Dupuytren's mistress.

*Dr. Bianchon*

Dr. Bianchon is for some the famous Dr. Bouillaud: their biographies and portraits are indeed quite similar. Prior to being an intern at Cochin Hospital, Bianchon was an unfortunate medical student, living in a miserable boarding house in the Latin Quarter, where he meets Father Goriot, and cares for him in his pain. Balzac had him born around the year 1800, son of a doctor at Sancerre. At the age of forty, he was a hospital doctor, officer of the Legion of Honor, and member of the Institute, representing the ultimate accolade for Balzac. He is described as slightly rotund, with an impassive face, large rounded forehead, and long hair; cheerful; devoted to his friends; and faithful. He is firm in his ideas and rigorous in his conduct.

Dr. Bianchon is interested in Gall's famous system. In *Le père Goriot* he examines the skull in an attempt to understand the enigma of the existence of this strange man. He jokes, however, about another resident: 'I have studied Gall's system, and I am sure she has the bump of Judas' [8], and about Father Goriot himself, 'there is only one bump – the bump of Paternity' [8].

Bianchon's scientific spirit is particularly well described, during Father Goriot's agony, when he sends instructions to Rastignac [8]. He tries to understand the disease: even if it does not help Father Goriot, the experience will be useful for other patients in the future. However, Bianchon maintains his respect for human beings, and time does not alter the quality of understanding attitude vis-à-vis the patient, and helps support his morbid condition.

He is also a man convinced of the strength of will on the body. Balzac makes him an advocate of magnetism and a great observer of diseases that now come under the psychosomatic and neurotic fields of expertise. Balzac adds brilliant intuition to his scholarly virtues making him a 'man of arts'. Moreover, he often identifies the psychology of his patients by somatic study and is not limited to only healing the body. Added to this is his natural goodness and perfect selflessness. Bianchon is irreproachable, unselfish, and has deep knowledge, accurate diagnoses, infallible prognoses, and an understanding of his patients, all of which embody the perfect doctor. He is open-minded and knows how to consider several possible explanations.

In a word, Bianchon has only virtues and throughout *La comédie humaine* he returns at each moment either to illuminate a difficult diagnosis or to represent a kind of goodness and medical kindness, or because Balzac needed a brilliant and witty storyteller to dissect the soul of humanity. Despite this profound understanding of human turpitude, or perhaps because of it, Bianchon retains a great indulgence for human weakness, kindness for suffering, and youthfulness in the midst of all this misery. Science, integrity, dedication, and deep philosophy – he is a synthesis of virtues that can develop the practice of the medical profession.

*Doctors Brisset, Caméristus, and Maugrédie*

These are three Parisian doctors who represent three different and opposing schools of thought at the Faculty of Medicine of Paris: organicism, vitalism, and experimental physiology. Balzac unites them in *La peau de chagrin* in order to pronounce their prognosis on Raphaël de Valentin, who is suffering from pulmonary tuberculosis.

Brisset is the leader of the organicists, undoubtedly the pseudonym of Dr. Broussais, whose name is barely disguised. It seems Balzac did not capture the nuance between the organicists and Broussais. The starting point of his medicine was very similar to that of the organicists in that he wanted to relate diseases to organic lesions visible on dissection. Broussais performed many autopsies on the battlefields, but the conclusions he drew from them led him to build what he called physiological medicine, where irritation of the stomach is the sole cause of all disease, and bleeding the only cure.

Caméristus, the fictional version of Dr. Récamier and head of the vitalists, is absolutely opposed to Brisset. During a consultation with Raphaël, he naturally gives a vitalist diagnosis [8]. Balzac summarizes the doctrine of Caméristus well: 'He discerned a lofty informing principle in human life, a mysterious and inexplicable phenomenon.' [9].

Balzac also depicts Caméristus as being religious and embodying spirituality. Récamier indeed distinguished himself by his very conservative views, and was himself a devout Catholic. This is why, via the doctrine of his vitalism, Récamier relied on divine power to explain the secrets of nascent physiology. Balzac then exaggerates this trait and makes him even a believer of mysticism. Here Balzac leaves his model of Récamier, as he was more of a positivist than Caméristus in that he was enthusiastic about new therapies. For Récamier, in contrast to Broussais, an identifiable organic lesion is at the root of a specific organic syndrome, thus requiring a specific treatment.

Maugrédie is neither a vitalist nor an organicist. This fictitious version of Dr. François Magendie is the third doctor called to Raphaël's bedside [9]. Via a brief description, the principles that guide the school of experimental medicine are traced. Most of it is made by observation, according to Magendie's medicine, and hence the rejection of any a priori assumptions before an experiment or patient. Even if he had no theory, he had an experimental method. Balzac does not grasp the importance of this and adopts an ironic tone. For him, he is merely a man without ideas, who adopts those of others. He does not clearly describe the treatment that Raphaël should follow. In the case of Magendie, Balzac did not understand that the denial of any preestablished principle was, in itself, a philosophy that would revolutionize medicine a few years later.

This famous consultation is a good example of medical indifference and cruelty, which for some seem to be attributes inherent in the profession. It remains one of the few medical caricatures that Balzac made in his work. He sometimes doubted the efficacy of medicine and often wished it to be less rational, but he almost never mocked or ridiculed the doctors. This consultation gives a striking picture of coldness and indifference of medical authorities before the tragedy of illness and death [9].

*The Unknown Doctors of Paris*

Medical greed is represented in *La comédie humaine* only by a single, foreign doctor: a Polish Jew, Dr. Halpersohn. This doctor, reputed to be an empiricist, became famous as a result of extraordinary cures that healed desperate patients. Who had Balzac wanted to describe? Was it one of the many foreign charlatans, who, relying on human credulity, were skilled enough to convince others of their knowledge and obtain exaggerated remuneration for their odious deceptions? The assumption could be made, however, that Balzac himself believed in Polish medicine. Balzac was treated for his heart disease by a physician, Dr. Knothe, who, although less avaricious, had much in common with Dr. Halpersohn.

### *The Country Doctor*

Dr. Benassis is the only representative of this type of doctor still unknown at the time. Balzac makes him a great organizer and above all a man of social and economic progress. Balzac did not really believe in the altruism and unselfishness that the exercise of this profession requires in the country. Benassis therefore has a secret, a mistake, a terrible remorse to atone for by choosing priesthood instead of focusing on a more glorious career in Paris for which he was destined [10]. However, in order to express his political views, Balzac needed a representative of progress, an active character affecting a society that Balzac considers to be sick, and the doctor therefore becomes a symbol [11].

This was an opportunity for Balzac to develop some ideas about the state of private and public hygiene in the nineteenth century, with his first fight against the stupidity that he attributed (as did the science of the time) to the lack of ventilation and sun in houses. Benassis fights against unsanitary conditions; builds a new village, bridges, and roads; cleans swamps; and becomes a symbol of socioeconomic development [11].

It is nevertheless true that in this book the doctor ceases to be merely an instrument. He has a full role [12] in executing a work of socioeconomic construction. Balzac idealizes this role by giving it to a simple country doctor. His social role is certainly predominant here, but probably unrealistic.

### *Military Doctors*

Balzac uses military doctors to describe specific situations that occurred in camps. Thus, in *La comédie humaine* the role of doctors is limited. Most representatives are not even in the army where Balzac introduces them, like Dr. Goddet, a former surgeon-major, who becomes the best doctor of Issoudun; Dr. Chardon, a former army surgeon of the armed forces of the Republic, established in Angoulême; or Dr. Vernon, formerly chief surgeon of the French Army between 1793 and 1815, who was retired when he appears in *La marâtre*. Balzac mostly made them narrators of dramatic adventures such as in *L'auberge rouge*.

## Conclusion

Balzac was more interested in the role of the doctor, his social position, and the ideological debates of the time, rather than the diseases themselves. He was the first in the history of the novel to introduce doctors in his work, and was guided along this new path by the particular realist vision he had of novels. He was thus the indisputable leader of the naturalist and realist schools. His view was to be adopted by all the novelists who followed, and who, repudiating romanticism, as well as classicism, or the implausibility of the sentimental and adventure novel, were the first to revive the nature of human beings and the environment in which they act.

For Balzac, the doctor is an 'active' observer of society in all social strata. The doctor is rarely the protagonist, but is always present in all human activities. Balzac, via his doctors, makes a grim clinical assessment of society. The main pathology of the human race is 'passion' in its most excessive and destructive sense: passion for money, fame, and love, pushed to the extreme. This passion crushes the individual who is trapped in society's 'plots,' a term frequently used in his work. Doctors are also Balzac's 'accomplices' in the observation of scientific developments and multiple theories that are current at the time.

The importance of the doctor became significant in nineteenth century society. He was 'the last priest, supreme faith, invincible superstition,' and Balzac was able to decrypt this emergence and predict its evolution determined by the development of medical science. It is through his doctors that all of society is described and, most importantly, through the lens of medicine that human nature is decoded.

However, we must not neglect Balzac's wider contribution to medicine. Through his personal experience and his perspicacity in detailing the symptoms and pathologies of his characters, the reader enters the field of mental illness without even realizing. In his work, parallel schools of thought are also well represented, such as phrenology and physiognomy, in order to create developed characters. He created mysterious illnesses in order to reinforce the dramatic destiny of his characters. With his sharpened perception of human nature, Balzac knew how to portray the full complexity of social interactions and their attendant behavioral disorders. By drawing together, according to his hypothetico-deductible method, the pathophysiological bases related to brain function, did Balzac not help lay the foundations for what would become neuropsychiatry?

## Acknowledgement

I would like to express my warm thanks to Holly Sandu for her contribution to and translation of this article.

## References

1 Caujole P: La médecine et les médecins dans l'oeuvre de H. de Balzac. Lyon, A. Storck & Cie, 1900.
2 Coursault R: La médecine en Touraine du Moyen Age à nos jours. Paris, Maisonneuve & Larose, 1991.
3 Cerfberr A, Christophe J: Répertoire de la comédie humaine de H. De Balzac. Avec une introduction par Bourget P. Paris, Calmann Lévy, 1887.
4 Taine H: Nouveaux essais de critique et d'histoire: Balzac, ed 2. Paris, L. Hachette, 1866.
5 Balzac H: Louis Lambert. Translated by Bell C, Waring J. University Park, Pennsylvania State University, 2002. http://www2.hn.psu.edu/faculty/jmanis/Balzac/Louis-Lambert.pdf (accessed July 30, 2012).
6 Balzac H: The Atheist's Mass. Translated by Bell C. University Park, Pennsylvania State University, 2002. http://www2.hn.psu.edu/faculty/jmanis/Balzac/Atheist-Mass.pdf (accessed July 25, 2012).
7 Balzac H: Modeste Mignon. Paris, Gallimard, 1982.
8 Balzac H: Father Goriot. Translated by Marriage E. University Park, Pennsylvania State University, 2002. http://www2.hn.psu.edu/faculty/jmanis/Balzac/Father-Goriot.pdf (accessed July 28, 2012).
9 Balzac H: The Magic Skin. Translated by Marriage E. University Park, Pennsylvania State University, 2002. http://www2.hn.psu.edu/faculty/jmanis/Balzac/magic-skin.pdf (accessed July 29, 2012).
10 Balzac H: Le Médecin de campagne. Paris, Gallimard, 1974.
11 Barberis P: Balzac et le mal du siècle: contribution à une physiologie du monde moderne. De la prise de conscience à l'expression 1830–1833. Paris, Folio-Gaillimard, 1990, vol 2.
12 Balzac H: La femme de trente ans. Préface de Barberis P. Paris, Folio-Gallimard, 1977.

Prof. Thierry Moulin
Service de Neurologie, CHU de Besançon
Hôpital Jean Minjoz, Boulevard Fleming
FR–25030 Besançon Cedex (France)
E-Mail thierry.moulin@univ-fcomte.fr

Bogousslavsky J, Dieguez S (eds): Literary Medicine: Brain Disease and Doctors in Novels, Theater, and Film.
Front Neurol Neurosci. Basel, Karger, 2013, vol 31, pp 236–244 (DOI: 10.1159/000343246)

# Doctor Chekhov's Doctors

Isabelle Crommelynck

Medical Doctor, Paris, France

**Abstract**

Anton Chekhov (1860–1904) was both a writer and a doctor, as well as a patient. In spite of his literary success, he did not turn away from medicine until 1897, at the age of 37, when his tuberculosis became too serious. During his medical studies in Moscow, he wrote short stories, at night, under various pseudonyms to provide money for his family; all his life, Chekhov was his parents' financial support. It was Alexei Suvorin (1834–1912), the powerful director of *Novoye Vremya* (New Times), and the well-known writer Dimitry Grigorovich (1822–1899) who persuaded him that he had exceptional literary talent and requested him to abandon pseudonyms and sign his articles. So, for all his life, he practiced medicine as a district doctor and wrote plays and short stories. In each of his plays, except *The Cherry Orchard,* Chekhov introduced characters of doctors, principally Yevgeny Konstantinovich Lvov in *Ivanov* and Mikhail Lvovich Astrov in *Uncle Vanya,* as well as Khrushchev in *The Wood Demon*, Dorn in *The Seagull*, Tcheboutykin in *The Three Sisters,* and Triletski in *Platonov*. In his countless short stories, there are numerous doctors, for instance Professor Stepanovich (*A Dreary Story*), Doctors Kirilov (*Enemies*), Sobol (*My Wife*), Outchinnikov (*An Inconvenience*), Dymov (*The Grasshopper*), Startsvev (*Ionitch*), and others. Chekhov's main interest in psychiatry was clearly visible in *The Nervous Breakdown*, *The Black Monk*, *The Man in a Case*, *A Doctor's Visit,* and *Ward No. 6* with Dr. Ragin. In his short stories as in his plays, Chekhov relied on his knowledge of provincial life; his doctor's characters were not professors, academicians, or Moscow's great physicians, but instead exhausted hard workers, with no effective diagnostic and therapeutic means, and poorly paid. Unlike himself, none of Chekhov's doctors was a writer or breadwinner, and Chekhov did not like to lay emphasis on the disease.



Anton Chekhov (1860–1904) [1–4], novelist, playwright, and founder of modern theater with Henrik Ibsen (1828–1906) and August Strindberg (1849–1912), was a doctor. All his life, however, he continued to write without giving up medicine: 'Medicine is my lawful wife, literature my mistress, when one bothers me, I will spend my night with the other' [5]. Unfortunately, he was also a patient, but he denied his tuberculosis until the spring of 1897, when he was hospitalized in Moscow for severe hemoptysis and was forced to turn away from medicine as his tuberculosis became too serious.

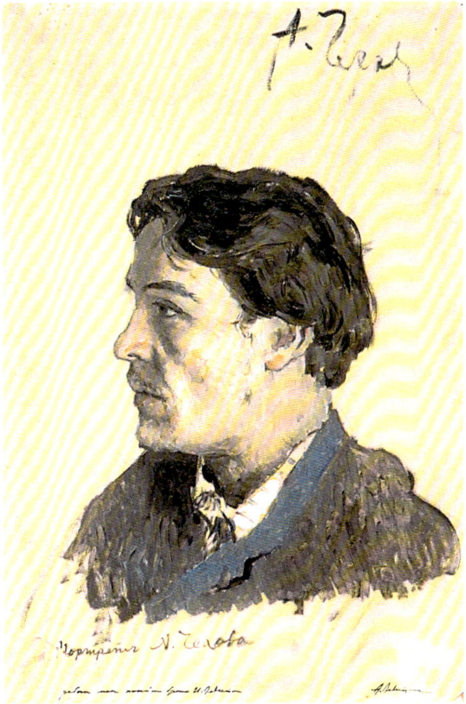

**Fig. 1.** Chekhov's Portrait (1886), by Isaak Levitan (1860–1900), Tretyakov Gallery, Moscow, Russia, with kind permission.

### Anton Pavlovich Chekhov, Doctor

Born in Taganrog, a small port on the Sea of Azov, he was the third child in a family of six: five boys and one girl. His mother was a housewife. His father, the son of a freed serf, was a wholesaler, and was authoritarian and brutal with his children. In 1876, he was declared bankrupt and left for Moscow to escape imprisonment for debt. Anton, only sixteen, was forced to work to provide for the family. In 1879, he arrived in Moscow and began his medical studies; at night he wrote short stories to earn money for his family under various pseudonyms.

After completing his medical studies, he began to practice in the district hospitals of Moscow (fig. 1). That same year, hemoptysis announced the tuberculosis which would mark his existence, but which he denied for years. Chekhov consulted and treated patients, and performed autopsies. After briefly settling down in Moscow, he took a provincial medical position at Melikhovo, in the Serpoukhov district. This provincial life allowed him to observe countless characters: government officials, soldiers, country doctors, patients, miserable peasants, vagabonds, and travelers. With few exceptions, his doctor characters were only rural physicians.

He used his experience to depict portraits of doctors in his plays [6–8] and numerous short stories [7, 9–12] (table 1). In 1889, he wrote to his friend Dr. Gregory Rossolimo (1860–1928) [13]: 'I have no doubt that my study of medicine has got a

**Table 1.** Some of the Chekhov's doctors in plays and short stories

| | Year | Title | Doctors | Diseases |
|---|---|---|---|---|
| Plays | 1881 | *Platonov* | Dr. Nikolai Ivanovich Triletski | |
| | 1887 | *Ivanov* | Dr. Yevgeny Konstantinovich Lvov | tuberculosis |
| | 1889 | *The Wood Demon* | Dr. Mikhail Lvovich Khrushchev | hypochondriasis |
| | 1890 | *A Marriage Proposal* | | hypochondriasis |
| | 1896 | *The Seagull* | Dr. Yevgeny Sergeevich Dorn | young Treplev's |
| | 1897 | *Uncle Vanya* | Dr. Mikhail Lvovich Astrov | hypochondriasis |
| | 1901 | *The Three Sisters* | Dr. Ivan Romanovich Tcheboutykin | |
| Short stories | 1882 | *Late-Blooming Flowers* | Dr. Toporkov | tuberculosis |
| | 1884 | *Perpetuum Mobile* | Dr. Stiviski | |
| | 1885 | *The Nerves* | | anxiety |
| | 1886 | *Excellent People* | Vera, a female doctor | 'fixed ideas' |
| | 1886 | *Martyrs* | a doctor | hysteria |
| | 1886 | *Anyuta* | Stepan Klotchkov, a medical student | |
| | 1886 | *The Chemist's Wife* | a doctor | |
| | 1887 | *The Doctor* | Dr. Tsvyetkov | brain tumor |
| | 1887 | *The Judge* | a doctor | |
| | 1887 | *Enemies* | Dr. Kirilov | diphteria |
| | 1887 | *Intrigues* | Dr. Chelestov | |
| | 1887 | *An Inconvenience* | Dr. Outchinnikov | |
| | 1887 | *Darkness* | a doctor | |
| | 1887 | *Typhus* | a doctor | typhoid fever |
| | 1888 | *The Nervous Breakdown* | a doctor | panic attack |
| | 1889 | *A Dreary Story* | Prof. Nikolai Stepanovich | depression |
| | 1889 | *The Princess* | Dr. Ivanovitch | |
| | 1891 | *The Duel* | Dr. Alexei Samoylenko | |
| | 1892 | *Ward No. 6* | Dr. Ragin and Dr. Khobotov | paranoia |
| | 1892 | *The Grasshopper* | Dr. Ossip Dymov | diphteria |
| | 1892 | *My Wife* | Dr. Sobol | |
| | 1894 | *The Black Monk* | a doctor | hallucinations |
| | 1894 | *Head Gardener's Story* | Dr. Thomson | |
| | 1895 | *The Wife* | a doctor | tuberculosis |
| | 1895 | *Three Years* | Dr. Sergueï Borrisytch | breast cancer |
| | 1896 | *My Life* | Dr. Vladimir Blagovo | |
| | 1898 | *Ionitch* | Dr. Ionitch Startsvev, | |
| | 1898 | *The Man in a Case* | Tchimcha-Himalaïski, a veterinarian! | obsessive personality |
| | 1898 | *A Doctor's Visit* | Korolev, a resident | anxiety |
| | 1899 | *An Official Duty* | Dr. Strarchenko | |
| | 1882 | *Village Doctors* | quacks | |
| | 1884 | *Surgery* | | |
| | 1885 | *Malingerers* | | |
| | 1885 | *A Cure for Hard Drinking* | | |
| | 1885 | *A Horsey Name* | | |
| | 1886 | *The Night Before the Trial* | | |
| | 1887 | *First Aid* | | |

serious influence on my literary activity. It had significantly expanded the scope of my observations. It had enriched my knowledge, whose value, for me as a writer, could be understood only by a writer who would be himself a physician.' This most likely produced the mixture of empathy combined with distance found in his works.

## Doctor Chekhov's Interest in Psychiatry and Psychopathology

In 1892, Chekhov confided to one of his friends: 'I am extremely interested in any deviations from what is called the soul and if I had not become a writer I would surely have been a psychiatrist' [7, p. XXXVIII]. Indeed, he was very interested in psychiatry, and he kept himself regularly informed of Freud's works. His famous short story *Ward No. 6* depicts the arrival of Dr. Ragin in a district hospital, whose deplorable state struck him. The worst thing was the condition of insane patients 'who had this particular air of sadness and malediction that can be seen only in hospitals and prisons.' Honest and with a scrupulous medical competence, he loses heart over the years and begins to attend Ward No. 6. He develops a taste for talking with a patient, Ivan Gromov, who suffers from persecution mania. As a result, he neglects his consulting hours in order to meet Gromov every day. His colleague, Dr. Khobotov, finally says: 'I feel that our old man has become crazy.' He has him interned in Ward No. 6, where the unfortunate Dr. Ragin soon dies.

The same tone can be seen in *The Nervous Breakdown*. In this story, a young man is taken to brothels by his fellow students, particularly Mayer, a medical student. Afterwards, he is seized with such anxiety that he considers killing himself. His friends take him to a psychiatrist who questions him at length about his personal and family history, performs neurological examination, and prescribes bromide and morphine. It is about this short story that Chekhov wrote: 'As a doctor, I think I have correctly depicted mental illness, according to all psychiatric science rules' [14]. In *A Dreary Story*, Nikolai Stepanovich, a professor of medicine close to retirement, has done everything in his profession: teaching and research, all without neglecting his family. He feels old, becomes an insomniac, and is intellectually less alert. He thinks of his past with nostalgia. Only his adopted daughter brings him joy. But she wants to become an actress and leaves. As we would say nowadays, it seems that this man is deeply depressed.

Chekhov's inclination for psychiatry is also evident in *The Black Monk*, in which the main character is a victim of hallucinations, and in *The Man in a Case* which depicts an obsessive personality, as well as in *The Nerves*, where, coming back from a spiritism session, an architect has an anxiety attack. In *Martyrs*, a hysterical woman exhausts her husband. In *Excellent People*, Vera, a female doctor, is facing fixed ideas after a funeral, with her brother commenting: 'she is crazy to her bone marrow'. And Ivan Vassilievitch Lomov was a hypochondriac in *A Marriage Proposal*, a farce in one act.

### Competent, Empathic: Chekhov's Doctors

In each of his plays, with the exception of *The Cherry Orchard,* Chekhov introduced doctors. In *Ivanov*, Yevgeny Konstantinovich Lvov is the young doctor of the district. Honest and competent, he has serious concerns regarding the health of Anna Petrovna, Ivanov's wife, who has tuberculosis, and he is critical of Ivanov who neglects her. In a letter to Alexei Suvorin, Chekhov wrote: 'Lvov is the type of honest and upright man full of passion but limited. . .; he is made to punish the forces of evil' [15]. For Chekhov, Ivanov belongs to 'the category of broken, misunderstood people' [15]. We would say today that he was deeply depressed. Indeed, at the end of the play, after Lvov calls him a bastard, Ivanov shoots himself.

In *The Seagull,* Yevgeny Sergeevich Dorn is a retired doctor. In Act I, he recalls, 'Ten or fifteen years ago, I was, if you remember, the only serious obstetrician in the region'. He is humorous, but pays attention to the health of people around him: he disapproves of Masha's snuff-taking, and advises Sorin to stop smoking and drinking. Sensitive to young Treplev's disarray, he senses his suicide when a gunshot rings out at the end of the play.

Sometimes one has the feeling of following Dr. Chekhov at work. This is the case in *A Doctor's Visit.* In this short story, a professor of medicine is called for a consultation in the vicinity of Moscow, to which he sends Korolev, his resident. There, Korolev meets a young girl, the 20-year-old Lisa Lyalikov, who has such violent palpitations that she cannot sleep and is afraid of dying. Full of empathy, Korolev listens to her, examines her, and makes her realize that it is her living conditions which are the cause. It is also the case in *An Official Duty*, where a doctor and a judge go to perform an autopsy in a snowstorm, and in *The Judge*, where a doctor rationally decrypts the story of a judge whose wife died after giving birth.

In *Ionitch,* Chekhov recounts the life of Dr. Ionitch Startsvev, who has a successful medical career but whose love life is a failure. In *The Grasshopper,* Ossip Dymov is a hard-working and talented doctor who dies of diphtheria he contracts while caring for a child. His wife was deceitful, but she then misses this remarkable man. *The Wife* is the story of a competent physician, who has tuberculosis and is cheated on by his wife. In *Late-Blooming Flowers,* Dr. Toporkov, a man of humble origins, succeeds through hard work and deprivation. He treats a young tuberculous woman and takes her to the Riviera, where she dies three days later. In the short story *The Doctor,* Dr. Tsvyetkov is called by his friend Olga, whose son has a brain tumor. He has to tell her that there is no hope, and it turns out that the child may be his own son. In *The Princess,* Dr. Ivanovitch criticizes Princess Gravilovna, who loves devotion but treats her servants 'as cannon fodder'. The generous and beloved Dr. Thomson in *Head Gardener's Story* must also be mentioned as well as the vain and warm Dr. Alexei Samoylenko in *The Duel,* and of course Dr. Vladimir Blagovo in *My Life.*

## Chekhov's Exhausted Doctors

Mikhail Lvovich Astrov, the doctor in *Uncle Vanya*, is very different from Dr. Lvov. He has been practicing medicine in the countryside for ten years and feels old and disillusioned. He is overworked, wakes at night, and is called to fight against epidemics or to operate on wounded people 'who die under chloroform'. He notes: 'My feelings are blur. I want nothing, I don't need anything, I love nobody.' He sometimes drinks vodka to excess. Exhausted by his work, he takes refuge in his passion of fighting deforestation, burning peat instead of wood, protecting wildlife, and not disrupting the climate. He carefully prepares maps showing the district forest loss of the last fifty years. Astrov is perhaps the doctor who most resembles Chekhov, who saw up to a thousand patients a year in Melikhovo and, urged by the district health authorities, was so exhausted by the fight against famine and epidemics that he could not find time to write. In the play *The Wood Demon* [16], one can see a first sketch of Uncle Vanya, but the doctor, Mikhail Lvovich Khrushchev, is young, full of energy, and allows more time to the preservation of forests than to his job. 'He knows about medicine as I do about astronomy', Professor Serebryakov said of him.

Most district doctors had an exhausting life. In *Enemies*, Dr. Kirilov's doorbell rings one night at ten o'clock; his son had just died of diphteria and he had not slept for three nights. In *My Wife*, Dr. Sobol explains how he is exhausted by the hospital, visits, the fight against typhus, and famine: 'I became a savage in this hole, a lout.' You would think you could hear Astrov. Some of them were losing their self-control. Thus, in *An Inconvenience*, Dr. Outchinnikov, exasperated by the incompetence of his nurse, in addition to being drunk, punches her in the face. In *Darkness*, the doctor, unable to answer the request of an unhappy supplicant is totally discouraged.

## Chekhov's Incompetent Doctors

In *The Three Sisters*, Ivan Romanovich Tcheboutykin is a military physician in a provincial city close to retirement. He considers himself lazy and is aware of his ignorance: 'Since I left University, I have done nothing, not even read, not a single book, nothing except newspapers.' Nikolai Ivanovich Triletski, the young doctor in *Platonov*, avoids any professional commitment, is always partying, and is in debt. In *Three Years*, while doctor Sergueï Borrisytch is treating the breast cancer of Nina, the burghers of the city believe that all their doctors have made a fortune but are incompetent and 'do not know anything, do not understand anything'. In *Intrigues*, Dr. Chelestov, amazed by the low level of his colleagues, reviews their medical errors and notes that out of thirty-two doctors, the majority of them had less knowledge than a first-year medical student.

### Humorous Portraits of Doctors

Chekhov often showed a humor either tender or fierce: 'I will start soon writing humorous stories, because my entire psychopathological repertoire is exhausted' [17]. In *Typhus*, the doctor talks to his patient, lieutenant Klimov, as if he were a child. In *Anyuta*, Chekhov depicts Stepan Klotchkov, a young medical student, as being unscrupulous toward his girlfriend. In *The Chemist's Wife*, he mocks a doctor and the spinelessness of the chemist, nicknamed 'black muzzle'. Homeopathy is ironically but severely criticized In *Malingerers* and in *The Night before the Trial*. The quackery is deeply ridiculed in *A Horsey Name*, *A Cure for Hard Drinking*, *Surgery*, *Village Doctors*, and *First Aid*.

On the contrary, it is Chekhov's empathy which is manifested in *Misery*, when after nobody listens to a poor driver who had lost his son, he finally confides in his horse. In *Nightmare*, the village doctor is so poor that his wife washes their clothes in the icy water of the river. This look, full of pity for human misery, is a trademark of the author.

### Dr. Anton Chekhov versus Chekhov's Doctors

Chekhov's ambivalence between medicine and literature is not easily discernible initially. During his medical studies, his literary beginnings were meant only to put food on the table. He was not aware of his literary talent. At the end of 1885, he was noticed by Alexei Suvorin, the powerful director of *Novoye Vremya* (New Times), the largest Russian newspaper. Soon after, the writer Dimitry Grigorovich (1822–1899) wrote him that he had exceptional talent and requested him to abandon pseudonyms and sign his articles. An author of serial stories, Chekhov awoke as a writer, but continued to practice medicine. In 1890, Chekhov visited the prison on Sakhalin island. The journey was exhausting; he had already been struck by hemoptysis. Chekhov stayed on the island for three months and interviewed each convict; during this time, he wrote ten thousand pages about his time there. From this experience, he wrote a book entitled *The Island Sakhalin*.

Back in Moscow, Chekhov returned to his literary activities (fig. 2). He portrayed his characters after his heavy experience as a district doctor and was not interested in the medical celebrities of his time. He did not see the rich and distinguished Moscow doctors, but only the poor district doctors, like himself. But he had no friends among them. His numerous friends belonged to the cultural world, which included the painter Isaac Levitan (1860–1900), Pyotr Tchaikovsky (1840–1893), Maxim Gorky (1868–1938), Sergei Rachmaninov (1873–1943), Leo Tolstoy (1828–1910), Ivan Bounin (1870–1953) [18], and others.

A very sociable but secret, indefatigable observer, what did Chekhov confide about himself through his doctor's characters? Unlike himself, none of Chekhov's doctors

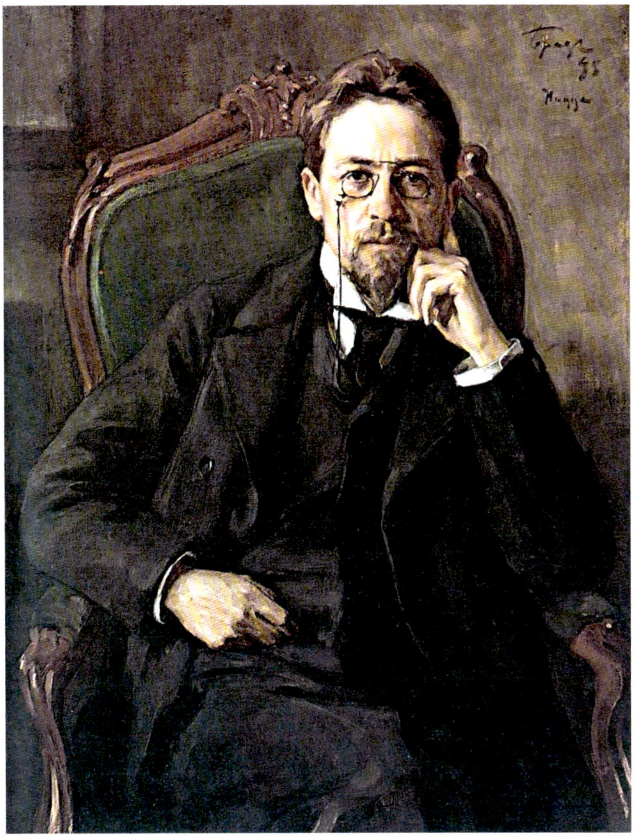

**Fig. 2.** Portrait of Anton Pavlovich Chekhov (1898), by Osip Braz (1873–1936), Tretyakov Gallery, Moscow, Russia, with kind permission.

was a breadwinner, a writer, or suffered from tuberculosis (except the doctor in *The Wife*). Most often, Chekhov did carefully observe and depict the district doctors close to him in his plays and short stories. Except for the unfortunate professor in *A Dreary Story,* his characters are not professors, academicians, or Moscow's great physicians, they are exhausted hard workers, with no effective diagnostic and therapeutic means, and to top it off, poorly paid. If Chekhov portrayed himself at times, it was only with small touches, as he is quoted as saying: 'We should not write a lot about ourselves ...' [19].


## Acknowledgments

I am greatly indebted to Aline Poirier for supervision of the English language and to Jacques Poirier for his comments and constructive criticism.

## References


1 Rayfield D: Anton Chekhov: A Life. Evanston, Northwestern University Press, 2000.
2 Darnal-Lesné F: Chekhov Dictionary (Le dictionnaire Tchekhov). Paris, L'Harmattan, 2010.
3 Grenier R: Watch Snow Falling (Regardez la neige qui tombe) (folio). Paris, Gallimard, 1992.
4 Chainet P: Anton Chekhov or the doctor in spite of himself (Anton Tchékhov ou le Médecin malgré lui). Médecine, revue mensuelle (Paris), February 1967.
5 Tanase V: Tchékhov. Letter to A. Souvorine (1834–1912), November 15, 1888. Folio Biographies. Paris, Gallimard, 2008, p 149.
6 Henry P (ed): Chekhov in English, 1998–2008. Oxford, Northgate Books, 2008.
7 Tchékhov A: Œuvres. Bibliothèque de la Pléiade. Paris, Les Éditeurs Français Réunis and Gallimard, 1967, vol I.
8 Tochet M: Physicians and Medicine in Chekhov's Work (Médecins et médecine dans l'œuvre de Tchékhov): mémoire de maîtrise. Université de la Sorbonne nouvelle, Paris III, 1988.
9 Rusk J: 201 Stories by Anton Chekhov. Eldritch Press. http://www.eldritchpress.org/ac/jr/index.htm.
10 Tchékhov A: Œuvres. Bibliothèque de la Pléiade. Paris, Les Éditeurs Français Réunis and Gallimard, 1970, vol II.
11 Tchékhov A: Œuvres. Bibliothèque de la Pléiade. Paris, Les Éditeurs Français Réunis and Gallimard, 1971, vol III.
12 Coulehan J (ed): Chekhov's Doctors: A Collection of Chekhov's Medical Tales. Foreword by Robert Coles. Kent, Kent State University Press, 2003.
13 Letter from Chekhov to Gregory Rossolimo, October 11, 1899, quoted by Gottlieb V. Chekhov and the Vaudeville. New York, Cambridge University Press, 1982.
14 Tchekhov A: Correspondence 1877–1904. Letter to A.N. Pletcheïev (1857–1918), November 13, 1888. Paris, Les Éditeurs Français Réunis, 1966, p 215.
15 Tchekhov A: Correspondence 1877–1904. Letter to A. Souvorine, December 30, 1888. Paris, Les Éditeurs Français Réunis, 1966, pp 226–229.
16 Tchekhov A: The Cherry Orchard, The Wood Demon, Uncle Vanya and Nine Plays in One Act (La cerisaie, le sauvage, oncle Vania et neuf pièces en un acte) (folio). Paris, Gallimard, 1974.
17 Tchekhov A: Correspondence 1877–1904. Letter to Mrs. E.M. Chavrova, 28 February 1895. Paris, Les Éditeurs Français Réunis, 1966, p 425.
18 Bounine I: Tchekhov (1952) (French translation by Claire Auchard). Monaco, Éditions du Rocher, 2004.
19 Tchekhov A: Correspondence 1877–1904. Letter to Mrs. R.F. Bachtchouk, 27 March 1897. Paris, Les Éditeurs Français Réunis, 1966, p 24.



Isabelle Crommelynck, MD
40 rue d'Alleray
FR–75015 Paris (France)
E-Mail isabelle.crom@gmail.com

Bogousslavsky J, Dieguez S (eds): Literary Medicine: Brain Disease and Doctors in Novels, Theater, and Film.
Front Neurol Neurosci. Basel, Karger, 2013, vol 31, pp 245–254 (DOI: 10.1159/000343240)

# Marcel Proust's Fictional Diseases and Doctors

Julien Bogousslavsky

Center for Brain and Nervous System Diseases, GSMN Neurocenter, Clinique Valmont, Glion/Montreux, Switzerland

**Abstract**

Marcel Proust (1875–1922), the son and brother of famous physicians, had close and continuous contact with medicine and doctors in connection with chronic asthma, neurasthenia, medical 'tourism', and self-medication. This proximity to medical issues is obvious in his work, particularly his novel *In Search of Lost Time*, which today is still considered one of the most important literary works ever. In this novel, medicine, patients, and doctors are everywhere, and it can be claimed that while it is often considered to be the great novel of memory, medicine in itself also can be seen as a true character of the story, in which Proust displays surprisingly extensive knowledge. Neurasthenia and asthma (i.e. Proust's diseases), as well as specific neurological disorders, such as stroke, migraine, epilepsy, and dementia, appear in the novel. The disease of the narrator's grandmother remains a piece of anthology, and probably remains the best literary report of a progressive stroke leading to death. Proust also quoted neurological conditions which were virtually unreported in his time, such as phantom limb syndrome and poststroke depression associated with aphasia in Baron Charlus. Doctors are nearly systematically depicted as incompetent and superficial, characteristics which appear to increase with academic titles and glory. The main physician of the novel, Professor Cottard, even ends up writing fake certificates for his rich friend Mrs. Verdurin during World War I so that she can obtain fresh croissants for breakfast, while poor people around her are starving. When called to examine a dying patient, one of the real doctors of the novel, Professor Dieulafoy, says and does nothing except ask for his fees. This defiance and criticism of physicians were indeed those of Proust in real life.


The main novel of Marcel Proust (1875–1922; fig. 1), *In Search of Lost Time* (published over more than a decade, beginning in 1913) [1], is considered as the most important French literary work of the twentieth century. Through the description of the life of a writer-to-be (the 'narrator') in fin de siècle ambiance, it is largely centered on a detailed analysis of memory, especially involuntary memory. The episode recounting the surge of old, apparently forgotten memories while eating a 'petite madeleine' (a kind of cookie) has remained famous much beyond Proust's novel. In

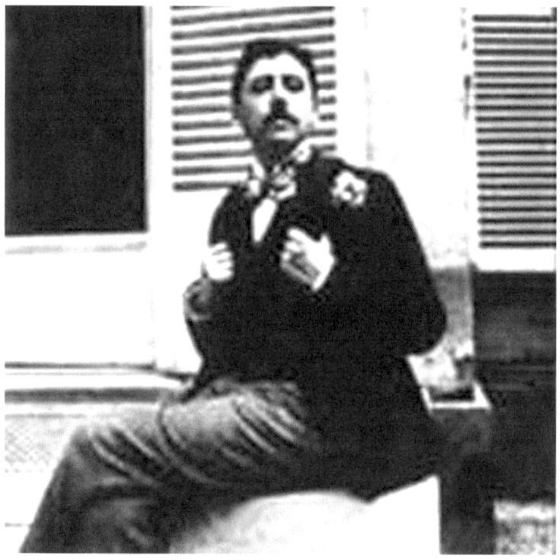

**Fig. 1.** Marcel Proust (1875–1922; first appeared in Abraham [18]).

a previous study, we found that memory issues are mentioned over 1,200 times in the 3,000 pages of the novel, with a specific emphasis on associations, time perception, forgetting, emotions, and the reconstructed structure of memory, in addition to involuntary reminiscence [2]. In Proust's view, involuntary surges of remembering are the cause of a specific feeling of happiness because they are the only mechanism which may make past and present experiences coincide in the same moment. In the novel, this phenomenon is indeed the key mechanism which leads the narrator to start a literary career in order to report such experiences. In writing, Proust displays an extensive knowledge of memory and other psychological phenomena, but also of more general medical issues. Indeed, another recurring theme in his novel is 'disease', largely as it is experienced by the main characters of the novel. Cerebral and mental disorders are repeatedly present throughout the novel, allowing Proust's leading expert Jean-Yves Tadié to entitle a chapter 'Proust the neurologist' [3].

## The Influence of Professor Adrien Proust and His Circle

Proust's father Adrien (1834–1903; fig. 2) was a physician who worked as Chief of Service at Lariboisière and La Charité, and was elected to the Chair of Hygiene in 1885, where he established an institution which would become the precursor of the World Health Organization [4]. However, he also published several works on neurological and psychiatric topics, such as aphasia, pseudobulbar palsy, hysteria, and behavioral disorders [5]. His professorship thesis in 1862 was on the different forms of ischemic stroke [6]. In his work on neurasthenia with Charcot's pupil Gilbert Ballet, it is obvious that he makes reference to his own son Marcel, who was diagnosed with this condition, along with asthma [7]. Through his father, Proust

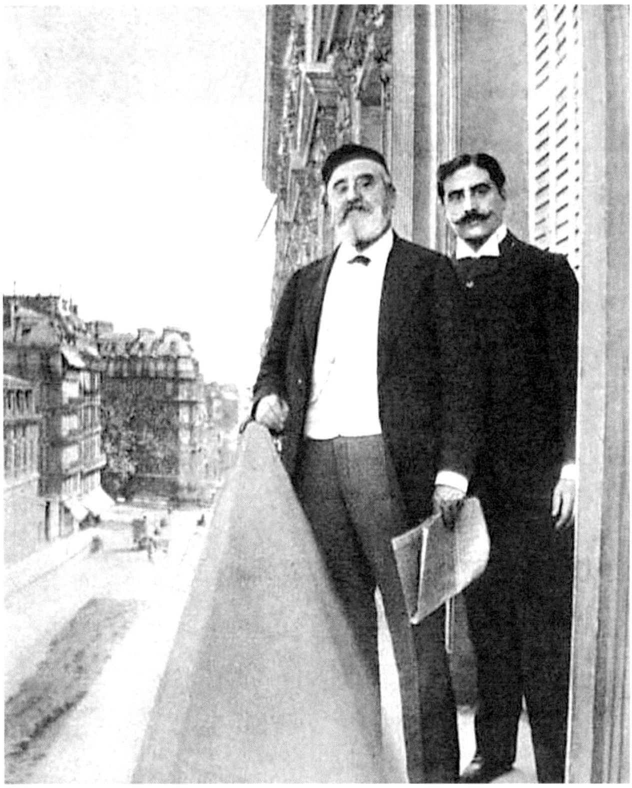

**Fig. 2.** Professor Adrien Proust with his son Robert, who became a urologist (first appeared in Abraham [18]).

met several famous doctors of the time, and he also contributed to discussions at family meals. Proust's younger brother Robert followed a medical track and later became a famous urologist [8]. Proust was also exposed to brain disease when his father died of an acute stroke in 1903, and his mother of uremia, probably also with a stroke, in 1905. In fact, this death was the trigger for Proust to be admitted to hospital for an 'isolation cure', a usual treatment for neurasthenia at the time. After envisioning this therapy with Jules Déjerine in Paris, Paul Dubois in Bern, or Auguste Widmer in Valmont, Proust finally selected Paul Sollier's clinic in Boulogne-Billancourt, upon Brissaud's advice [9]. He spent several weeks there between the end of 1905 and the beginning of 1906. Although he reported this stay to be useless, it in fact became instrumental in the genesis of his novel. Indeed, Sollier, who was described by Léon Daudet as the best follower of Jean-Martin Charcot, along with Joseph Babinski [10], was a major scientific expert on memory. He had written two important books on this topic, and dedicated a copy of the second one to his famous inpatient on Christmas Day 1905 (fig. 3). This work obviously had a critical influence on Proust since it largely focused on involuntary memory and what the author called 'emotional revivals' triggered by apparently futile perceptions [2]. While Proust never frankly acknowledged this influence,

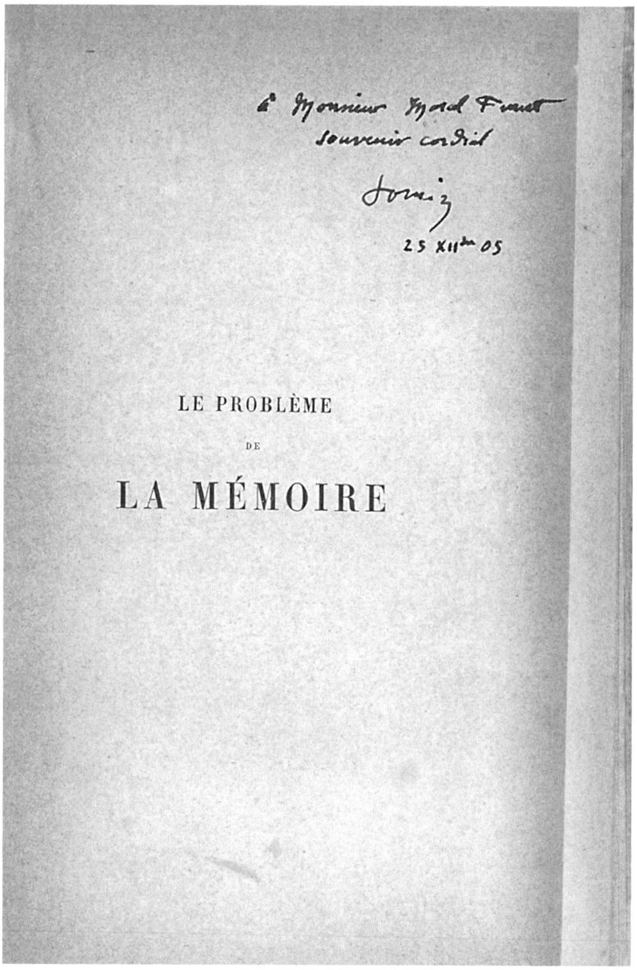


**Fig. 3.** Dedication of Paul Sollier to Marcel Proust of his book 'Le problème de la mémoire' (published 1900) on Christmas day, 1905, while Proust had just entered the Boulogne-Billancourt clinic for an 'isolation cure' under the care of Sollier (private collection).

there are some parts in his novel which seem to have been directly taken from Sollier's work [2]. During the rest of his life, Proust continued to see many doctors for his condition, including Babinski when he was afraid he had developed aphasia [8]. In 1922, Babinski came to examine him at home a few hours before he died from pulmonary infection, upon request of Robert Proust [4, 5, 8].

## Brain and Neurological Diseases in *In Search of Lost Time*

A specific mention of the brain can be found nearly 50 times in the novel, in which Proust also mentions the 'nervous system' and 'nervous cells' [2]. Proust acknowledges the highest role of the brain over other organs, and states that 'to each alteration of the brain corresponds a fragment of death' [IV/374; quotations from Proust's novel are mentioned following the French Folio edition (see [1]), with volume (I-VII) and corresponding pages]. It is striking that certain remarks seem more intuitive than based on current knowledge of the time, for instance when the narrator states that there is some distance between the two parts of his brain, which correspond to two different emotional perceptions (I/133), while virtually nothing was known on right-left hemisphere specificities and disconnection.

Proust used the adjective 'nervous' to refer to neurasthenia, the very condition that his father had diagnosed in him. Along with asthma (from which Proust also suffered) and stroke (the condition which he was afraid of developing, as both his mother and father died of it), neurasthenia (defined as a neurosis including respiratory and cardiac symptoms, insomnia, melancholy, dizziness, and 'disease of doubt') is the most frequently mentioned disease in Proust's novel [11]. Nowadays this condition has disappeared from the medical lexicon. Although it is clear that there was a cultural factor ('mal du siècle'), neurasthenia mainly corresponds to what we now would call somatization or psychosomatic disorders. On occasions, Proust uses other terms for this condition which are more familiar to us today, such as 'neurovegetative dystonia' in Andrée, Albertine's friend. Proust was particularly familiar with it since his father had written a famous book on the topic, *L'hygiène du neurasthénique* [7], underscoring that the condition is largely influenced by a too-close proximity between patient and mother, and obviously taking his own son as a typical example [12].

Migraine, with its female preponderance, is also quoted by Proust twelve times (I/186, 268; III/31, 326; IV/285; V/218, 237, 433; V/77, 337; and VII 36, 80). Neuralgias (I/36, 203; IV/298, 349), epilepsy (IV/349; V/262; VII/106), dementia or arteriosclerosis (IV/292; VII/145, 244), and several manifestations of syphilis, including general paresis with dysarthria (IV/356), loss of pupillary reflex (IV/439), tabetic ataxia (II/98; IV/284), and neuroarthritic disease (I/98; IV/284; V/201) are also present in *In Search of Lost Time*.

Stroke is the most frequently quoted organic brain disease, being absent only in volume two. Proust speaks of 'apoplexy attack' (V/174; VII/166), 'cerebral hemorrhage' (II/340), 'cerebral accident' (VII/342), 'hemiplegia' (VI/66), 'paralysis attack' (VI/196), 'brain congestion' (III/323), 'small stroke' (III/302; V/347), or simply 'stroke' ('attaque' in French; I/305–8; IV/41, 153, 239, 336; V/112, 114, 254, 312; VII/348). Four main characters of the novel are affected by it: the grandmother, Bergotte (the writer), Saniette (a member of the Verdurin circle), and Baron Charlus. The descriptions of stroke in the grandmother and Charlus are especially accurate and detailed, with an emphasis on 'uremia' (the main cause of arterial hypertension at the time, like in Proust's mother's stroke; III/308–10; V/174–6), through a 'small rupture or obstruction of a vessel'. The former mechanism, with subsequent hemorrhage (as compared to brain 'softening'), is critically underlined by Proust (VI/173; VII/344). Paralyses and language dysfunction are the main stroke manifestations mentioned by Proust, who somewhat confuses alexia and agraphia (IV/336); however, a specific consequence should be mentioned:

poststroke 'mental depression' in Baron Charlus after he developed aphasia (VII/171). This report precedes by several decades the scientific description of depression after stroke in medical literature, a complication which is now known to be closely associated with left hemisphere involvement with aphasia.

Two other conditions warrant a special mention since they were not well described in Proust's time: firstly, Proust describes the phantom limb syndrome, in which 'by certain weather changes, amputees have pain in the leg which they have lost' (VI/173); and secondly, the violinist Morel develops a musician's cramp in his hand, which limits his performance skills (V/44).

Finally, we are left with the paradox that while Proust's book remains the great novel about memory, memory dysfunction is hardly mentioned in it. While forgetting is not included by Proust into memory dysfunction, but instead into normal useful memory processes, memory loss appears only twice (IV/172; V/112). Proust mentions the possibility of memory impairment in stroke (V/112; VI/173; VII/167), but he also rightly emphasizes the preservation of memory in Baron Charlus who was struck with aphasia (VII/168). This lack is somewhat frustrating, especially since Proust stated that memory impairment may in fact be a useful stimulus to study the mechanisms of memory (IV/52; VII/347), particularly in association with the 'intermittences of the heart' (IV/152–5).

Contrary to certain claims [13], I do not think that Proust should be considered a 'neuroscientist'. This kind of statement is fashionable nowadays, but Proust did not discover brain or neural mechanisms. On the other hand, he reported and analyzed with extreme finesse several diseases and cognitive and psychological phenomena, which makes him one of the most 'modern' writers on human life.

## Fictional Patients

Over 25 minor characters in Proust's novel have various diseases. In addition, Proust also occasionally quotes real patients from the medical literature, such as his father's case report of 'Émile X' about an honest man with duplication of personality making him steal objects [14], which is quoted by professor Cottard in the novel. Proust also uses disease to qualify nonmedical features, such as the 'sickly aspect' of Odette's face or the mundanity of Mrs. Verdurin.

But disease itself is one of the main characters of the novel, conveyed through eight people: the narrator, Baron Charlus, La Berma, Swann, Bergotte, Saniette, the grandmother, and aunt Léonie [11]. The narrator is the typical neurasthenic, as Proust himself was, and the disease makes him stay twice, for 'several years', in a clinic (Proust only stayed in a clinic for a few weeks). Only at the end of the novel does he seem to emerge from his recurrent symptoms, when he joins the Princess of Guermantes' party (the old Mrs. Verdurin) and observes in a rather detached way this sort of geriatric club now formed by his former acquaintances.

Charlus is a caricature of a 'mad', unpredictable, highly emotional, masochistic, homosexual psychopath, in whom Proust, himself a homosexual, presents homosexuality as a clearly pathological 'inversion'. At the end of the novel, Professor Brichot even proposes him for a virtual 'Chair of Homosexuality'. Charlus also develops a stroke triggered by a strong emotional factor (when his lover Morel leaves him). He becomes aphasic after a period of aphonia, associated with motor incoordination and transient blindness (posterior circulation infarction?), leading to deep depressive phases. Proust compares him to King Lear in that his downfall seems to magnify him.

The actress 'La Berma' has a lethal disease, which remains unclear, although she has kidney involvement and spits blood, due to severe overwork stimulated by her family. Like in Swann and Saniette, for Proust severe disease symbolically means mischief and incomprehension by others [11]. In Swann, a first disease (his incurable love for Odette) is replaced by another one, also incurable (a malignant abdominal tumor), which both 'torture' him and leave him affectively and mentally alone.

The writer Bergotte, which was inspired by many contemporary writers but also by Proust himself, suffers like him from dizzy spells and insomnia, which he treats with self-medication. This leads to substance abuse, worsening the condition, which worsens even more when he tries to interrupt the medications. His death may have been a phantasm of Proust for himself since he dies after two recurrent strokes while admiring a Vermeer painting in a museum, and is survived by his literary work and glory.

Saniette represents the shy, innocent, simple person who is the victim of other people's aggression, with subsequent stress ending up with cardiovascular dysfunction, dyspnea, and two strokes.

Aunt Léonie (responsible for the famous 'petite madeleine' reminiscence episode) has a worse case of neurasthenia than the narrator. She states to herself that she must remember that she did not sleep, so that she can complain about it. She dreams that her late husband wanted to have her go outside for a walk: this is such a nightmare for her, that she never leaves her bed anymore. However, after she finally died, people wonder whether she was not suffering from an organic disease, which had been misdiagnosed.

Finally, the narrator's grandmother provides Proust with the opportunity to write one of the best literary descriptions of a stroke, starting with transient episodes, continuing with a detailed picture of a progressing stroke, and ending up with death, while five doctors, each more ineffective than the other, come and go around the patient: Dr. Cottard looks stupid and makes unwarranted jokes; Dr. du Boulbon nearly does not look at the patient and theatrically speaks of literature and neurasthenia, making inappropriate diagnoses; Dr. Dieulafoy (who really existed and was a famous professor) says and does nothing but ask for his fees; an ENT doctor makes a diagnosis of a nose problem; and Professor E looks bothered because he was just putting on gala clothes to go out to a special party, and quickly concludes:

'Your grandmother is lost'. Contrary to Aunt Léonie and Proust himself, the grandmother 'does not listen to herself', one of the reasons for her severe disease, but like Proust, she is suspicious of doctors in general. Her death corresponds to the disappearance of one of the narrator's 'intimate identities' [11], like for Proust his mother's death in 1905.

## Fictional Doctors

In the novel, disease appears on page 2, and the first doctor on page 22. At least 20 doctors are in the novel, the main ones being Dr. Cottard and Dr. du Boulbon. Proust also introduces real famous practitioners, such as Dieulafoy and Potain, but also less known doctors, who he selected for their comical name (Bouffe de Saint-Blaise and Courtois-Suffit). A constant feature is the inefficacy of their practice, from Dr. Percepied in the village of Combray to famous professors in Paris.

Dr. du Boulbon has a great reputation, and indeed Charcot predicted that he would 'reign over neurology and psychiatry'. He has certain human qualities, but at the expense of poor diagnostic skills, and his consultation of the dying grandmother is a catastrophe. Édouard Brissaud, the interim successor at Charcot's chair for one year [15], seems to have been Proust's main inspiration for this character [4, 8]. His father knew him well, and he wrote the preface to his book, *Hygiène des asthmatiques* [15, 16], which was not without interest to the young Marcel.

Dr. (and later professor) Cottard is Proust's most important fictional doctor, and is present throughout the novel. Béhar calls him a 'peasant in Paris' [11]. He is naive, uncultivated, and does not perceive properly the social relationships, but he is ambitious; he hides his lack of mundanity and education behind jokes and play of words, without refraining to speak badly of his colleagues. Proust emphasizes the contrast between his stupidity and his diagnostic skills, which makes him a 'great clinician', except with the grandmother. Mrs. Verdurin calls him 'Dr. God'. However, he is not really conscientious, and sometimes can even be a bad guy. For example, he would miss a party at the Verdurin's only for a 'minister's coryza', and would not care for a worker with a stroke. He also refuses to attend a servant because he has already put on his white waistcoat for a party, and he expels a peasant out of his train compartment while stating all his titles. Finally, during the war he writes a fake certificate for Mrs. Verdurin so that she can get fresh croissants for breakfast, while others are starving. Misleading information about him continues after his death since people think he was killed by the enemy while on duty at the front, while in fact he died peacefully at home in his bed. Dr. Cottard's models include several physicians of the time, including Adrien Proust himself. The name 'Cottard' was derived from 'Cotard', a friend of Adrien Proust, who made his thesis with Charcot on brain hemiatropy, and later wrote a famous paper, 'Délire des négations' [17], which is still called Cotard syndrome today (fig. 4).

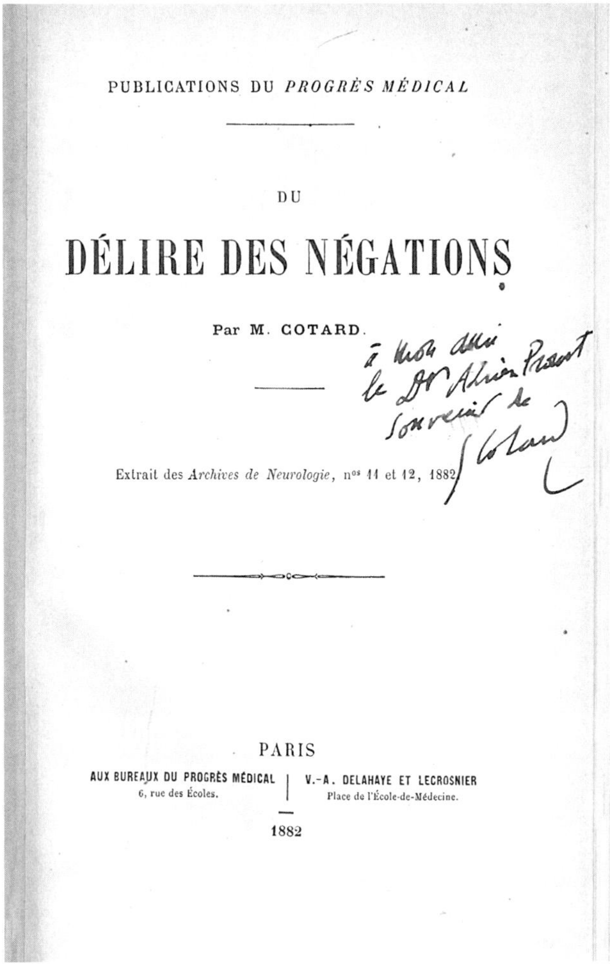
PUBLICATIONS DU *PROGRÈS MÉDICAL*

DU

DÉLIRE DES NÉGATIONS

Par M. COTARD.

à mon ami
le Dr Adrien Proust
souvenir de
J Cotard

Extrait des *Archives de Neurologie*, nos 11 et 12, 1882

PARIS

AUX BUREAUX DU PROGRÈS MÉDICAL | V.-A. DELAHAYE ET LECROSNIER

6, rue des Écoles. | Place de l'École-de-Médecine.

1882

**Fig. 4.** Adrien Proust's personal copy of the 'Délire des négations' paper by his colleague and friend Jules Cotard, with inscription (private collection).

Finally, the only doctor who Proust depicts as a good and honest practitioner is the modest doctor in Balbec, who contrary to Cottard makes a good diagnosis of a simple problem in a VIP with an eye irritation.

## Conclusion

*In Search of Lost Time* not only is the great novel of involuntary memory, it is also a 'novel of disease, patients and doctors', where Proust used his personal experience both as the son of a famous professor of medicine and as a patient himself. Since disease, fear of the incompetence of doctors, and self-medication ruled a major part of his life, Proust transcribed his feelings and reflections into most of his novel's characters, leading to a masterly depiction of the complex human relationships which develop around disease.

## References


1 Proust M: À la recherche du temps perdu. Bibliothèque de la pléiade et collection Folio. Paris, Gallimard, 1987–1990.

2 Bogousslavsky J: La mémoire de Proust. Vevey, Le Cadratin, 2009.

3 Tadié JY: Marcel Proust. Biographies. Paris, Gallimard, 1996.

4 Bogousslavsky J: Marcel Proust's diseases and doctors: the neurological story of a life; in Bogousslavsky J, Hennerici MG (eds): Neurological Disorders in Famous Artists – Part 2. Front Neurol Neurosci. Basel, Karger, 2007, vol 22, pp. 89–104.

5 Bogousslavsky J: Marcel Proust's lifelong tour of the Parisian neurological intelligentsia: from Brissaud and Dejerine to Sollier and Babinski. Eur Neurol 2007;57:129–136.

6 Proust A: Des différentes forme de ramollissement du cerveau. Paris, Thèse d'agrégation, 1866.

7 Proust A, Ballet G: L'hygiène du neurasthénique. Paris, Masson, 1897.

8 Tadié JY: Nouvelles recherches sur la mémoire proustienne; in: De Proust à Dumas. Paris, Gallimard, 2006.

9 Walusinski O, Bogousslavsky J: À la recherche du neuropsychiatre perdu: Paul Sollier (1861–1933) (in French). Rev Neurol (Paris) 2008;164:F238–F247.

10 Daudet L: Devant la douleur; in Daudet L (ed): Souvenirs et polémiques. Paris, Bouquins, Robert Laffont, 1992.

11 Béhar S: L'univers médical de Marcel Proust. Cahiers Marcel Proust. Paris, NRF, Gallimard, 1970.

12 Tadié JY (ed): Proust: L'écriture et les arts. Bibliothèque Nationale de France-Réunion des Musées Nationaux. Paris, Gallimard, 1999.

13 Lehrer J: Proust Was a Neuroscientist. Boston, Houghton Mifflin, 2008.

14 Proust A: Cas curieux d'automatisme ambulatoire chez un hystérique. Tribune Médicale 1890;13: 202–203.

15 Brissaud É: L'hygiène des asthmatiques. Paris, Masson, 1896.

16 Poirier J: Édouard Brissaud. Un neurologue d'exception dans une famille d'artistes. Paris, Hermann, 2010.

17 Cotard J: Le délire des négations. Arch Neurol 1882;4:152–170, 282–296.

18 Abraham P: Proust. Paris, Les Editiones Rieder, 1930.



Julien Bogousslavsky, MD
Center for Brain and Nervous System Diseases
GSMN Neurocenter, Clinique Valmont
CH–1823 Glion/Montreux (Switzerland)
E-Mail jbogousslavsky@cliniquevalmont.ch

# Author Index

# Subject Index